Hematologic Disorders in Pregnancy

Guest Editor

JEAN M. CONNORS, MD

HEMATOLOGY/ONCOLOGY CLINICS OF NORTH AMERICA

www.hemonc.theclinics.com

Consulting Editors
GEORGE P. CANELLOS, MD
NANCY BERLINER, MD

April 2011 • Volume 25 • Number 2

SAUNDERS an imprint of ELSEVIER, Inc.

W.B. SAUNDERS COMPANY
A Division of Elsevier Inc.

1600 John F. Kennedy Blvd. ● Suite 1800 ● Philadelphia, PA 19103-2899

http://www.theclinics.com

HEMATOLOGY/ONCOLOGY CLINICS OF NORTH AMERICA Volume 25, Number 2
April 2011 ISSN 0889-8588, ISBN 13: 978-1-4557-0459-0

Editor: Patrick Manley

Photocopying
Single photocopies of single articles may be made for personal use as allowed by national copyright laws. Permission of the Publisher and payment of a fee is required for all other photocopying, including multiple or systematic copying, copying for advertising or promotional purposes, resale, and all forms of document delivery. Special rates are available for educational institutions that wish to make photocopies for non-profit educational classroom use. For information on how to seek permission visit www.elsevier.com/permissions or call: (+44) 1865 843830 (UK)/(+1) 215 239 3804 (USA).

Derivative Works
Subscribers may reproduce tables of contents or prepare lists of articles including abstracts for internal circulation within their institutions. Permission of the Publisher is required for resale or distribution outside the institution. Permission of the Publisher is required for all other derivative works, including compilations and translations (please consult www.elsevier.com/permissions).

Electronic Storage or Usage
Permission of the Publisher is required to store or use electronically any material contained in this journal, including any article or part of an article (please consult www.elsevier.com/permissions). Except as outlined above, no part of this publication may be reproduced, stored in a retrieval system or transmitted in any form or by any means, electronic, mechanical, photocopying, recording or otherwise, without prior written permission of the Publisher.

Notice
No responsibility is assumed by the Publisher for any injury and/or damage to persons or property as a matter of products liability, negligence or otherwise, or from any use or operation of any methods, products, instructions or ideas contained in the material herein. Because of rapid advances in the medical sciences, in particular, independent verification of diagnoses and drug dosages should be made.

Although all advertising material is expected to conform to ethical (medical) standards, inclusion in this publication does not constitute a guarantee or endorsement of the quality or value of such product or of the claims made of it by its manufacturer.

Hematology/Oncology Clinics (ISSN 0889-8588) is published bimonthly by Elsevier Inc., 360 Park Avenue South, New York, NY 10010-1710. Months of issue are February, April, June, August, October, and December. Business and Editorial Offices: 1600 John F. Kennedy Blvd., Ste. 1800, Philadelphia, PA 19103—2899. Customer Service Office: 3251 Riverport Lane, Maryland Heights, MO 63043. Periodicals postage paid at New York, NY and at additional mailing offices. Subscription prices are $327.00 per year (domestic individuals), $541.00 per year (domestic institutions), $160.00 per year (domestic students/residents), $371.00 per year (Canadian individuals), $662.00 per year (Canadian institutions) $442.00 per year (international individuals), $662.00 per year (international institutions), and $216.00 per year (international and Canadian students/residents). International air speed delivery is included in all *Clinics* subscription prices. All prices are subject to change without notice. **POSTMASTER:** Send address changes to *Hematology/Oncology Clinics of North America*, Elsevier Health Sciences Division, Subscription Customer Service, 3251 Riverport Lane, Maryland Heights, MO 63043. Customer Service (orders, claims, online, change of address): Elsevier Health Sciences Division, Subscription Customer Service, 3251 Riverport Lane, Maryland Heights, MO 63043. Tel: 1-800-654-2452 (U.S. and Canada); 314-447-8871 (outside U.S. and Canada). Fax: 314-447-8029. E-mail: journalscustomerservice-usa@elsevier.com (for print support); journalsonlinesupport-usa@elsevier.com (for online support).

Reprints. For copies of 100 or more, of articles in this publication, please contact the Commercial Reprints Department, Elsevier Inc., 360 Park Avenue South, New York, New York 10010-1710; Tel.: 212-633-3813, Fax: 212-462-1935, E-mail: reprints@elsevier.com.

Hematology/Oncology Clinics of North America is covered in *MEDLINE/PubMed (Index Medicus), EMBASE/ Excerpta Medica, and BIOSIS.*

Printed and bound by CPI Group (UK) Ltd, Croydon, CR0 4YY

Transferred to Digital Print 2011

Contributors

CONSULTING EDITORS

GEORGE P. CANELLOS, MD
William Rosenberg Professor of Medicine, Department of Medical Oncology, Dana-Farber
Cancer Institute, Boston, Massachusetts

NANCY BERLINER, MD
Chief, Division of Hematology, Brigham and Women's Hospital; Professor of Medicine,
Harvard Medical School, Boston, Massachusetts

GUEST EDITOR

JEAN M. CONNORS, MD
Assistant Professor of Medicine, Harvard Medical School; Medical Director,
Anticoagulation Management Services, Division of Hematology, Department of Medicine,
Brigham and Women's Hospital, Dana Farber Cancer Institute, Boston, Massachusetts

AUTHORS

URI ABADI, MD
Senior Physician, Hematology Institute, Department of Medicine, Meir Medical Center,
Kfar Saba, Israel

E.M. BATTINELLI, MD, PhD
Instructor of Medicine, Division of Hematology, Brigham and Women's Hospital, Harvard
Medical School, Boston, Massachusetts

K.A. BAUER, MD
Professor of Medicine, Division of Hematology/Oncology, Beth Israel Deaconess Medical
Center; Department of Hematology/Oncology, Veterans Affairs Boston Healthcare
System, Harvard Medical School, Boston, Massachusetts

PAULA L. BOCKENSTEDT, MD
Clinical Associate Professor of Medicine; Director of the Adult Coagulation Disorders
Program, Division of Hematology/Oncology, University of Michigan Medical Center,
Ann Arbor, Michigan

PAULA H.B. BOLTON-MAGGS, DM, FRCP, FRCPath
Consultant Haematologist and Honorary Senior Lecturer in Medicine, Department
of Clinical Haematology, Manchester Royal Infirmary, Manchester, United Kingdom

WILLIAM R. CAMANN, MD
Department of Anesthesiology, Perioperative and Pain Medicine, Associate Professor
of Anesthesia, Harvard Medical School; Director of Obstetric Anesthesia, Brigham and
Women's Hospital, Boston, Massachusetts

LORRAINE CHOW, MD, FRCPC
Department of Anesthesiology, Perioperative and Pain Medicine, Clinical Fellow
of Obstetric Anesthesia, Harvard Medical School, Brigham and Women's Hospital,
Boston, Massachusetts

JEAN M. CONNORS, MD
Assistant Professor of Medicine, Harvard Medical School; Medical Director,
Anticoagulation Management Services, Division of Hematology, Department of Medicine,
Brigham and Women's Hospital, Dana Farber Cancer Institute, Boston, Massachusetts

MAURA A. DUMAS, RN, MSN
Clinical Nurse Specialist, Hemophilia and Thrombosis Center, Section of Hematology/
Oncology, Dartmouth-Hitchcock Medical Center, Lebanon, New Hampshire

KATHERINE E. ECONOMY, MD, MPH
Instructor, Division of Maternal Fetal Medicine, Department of Obstetrics and
Gynecology, Brigham and Women's Hospital, Harvard Medical School, Boston,
Massachusetts

MICHAELA K. FARBER, MD
Department of Anesthesiology, Perioperative and Pain Medicine, Instructor of Anesthesia,
Harvard Medical School; Fellowship Director, Obstetric Anesthesia, Brigham and
Women's Hospital, Boston, Massachusetts

ANNEMARIE E. FOGERTY, MD
Department of Hematology/Oncology, Massachusetts General Hospital Cancer Center;
Instructor in Medicine, Harvard Medical School, Boston, Massachusetts

CLAIRE N. HARRISON, DM, FRCP, FRCPath
Consultant Haematologist, Department of Haematology, Guy's and St Thomas' NHS
Foundation Trust, Guy's Hospital, Great Maze Pond, London, United Kingdom

ALFRED IAN LEE, MD, PhD
Clinical Fellow, Department of Medical Oncology, Dana-Farber Cancer Institute, Harvard
Medical School, Boston, Massachusetts

RICHARD M. KAUFMAN, MD
Assistant Professor of Pathology, Harvard Medical School; Medical Director, Adult
Transfusion Service, Brigham and Women's Hospital, Boston, Massachusetts

GIDEON KOREN, MD
Professor of Pediatrics, Pharmacology, Pharmacy, and Medical Genetics, University
of Toronto; Director of the Motherisk Program, Hospital for Sick Children, Toronto,
Ontario, Canada

BREA C. LIPE, MD
Fellow, Section of Hematology/Oncology, Dartmouth-Hitchcock Medical Center,
Lebanon, New Hampshire

MICHAEL LISHNER, MD
Professor of Medicine, Sackler Faculty of Medicine, Tel Aviv University,
Ramat Aviv, Tel Aviv; Director of Internal Medicine Ward A, Meir Medical Center,
Kfar Saba, Israel

MAUREEN M. OKAM, MD, MPH
Instructor in Medicine, Harvard Medical School; Attending Physician, Division of Hematology, Brigham and Women's Hospital, Boston, Massachusetts

DEBORAH L. ORNSTEIN, MD
Medical Director, Hemophilia and Thrombosis Center, Section of Hematology/Oncology, Dartmouth-Hitchcock Medical Center, Lebanon; Associate Professor of Medicine and Pathology, Department of Medicine, Dartmouth Medical School, Hanover, New Hampshire

MICHAEL J. PAIDAS, MD
Associate Professor, Co-Director, Yale Women and Children's Center for Blood Disorders; Associate Professor, Co-Director, National Hemophilia Foundation-Baxter Clinical Fellowship Program at Yale; Division of Maternal Fetal Medicine, Department of Obstetrics, Gynecology and Reproductive Sciences, Yale University School of Medicine, New Haven, Connecticut

SALLEY G. PELS, MD
Instructor, National Hemophilia Foundation-Baxter Clinical Fellow, Section of Hematology Oncology, Department of Pediatrics, Yale University School of Medicine, New Haven, Connecticut

GILLIAN N. PIKE, MBChB, MRCP
Specialist Registrar in Haematology, Department of Clinical Haematology, Manchester Royal Infirmary, Manchester, United Kingdom

SUSAN E. ROBINSON, MSc, MRCP, FRCPath
Consultant Haematologist, Department of Haematology, Guy's and St Thomas' NHS Foundation Trust, Guy's Hospital, Great Maze Pond, London, United Kingdom

NICOLE A. SMITH, MD, MPH
Clinical Fellow in Obstetrics, Gynecology and Reproductive Biology, Division of Maternal Fetal Medicine, Department of Obstetrics and Gynecology, Brigham and Women's Hospital, Harvard Medical School, Boston, Massachusetts

Contents

> Anemia in pregnancy is a global health problem affecting nearly half of all pregnant women worldwide. High fetal demands for iron render iron deficiency the most common cause of anemia of pregnancy, with other micronutrient deficiencies contributing less frequently. In certain geographical populations, human pathogens such as hookworm, malarial parasite and human immunodeficiency virus are important factors in anemia of pregnancy. The hemoglobinopathies, sickle cell disease and thalassemia, represent diverse causes of anemia of pregnancy, requiring specialized care. Aplastic anemia is a rare, morbid cause of anemia of pregnancy and is managed with transfusions until the completion of pregnancy.

> This article reviews pregnancy outcome in women diagnosed with a myeloproliferative neoplasm (MPN), and discusses possible risk markers and the pathogenesis of poor pregnancy outcome. An outline of the key factors regarding the diagnosis and management of MPN in women of reproductive potential is followed by a description of the authors' management strategy for standard and high-risk pregnancy in MPN patients.

> Treatment of pregnant women with chemotherapy may pose a risk to the fetus, raising therapeutic, ethical, moral, and social dilemmas. Publications on this issue are limited to retrospective series and case reports, thus further complicating decision making. Diagnosis and staging are usually performed as in nonpregnant women, but procedures that expose the fetus to radiation are excluded. Chemotherapy is not recommended in the first trimester to avoid fetal malformations. Thus, the option is either treatment delay or pregnancy termination. Later in pregnancy, treatment is often initiated without delay, with no apparent evidence of teratogenicity.

> Thrombocytopenia in pregnancy is most frequently a benign process that does not require intervention. However, 35% of cases of thrombocytopenia in pregnancy are related to disease processes that may have serious bleeding consequences at delivery or for which thrombocytopenia may be an indicator of a more severe systemic disorder requiring emergent

maternal and fetal care. Thus, all pregnant women with platelet counts less than 100,000/μL require careful hematological and obstetric consultation to exclude more serious disorders.

Microangiopathic disorders present with thrombocytopenia, hemolytic anemia, and multiorgan damage. In pregnancy, these disorders present a challenge both diagnostically and therapeutically, with widely overlapping clinical scenarios and disparate treatments. Although rare, a clear understanding of these diseases is important because devastating maternal and fetal outcomes may ensue if there is misdiagnosis and improper treatment. Microangiopathic disorders presenting in pregnancy are thus best assessed and treated by both obstetric and hematology teams. As a better understanding of the pathophysiology underlying each of the disease processes is gained, new diagnostic testing and therapies will be available, which will lead to improved outcomes.

Thrombophilic conditions are associated with an increased risk of venous thromboembolic events (VTE) during pregnancy. Thrombophilic disorders are either acquired, as in antiphospholipid syndrome, or inherited, as in factor V Leiden. Both are associated with VTE but acquired disorders can also increase the risk of arterial events. However, there is controversy as to whether they may adversely affect other pregnancy outcomes including pregnancy loss, placental abruption, severe preeclampsia, and stillbirth. This article discusses the effect of thrombophilias on pregnancy.

Because von Willebrand factor (VWF) levels increase during pregnancy, many women with VWD, though not requiring support with hemostatic agents, are at increased risk for delayed postpartum hemorrhage as coagulation factor levels fall to their prepregnancy levels in the puerperium. Women with moderate or severe disease or complicated pregnancies are best served by delivering at a center with an obstetrician, hematologist, and anesthesiologist experienced in managing coagulation disorders. In addition, on-site laboratory facilities with specialized coagulation testing capability, pharmacy, and blood bank support are critical for success. Ensuring optimal outcomes for pregnant women with VWD requires a multidisciplinary approach.

Pregnancy, childbirth, and the puerperium are hemostatically challenging to women with bleeding disorders. This article provides general recommendations for the management of pregnant women with inherited coagulation disorders. Each factor deficiency is discussed, providing an up-to-date review of the literature and, where possible, guidance about how to manage patients throughout pregnancy, delivery, and the puerperium. The factor deficiencies covered are inherited abnormalities of fibrinogen; deficiencies of prothrombin, factor (F)V, FVII, FX, FXI, FXIII; combined deficiencies of FV and FVIII; and the inherited deficiency of vitamin K–dependent clotting factors. The management of carriers of hemophilia A and B is also discussed.

to a decline in maternal morbidity and mortality, the presence of uncorrected coagulopathy or the use of anticoagulant or antithrombotic medications pose a special risk for the rare complication of an epidural hematoma after neuraxial anesthesia. This article briefly reviews the common principles of anesthesia for obstetric patients, provides an obstetric anesthesiologist's perspective on the implications of regional anesthesia in obstetrics, and enhances communication between the specialties.

THE CLINICS ARE NOW AVAILABLE ONLINE!

Access your subscription at:
www.theclinics.com

Preface

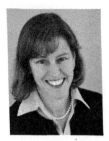

Jean M. Connors, MD
Guest Editor

Pregnancy is a unique physiologic state in which the mother supports the developing fetus until it is ready to be delivered into the external environment. The process of creating another human being is overwhelmingly complex. Significant stress is placed on the mother's body during this time, and almost all major organ systems are affected by pregnancy.

In a normal pregnancy, the components of the hematologic system, including hematopoiesis and hemostasis, undergo substantial change in response to the demands of pregnancy. Although red cell mass increases, a physiologic anemia occurs in pregnancy as there is an even greater increase in plasma volume. The platelet count often drops slightly, with an accepted lower limit of normal range in pregnancy, while white cell count increases due to an increase in circulating neutrophils. Changes occur in the coagulation system, with increased procoagulant activity, decreased natural anticoagulant activity, and decreased fibrinolysis, resulting in a prothrombotic state.

In a woman with a preexisting hematologic disorder, the normal physiologic changes that occur in pregnancy can exacerbate the underlying disease process, resulting in increased symptoms, increased need for treatment, and often increased risk for the mother and fetus. The development of a new hematologic disorder during pregnancy poses many challenges. Both "benign" and "malignant" hematologic disorders that develop during pregnancy can be more difficult to diagnose given the expected physiologic changes and can require treatments that may pose significant risk to mother or fetus. Disorders unique to pregnancy affecting the hematologic system can occur that can also be difficult to diagnose and can be severe and even life-threatening. The risks and benefits of treatment, or withholding treatment, and the impact on mother and fetus, must be carefully evaluated.

The primary care of a pregnant woman resides with the obstetrician but significant collaboration between hematologist and obstetrician is required to provide optimal care for any patient with a hematologic disorder. Anesthesiologists play a significant role during labor and delivery. Early consultation with anesthesia in advance of the delivery date is important to facilitate a smooth delivery. A well-thought-out, detailed, and documented plan for treatment at labor and delivery for the patient with a hematologic disorder, especially a coagulation disorder, can be of enormous benefit when the

Hematol Oncol Clin N Am 25 (2011) xiii–xiv
doi:10.1016/j.hoc.2011.03.001
0889-8588/11/$ – see front matter © 2011 Elsevier Inc. All rights reserved.

hemonc.theclinics.com

woman presents in labor. Transfusion medicine physicians may also need to be consulted during pregnancy or during labor and delivery. The collaborative management of a pregnant patient with a hematologic disorder through pregnancy and delivery is a multidisciplinary accomplishment.

This is the first volume of *Hematology/Oncology Clinics of North America* to address hematologic disorders in pregnancy. The authors of the articles in this issue are international leaders who present the current understanding of the pathophysiology and management of these diseases in pregnancy. Both common hematologic disorders, such as iron deficiency anemia, as well as less frequent hematologic disorders that have significant impact on pregnancy, such as myeloproliferative disorders and factor deficiencies, are reviewed. Articles by high-risk obstetricians, anesthesiologists, and transfusion medicine experts are included to provide their approach to the management of the pregnant patient with a hematologic disorder.

The desired primary outcome of any pregnancy is a healthy mother and a healthy baby. In the woman with a previously or newly diagnosed hematologic disorder careful diagnosis and management are needed to achieve this outcome. We hope that the readers will find this volume of *Hematology/Oncology Clinics of North America* informative, practical, and useful in achieving this goal.

Jean M. Connors, MD
Division of Hematology, Department of Medicine
Brigham and Women's Hospital
75 Francis Street
Boston, MA 02115, USA

E-mail address:
jconnors@partners.org

Anemia in Pregnancy

Alfred Ian Lee, MD, PhD[a], Maureen M. Okam, MD, MPH[b],*

KEYWORDS

• Anemia • Pregnancy • Iron deficiency • Folate • B_{12} deficiency

"A person, ordinarily in good health … suddenly becomes pale, the surface of the body being waxy and bloodless; she is faint and fatigued; capable of great bodily efforts which, however, produce palpitations and distress; she has pain in the head, impatience of light, throbbing at the temples, and sometimes an universal throbbing, slight confusion in the mind, and a sense of total and extreme prostration. At the same time the pulse is frequent, large, strong and hard; at least, an observer who should not see the pallid face and miserable look of the patient, would pronounce it to be hard…. Still every surface which can be examined during life, is destitute of blood. And after death, the only remarkable appearance is the bloodlessness of the tissues."

> *Walter Channing, 1842*

In 1842, Walter Channing, Dean of Harvard Medical School, published the first documented account of puerperal anemia in his narrative of Mrs H, who developed a fatal nonhemorrhagic anemia shortly after delivery.[1] Addison soon followed with his report of idiopathic anemia, later renamed pernicious anemia owing to its grim prognosis, with the term "pernicious anemia of pregnancy" coined to describe the Channing disease. Landmark advances in the early part of the twentieth century uncovered the pathologic basis of classic pernicious anemia, demonstrating the therapeutic potential of parenteral liver extract and the central role of gastric intrinsic factor in cobalamin (vitamin B_{12}) absorption.[2] Pernicious anemia of pregnancy was shown to be primarily caused by a deficiency of folate rather than vitamin B_{12}, based on the observations that affected women lacked gastric achlorhydria and exhibited a slow or absent response to liver supplementation.

Anemia of pregnancy is currently recognized as a major global health problem, affecting nearly half of all pregnant women worldwide.[3] The pernicious anemia of Channing, once regarded as a model for puerperal and gestational anemia, has been shown to be rare, accounting for only 1 of 200 to 1 of 1000 cases. Hydremia of pregnancy, a gestational decrease in hemoglobin levels because of

The authors have nothing to disclose.

[a] Department of Medical Oncology, Dana-Farber Cancer Institute, Harvard Medical School, 44 Binney Street, Smith 353, Boston, MA 02118, USA

[b] Division of Hematology, Brigham and Women's Hospital, Harvard Medical School, 75 Francis Street, Mid-campus 3, Boston, MA 02115, USA

* Corresponding author.

E-mail address: mokam@partners.org

Hematol Oncol Clin N Am 25 (2011) 241–259

doi:10.1016/j.hoc.2011.02.001

0889-8588/11/$ – see front matter © 2011 Published by Elsevier Inc.

hemonc.theclinics.com

a disproportionate increase in plasma volume, is the major physiologic contributor to anemia of pregnancy.[4] Globally, the most important pathologic cause of anemia of pregnancy is iron deficiency, arising as a consequence of increased fetal use of iron. In nonindustrialized countries, hookworm, malarial parasite, human immunodeficiency virus (HIV), and deficiencies in folate and other micronutrients may contribute to anemia of pregnancy. Pregnancy-associated complications, including sepsis, infection, preeclampsia, malignancy, marrow failure, can also precipitate anemia.[5]

ANEMIA OF PREGNANCY: DEFINITIONS AND EPIDEMIOLOGY

The World Health Organization (WHO) defines anemia of pregnancy as a hemoglobin level of less than 11 g/dL, or hematocrit less than 33%, at any point during pregnancy.[3] The US Centers for Disease Control and Prevention (CDC) defines anemia of pregnancy as a hemoglobin level of less than 11 g/dL, or hematocrit less than 33%, in the first or third trimester or hemoglobin less than 10.5 g/dL, or hematocrit less than 32%, in the second trimester.[6]

- *Anemia of pregnancy primarily affects women of low socioeconomic status.* Globally, by WHO criteria, 52% of pregnant women from undeveloped or developing countries are anemic compared with 20% from industrialized nations.[3] The highest prevalence is among pregnant women in India (88%), followed by Africa (50%), Latin America (40%), and the Caribbean (30%).
- *The risk of anemia of pregnancy increases with progression of pregnancy.* By CDC criteria, among low-income pregnant women in the United States, 8% are anemic in the first trimester, 12% in the second, and 34% in the third.[7] The prevalence of third-trimester anemia is viewed by the US Department of Health and Human Services (DHHS) as a major indicator of reproductive health among low-income women, with the highest prevalence in African Americans (48.5%), followed by American Indians and Alaska Natives (33.9%), Hispanics and Latinas (30.1%), Asians, Native Hawaiians, and other Pacific Islanders (29%), and Whites (27.5%). The Healthy People 2010 initiative, launched in 2000 by the DHHS, proposed to reduce the prevalence of third-trimester anemia among low-income women to 20% or less during the subsequent decade[7]; however, as of 2008, the overall prevalence had increased compared with previous years, with only 1 state achieving DHHS goals (Montana, with 15.4% of low-income pregnant women classified as anemic in the third trimester).

IRON HOMEOSTASIS

Dietary iron is absorbed by intestinal epithelial cells in the duodenum and jejunum.[8,9] Absorption depends on gastric acid, which maintains iron in its soluble ferrous (Fe^{2+}) form rather than the insoluble ferric (Fe^{3+}) form. Intracellular iron within macrophages is liberated from senescent erythrocytes during erythrophagocytosis. Iron from both intestinal epithelial cells and macrophages is transported, via ferroportin channels, to the circulation, where it is bound to serum transferrin, which carries the bound iron to target cells (**Fig. 1**). Transferrin receptors on the surfaces of erythroid progenitors, lymphocytes, and other proliferating cells bind and internalize the transferrin-iron complex, releasing iron intracellularly through the transferrin cycle. Ferritin, an intracellular protein that binds and sequesters iron, is leaked into the circulation in small levels; serum ferritin levels are an accurate indicator of total body iron stores, although the function of intracellular ferritin is unknown.

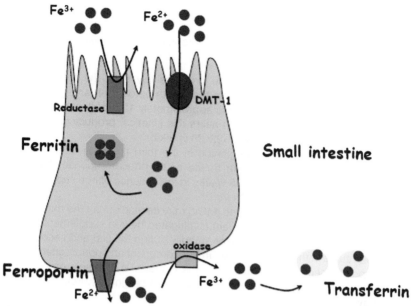

Fig. 1. Iron metabolism. Absorption of dietary iron by duodenal and jejunal epithelial cells is dependent on gastric acid, which maintains iron in its soluble ferrous (Fe^{2+}) form rather than the insoluble ferric (Fe^{3+}) form. Intestinal ferric reductase reduces any remaining ferrous iron before intestinal epithelial cell uptake. Ferric iron is transported into intestinal epithelial cells via divalent metal transporter (DMT-1) receptors. Within the intestinal epithelial cell, some iron becomes bound by intracellular ferritin, whereas the remainder is secreted via ferroportin channels into the circulation and bound by serum transferrin. Hepcidin (not shown) regulates iron metabolism by binding ferroportin, inducing its endocytosis and degradation in lysosomes.

The primary regulator of iron use is hepcidin, which binds ferroportin and induces its endocytosis and degradation in lysosomes.[8,9] High hepcidin levels cause intracellular accumulation of iron and impairment of iron use, as seen in anemia of inflammation; by contrast, hepcidin deficiency, seen in hemochromatosis, results in uncontrolled release of iron into the circulation. Transferrin, ferritin, and hepcidin are produced by the liver. The latter 2 are acute phase reactants, and their levels may be elevated during infection, inflammation, or stress.

Iron Requirements During Pregnancy

Approximately 1190 mg of iron is required to sustain pregnancy from conception through delivery.[10] Processes such as maternal and fetal erythropoiesis, as well as blood loss during labor and delivery, consume iron, whereas cessation of menses during pregnancy and lactation conserve iron. The net iron balance during pregnancy, delivery, and the postpartum period is a deficit of 580 mg. When averaged over a gestational period of 290 days, the overall maternal iron deficit amounts to an iron requirement of 2 mg/d, in addition to the recommended daily allowance of 15 mg for women of childbearing age. By comparison, the average daily iron absorption from Western diets is 1 to 2 mg/d, or 3 to 5 mg/d from diets rich in iron-containing foods. Most women therefore cannot optimally maintain iron needs during pregnancy even under optimal dietary circumstances, accounting for the high incidence of pregnancy-associated anemia in nonindustrialized countries, where nutritional status is poor.

The kinetics of iron use over the course of pregnancy gives rise to predictable fluctuations in hematologic parameters[11]:

- Maternal hemoglobin levels decline progressively from the first to the ninth month of gestation, then increase in the month before delivery. In the absence of iron supplementation, the nadir is approximately 10.5 g/dL at 27 to 30 weeks of gestation. Iron supplementation alters this kinetics, producing a less-severe nadir (11.5 g/dL) occurring earlier (22–26 weeks).
- Serum ferritin levels decline beginning in the third trimester, then increase in the month before delivery owing to the acute phase response. The nadir is approximately 15 g/μL at 35 to 38 weeks in the absence of iron supplementation or 20 μ/L at 31 to 34 weeks with iron.
- Red cell mean corpuscular volume (MCV) may decline during the third trimester, although the magnitude of the effect is mitigated by iron supplementation.
- Serum erythropoietin levels increase steadily during the first and second trimesters, then surge in the third trimester. In both pregnant and nonpregnant patients, erythropoietin secretion, mediated by the kidneys, is inversely proportional to hemoglobin levels and blood oxygen content. In pregnancy, iron supplementation may lower peak erythropoietin levels.
- Maternal hepcidin levels are reduced at term to facilitate iron transfer and use.[12] Women with iron deficiency in pregnancy have more profound levels of hepcidin suppression at term than those in iron-replete women, although interpretation of such findings is complicated by hepcidin's role as an acute phase reactant, with increased levels at the time of labor.

Hemodynamic Changes During Pregnancy

Hydremia of pregnancy was first proposed by German and French physicians in the 1830s and formally demonstrated in 1934 by Dieckmann and Wegner,[4] who measured plasma volume, red cell mass, and hemoglobin levels at intervals throughout pregnancy and observed that although all 3 parameters increased with gestation, the increase in plasma volume was greater than that of red cell mass or hemoglobin levels. As a general rule, the total circulatory volumes during pregnancy increase by a factor of 30% to 50% compared with baseline, although in individual studies, considerable variation is reported, reflecting differences in study populations and in techniques used to measure plasma and cell volumes. During pregnancy, the following specific hemodynamic changes occur:

- Plasma volume decreases in the first 6 weeks of gestation, then expands from the sixth week to 34 to 36 weeks, achieving levels 50% above baseline.
- Red cell mass decreases in the first 12 weeks, then increases from 12 weeks to the third trimester, reaching levels that are 20% to 30% above baseline.
- Both plasma volume and red cell mass decline in the final month of gestation, returning to prepregnancy levels by 6 to 8 weeks post partum.

The increase in maternal circulatory volume during pregnancy is accompanied by a decrease in systemic vascular resistance and an increase in perfusion of the utero-placental and renal vascular beds, thought to be the effect of multiple hormones (eg, renin, angiotensin II, aldosterone, thromboxane A_2, cortisol, estrogens, progesterone, antidiuretic hormone, atrial natriuretic hormone, and prostacyclin).[13] Maternal expansion of plasma volume and red cell mass supports fetal amniotic fluid production, mitigates hemodynamic insults such as hemorrhage, enhances total blood oxygen binding capacity, and facilitates tissue oxygen delivery. The importance of maternal circulatory expansion is illustrated by the consequences of hypovolemia, which include reduction in maternal glomerular filtration rate and development of fetal oligohydramnios.[14]

IRON DEFICIENCY IN PREGNANCY

Clinicians long recognized that hydremia alone could not account for the hemoglobin levels of less than 7 g/dL in 10% to 70% of pregnant women reported in the early twentieth century studies. A central role for iron deficiency in anemia of pregnancy was demonstrated in the 1950s by the frequent finding of hypochromia, microcytosis, and anisocytosis in the blood smears of pregnant women with anemia, and the resolution of such abnormalities following iron supplementation.[15] Iron deficiency has since been recognized as the most common cause of anemia of pregnancy worldwide, manifesting predominantly in the third trimester, when iron is maximally accumulated to accommodate erythropoiesis in the growing fetus.[16]

Risk Factors

In addition to poor nutritional intake, factors that impair iron absorption may precipitate iron deficiency in pregnancy, including bariatric surgery, antacids, and deficiencies of micronutrients such as vitamin A, vitamin C, zinc, and copper.[17,18]

Clinical Manifestations

Fatigue, pallor, light-headedness, tachycardia, dyspnea, poor exercise tolerance, and suboptimal work performance have all been reported in pregnant or postpartum women with iron deficiency, as have postpartum depression, poor maternal/infant behavioral interactions, impaired lactation, low birth weight, premature delivery, intrauterine growth retardation, and increased fetal and neonatal mortality.[19–23] Although supplemental iron improves the hematologic abnormalities of iron deficiency in pregnancy, the therapeutic benefits to neonatal mortality, infant morbidity, and child development are uncertain.[11,19,21,22]

Diagnosis

By either the CDC or WHO criteria, the presence of anemia in combination with a low ferritin level (<15–20 μg/L) is considered diagnostic of iron deficiency in pregnancy.[24] Diagnosis is complicated by the increase in ferritin levels during the third trimester, when iron deficiency is most likely to be present. If ferritin levels are normal or elevated, hypochromia, microcytosis, or a reduced red cell MCV may support a picture of iron deficiency.[11] C-reactive protein is an alternate measure of inflammation; a normal or elevated ferritin level with a normal C-reactive protein level should prompt investigation for alternate causes of anemia, such as hemoglobinopathies.[24] Soluble transferrin receptor (sTfR) concentration, released into the circulation by transferrin receptor–expressing cells, correlates inversely with total body iron content and exhibits high sensitivity and specificity in the diagnosis of iron deficiency during pregnancy.[25] Because sTfR is not an acute phase reactant, its levels do not increase with inflammation, although they can be influenced by red cell mass or erythropoietic activity and are often low in early pregnancy, when erythropoiesis is reduced.

Prevention

The WHO, CDC, and US Food and Drug Administration (FDA) recommend that all pregnant women receive oral iron supplementation from the beginning of gestation to 3 months post partum, at doses of 27 mg/d (FDA), 30 mg/d (CDC), or 60 mg/d (WHO), although doses as low as 20 mg/d may be effective.[3,11,19,21,26] The major side effects of oral iron supplementation are gastrointestinal symptoms, which occur in a dose-dependent manner, primarily at doses of 200 mg/d or more.

Treatment

Patients with mild anemia (hemoglobin level, 9.0–10.5 g/dL) should receive oral iron at 160 to 200 mg of elemental iron daily, with an expected increase in hemoglobin levels of 1 g/dL after 14 days of therapy.[24] Compared with oral iron, parenteral iron demonstrates faster hematologic recovery, likely because of variations in oral iron tolerability, absorption, and compliance. Parenteral iron may be administered in the second or third trimester to patients who have moderate to severe anemia (hemoglobin <9 g/dL), who are intolerant to oral iron, or who fail to respond appropriately to oral therapy.[11,19,21,27–29] Four preparations of parenteral iron are available in the United States: iron dextran (low–molecular-weight InFeD and high–molecular-weight DexFerrum), sodium ferric gluconate (Ferrlecit), iron sucrose (Venofer), and ferumoxytol (Feraheme). Among pregnant women who received parenteral iron in published studies, 15% to 20% developed thrombosis, although the relationship between these factors is uncertain.[21] Administration of recombinant human erythropoietin, in combination with parenteral iron, may be an alternate therapy for pregnant women with anemia, who are refractory to oral iron.[30,31] Darbepoietin has been similarly used in a single case report of a pregnant woman with chronic kidney disease.[32] Larger studies are needed to confirm the appropriateness, safety, and feasibility of erythropoietic stimulating agents in anemia of pregnancy.

OTHER NUTRITIONAL DEFICIENCIES IN ANEMIA OF PREGNANCY

Folate and Cobalamin Deficiency

Folate deficiency is historically regarded as the second most common cause of anemia of pregnancy after iron deficiency, although in many modern series vitamin B_{12} deficiency may be more prevalent, particularly in underprivileged areas. In studies from India, Turkey, Africa, Newfoundland, and Venezuela, 10% to 100% of pregnant women have a diagnosis of folate deficiency (defined as a serum level of <2.5–3.0 ng/mL), whereas 30% to 100% have vitamin B_{12} deficiency (defined as a serum level of <160–200 pg/mL).[23,33–38] The prevalence of folate or vitamin B_{12} deficiency increases with gestation.[34]

Fetal growth depends on folate and vitamin B_{12} because both are involved in the synthesis of tetrahydrofolate, an integral component of deoxyribonucleic acid synthesis and nuclear maturation (**Fig. 2**). Dietary folate is absorbed in the jejunum; poor nutrition and intestinal malabsorption can precipitate folate deficiency in pregnancy. Oral vitamin B_{12} is absorbed in the ileum; R proteins (eg, haptocorrins, secreted by the salivary gland) bind vitamin B_{12} in the acid environment of the gastrium, transporting vitamin B_{12} to the duodenum where pancreatic proteases degrade the R proteins, releasing vitamin B_{12} for binding by intrinsic factor (from gastric parietal cells) and subsequent uptake by ileal enterocytes. Malabsorption, ileal resection, intestinal parasites, atrophic gastritis, antihistamines, and proton pump inhibitors can all increase the risk of vitamin B_{12} deficiency in pregnancy.[15]

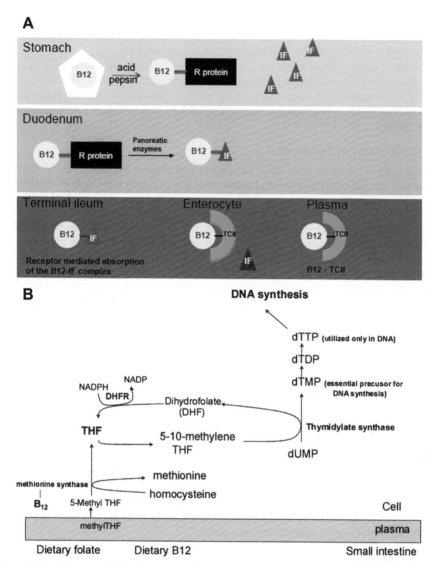

Fig. 2. Physiology and biochemistry of folate metabolism. (*A*) In the stomach, pepsin releases vitamin B_{12} from ingested food, and R proteins (eg, haptocorrin, secreted by the salivary gland) bind vitamin B_{12} and carry it to the duodenum, where pancreatic proteases degrade the R proteins, releasing vitamin B_{12} for binding by intrinsic factor (IF). The complex is carried to the terminal ileum, and vitamin B_{12} is transported into intestinal epithelial cells via the transcobalamin II (TCII) receptor. (*B*) Within cells, folate and vitamin B_{12} are required for synthesis of tetrahydrofolate (THF), which itself is required for the conversion of deoxyuridyl monophosphate to deoxythymidyl monophosphate, an essential precursor for DNA synthesis. DHFR, dihydrofolate reductase.

Most pregnant women with folate or vitamin B_{12} deficiency do not exhibit erythrocyte macrocytosis, although 2% to 5% of pregnant women with normocytic anemia have mild megaloblastic changes in the bone marrow that resolve with folic acid supplementation.[15] Elevation in homocysteine or methylmalonic acid levels accompanies most cases of clinically significant vitamin B_{12} deficiency in pregnancy. About 20% of pregnant women have a "physiologic" decline in vitamin B_{12} levels with no change in homocysteine or methylmalonic acid levels.[39,40]

The WHO recommends folate supplementation for all pregnant women at a dose of 400 μg/d from the beginning of pregnancy to 3 months post partum.[3] The US National Institutes of Health (NIH) recommends a higher daily allowance of vitamin B_{12} in pregnant women than in nonpregnant women (2.6 vs 2.4 μg/d) to support fetal neurologic development.

Other Micronutrient Deficiencies

Deficiencies in micronutrients other than folate and vitamin B_{12} remain the important causes of anemia of pregnancy worldwide, affecting primarily women from underprivileged areas. The prevalence of anemia due to specific micronutrient deficiencies is difficult to assess because multiple nutritional deficits may coexist within the same community.[34] Coinfection by human pathogens may compound the effects of micronutrient deficiency on pregnancy in certain populations.[33] Deficiencies in vitamin A, vitamin C, zinc, and copper have all been reported in association with anemia of pregnancy, possibly because of the inhibitory effects of such deficiencies on gastrointestinal iron absorption, although the interactions between specific micronutrients are complex and may be dose dependent.[41] Multimicronutrient supplementation may improve maternal anemia and other gestational and neonatal outcomes in specific populations, although the risks and benefits of individual micronutrients are uncertain, as are the magnitude of the observed hematologic and nonhematologic benefits compared with the combination of iron and folate alone.[42–44]

INFECTIOUS DISEASES AND ANEMIA OF PREGNANCY

In nonindustrialized countries, hookworm (*Ancylostoma*) infection and malaria are widespread and can cause anemia of pregnancy through nutrition depletion, gastrointestinal bleeding, and hemolysis. Whipworm (*Trichuris trichiura*) and roundworm (*Ascaris lumbricoides*) infections may also be associated with anemia in both pregnant and nonpregnant women. Coinfection with these organisms is common and can lead to complex physiologic interactions. For example, in a study of pregnant women along the Thai-Burmese border, hookworm infection increased the risk of malaria and anemia; ascariasis was protective against both malaria and anemia, whereas whipworm infection bore no association with either.[45]

Hookworm Infection

Among pregnant women with hookworm infection, the burden of infection is a strong predictor of maternal iron stores, with severity of anemia correlating with the number of hookworm eggs isolated from stool.[46–48] The WHO recommends universal deworming of pregnant women in hookworm-endemic areas with antihelminthic medications (eg, albendazole or mebendazole), in conjunction with iron and folate supplementation, although the hematologic benefits of deworming are uncertain.[48,49]

Malaria

In malaria-endemic regions, chronic malaria can cause acute hemolytic anemia during pregnancy, particularly in patients with coexisting nutritional deficiencies or hemoglobinopathies (eg, sickle cell disease).[50] Primigravidas are particularly prone, with a strong association of *Plasmodium falciparum* with severe anemia (defined as a hemoglobin level of <7 g/dL) and maternal death.[51] The relationship between severity of anemia and burden of parasitemia is uncertain.[47] For pregnant women in malaria-endemic areas, intermittent preventive treatment (IPT, typically using sulfa-doxine/pyrimethamine) is indicated, in conjunction with the use of insecticide-treated mosquito nets; the role of IPT in nonendemic areas (eg, Latin America) is uncertain.[52] Pregnant women with documented malaria should be treated according to the CDC guidelines based on geographic resistance patterns (eg, in Latin America, mefloquine/artesunate is used, although its efficacy in pregnancy has not been tested; in the United States, chloroquine or hydroxychloroquine is used for uncomplicated *Plasmodium malariae*, *Plasmodium vivax*, or *Plasmodium ovale* infection or quinine sulfate and clindamycin are used for uncomplicated, chloroquine-resistant *P falcipa-rum* infection).[53–55]

Human Immunodeficiency Virus (HIV)

In both pregnant and nonpregnant patients, HIV causes several hematologic manifes-tations, including immune thrombocytopenia, coagulopathy, and anemia; anemia is a consequence of inflammation, bone marrow suppression, hemolysis, parvovirus B19 coinfection, or antiretroviral therapy.[56] Globally, HIV infection is an independent risk factor for anemia of pregnancy in populations in which HIV infection, malaria, and nutritional deficiencies coexist.[57] In such populations, in HIV-infected pregnant women, the standard-dose IPT for malaria is more likely to fail and should receive higher dosing schedules.[52] Micronutrient supplementation with iron, folate, and vita-mins B, C, and E can delay progression of HIV infection in HIV-infected pregnant African women.[58]

HEMOGLOBINOPATHIES AND PREGNANCY

A total of 269 million individuals worldwide, or 5% of the world's population, are genetic carriers for or are affected by a hemoglobin disorder.[59] Each year 365,000 infants are born with either sickle cell disease (70%) or thalassemia (30%). Geographic distribution varies widely, with an incidence of 1 in 1000 in the United States compared with more than 20 in 1000 in parts of West Africa. Prenatal counseling and antenatal screening programs have been launched in Canada, the United Kingdom, and multiple other nations to identify parents with hemoglobinopathies.[60,61] Since 2006, all US states have instituted universal newborn screening for sickle cell disease,[62] and in 2010, the NIH and the CDC launched a cooperative initiative in several states to create surveillance programs for the detection of hemoglobinopathies.

Human Hemoglobins and Hemoglobinopathies

The human α-globin gene cluster is located on chromosome 16 and consists of 2 identical α-globin genes downstream of 1 embryonic ζ-globin gene (and other nonex-pressed sequences) (**Fig. 3**).[63] The β-globin locus is on chromosome 11 and contains 1 β-globin gene downstream of 1 embryonic ϵ-globin, 2 fetal γ-globins, and 1 δ-globin. Embryonic hemoglobin, the first hemoglobin expressed in fetal development, is composed of ζ- and ϵ-globin chains. Fetal hemoglobin (HbF, $\alpha_2\gamma_2$) is synthesized beginning in the sixth week of gestation and predominates through all of fetal life into the first few weeks after delivery. β-Globin expression begins shortly before birth, and by 6 weeks of life, adult hemoglobin A (HbA, $\alpha_2\beta_2$) is the dominant hemoglobin, with hemoglobin A_2 ($\alpha_2\delta_2$) produced in minor amounts. HbF differs from HbA in having a left-shifted hemoglobin-oxygen dissociation curve, allowing HbF to preferentially bind oxygen delivered by maternal HbA from the placental circulation.

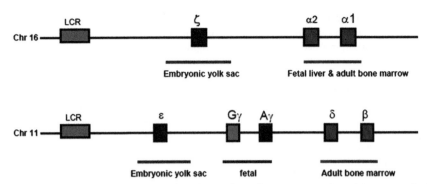

Fig. 3. Human α- and β-globin gene loci, located on chromosomes 16 and 11, respectively. Expression of both loci is regulated by enhancer elements known as locus control regions (LCRs). Embryonic hemoglobin is the first hemoglobin expressed in fetal development and is composed of ζ- and ε-globin chains. Beginning at 6 weeks of gestation and continuing into the first few weeks after delivery, fetal hemoglobin is synthesized, consisting of α- and γ-globin chains. Two forms of adult hemoglobin are synthesized shortly before birth: hemoglobin A, the major adult hemoglobin, consisting of α- and β-chains, and hemoglobin A_2, consisting of α- and δ-chains.

Sickle cell disease

Substitution of valine for glutamic acid (Glu→Val) in the sixth position of the β-globin chain generates sickle cell β-globin ($β^S$), which associates with α-globin to form tetrameric hemoglobin S (HbS, $α_2β_2$).[63] Homozygous sickle cell disease (SS) arises when both the β-globin alleles are $β^S$, leading to the exclusive production of HbS, which has a severe phenotype. Sickle cell trait occurs when one β allele is wild-type β and the other is $β^S$, leading to the production of both HbA and HbS, with a clinically indolent phenotype. A slightly different paradigm exists for hemoglobin C (HbC), which arises from a glutamic acid to lysine (Glu→Lys) substitution in the sixth position of the β-globin chain ($β^C$). Homozygous C (HbCC) has a mild phenotype, whereas HbC trait is clinically silent. Hemoglobin SC disease, in which both $β^S$ and $β^C$ alleles are present, carries a moderately severe phenotype. The difference in phenotypic severity of sickle cell trait compared with SC disease reflects the dependence of sickling on intracellular HbS concentration because $β^C$ promotes erythrocyte dehydration, leading to polymerization of HbS because of increased intracellular HbS concentrations, whereas the presence of HbA with HbS preserves intracellular HbS concentrations, preventing sickling.[64,65] The only FDA approved therapy for sickle cell disease in nonpregnant patients is use of hydroxyurea, which stimulates HbF production and the formation of HbS/HbF hybrid hemoglobin tetramers that inhibit HbS polymerization and erythrocyte sickling.

β-Thalassemia

More than 200 mutations in the β-globin gene have been described for β-thalassemia, which affects primarily the people of Mediterranean, African, Middle Eastern, East Asian, South Asian, and Latin American descent.[63,66] Mutations causing a reduction in β-chain synthesis are designated as $β^+$, whereas those causing a complete absence of β-chain expression are designated $β^0$. The β-thalassemias are classified as β-thalassemia minor, β-thalassemia intermedia, and β-thalassemia major, based on variations in phenotypic severity that arise from different combinations of $β^+$, $β^0$, and wild-type β. Heterozygosity for $β^S$ and β-thalassemia leads to the S/β-Thal phenotype, which can be severe, particularly if the β allele is $β^0$.

Hemoglobin E thalassemia

Hemoglobin E (HbE) arises from a missense (G-to-A) mutation in the 26th codon of the β-globin gene, encoding an unstable β-globin synthesized at reduced levels because of an abnormal messenger RNA splice site.[67] HbE thalassemia is one of the most common β-thalassemias, occurring in patients of East and South Asian descent. Similar to β[C], HbE trait and homozygous HbE (HbEE) are mild diseases, whereas heterozygosity for β[S] and HbE (HbSE) produces a severe phenotype.

α-Thalassemia

More than 40 different deletions and other mutations in the α-globin locus have been described for α-thalassemia.[68,69] Genotypes are classified as α^+ or α^0, based on whether α-globin gene expression is present or absent, respectively, in each of the 4 α genes. Phenotypic severity reflects the number of α genes expressed, with deletion of 1 α gene designated as a silent carrier state (α-thalassemia-2, or α-thalassemia trait); deletion of 2 α genes, α-thalassemia minor (α-thalassemia-1); deletion of 3 α genes, hemoglobin H (HbH) disease, characterized by accumulation of tetramers of β globin (β_4); and deletion of all 4 α genes, hemoglobin Bart's hydrops fetalis, with fatal accumulation of tetrameric fetal γ globin (γ_4) in utero.

Sickle Cell Disease in Pregnancy

Whereas some pregnant women with sickle cell disease experience periodic sickling crises throughout pregnancy, most pregnant women have sickle-related complications in the third trimester, at term, and in the puerperium.[70] Maternal complications from sickle cell disease include pulmonary embolism, acute chest syndrome, pneumonia, and severe pain crises. Prophylaxis of these complications is paramount because they may precipitate delivery. Cerebral vein thrombosis, stroke, venous thromboembolism, pulmonary hypertension, infection, postpartum hemorrhage, cardiomyopathy, pulmonary hypertension, and increased maternal mortality are additional maternal risks.[71] Fetal risks include preeclampsia, eclampsia, abruptio placentae (from placental necrosis following vascular thrombosis), preterm labor, premature or preterm premature rupture of membranes, intrauterine growth restriction, low birth weight, cesarean delivery, and increased rates of spontaneous abortion and perinatal mortality.[70–75] Worldwide, malaria is the major identifiable cause of acute anemia in pregnant women with sickle cell disease, with postpartum hemorrhage, preeclampsia, aplastic crisis (from parvovirus B19 infection), splenic sequestration (in patients with SC disease or S/β-Thal phenotypic disease, who have preexisting splenomegaly), and erythrocyte sickling being additional causes.[50,76]

Despite these risks, maternal and fetal outcomes in pregnancy complicated by sickle cell disease are generally favorable. In the landmark Cooperative Study of Sickle Cell Disease, 445 pregnancies in women with sickle cell disease (SS, SC, S/β[+], and S/β[0]) were followed up from 1979 to 1985 and 64% of the pregnancies were carried to term.[74,77] Pain crises occurred in half of the women with SS, S/β[+], or S/β[0] disease compared with 25% with SC disease. Acute chest syndrome occurred in 6%, preeclampsia in 14%, and eclampsia in 1%. Infants of SS mothers were twice as likely as those of SC mothers to be born preterm (27% vs 14%). One-fifth of the infants were small for gestational age (SGA), with preeclampsia and anemia being the major risk factors for SGA.

Although the fetus benefits from the increased oxygen affinity of HbF compared with maternal HbA, the placenta in sickle cell disease sustains considerable damage. Postpartum placental specimens from women with sickle cell disease show extensive evidence of hypoxemic injury, including vascular anomalies, thromboses, excess fibrin deposition, syncytial changes with knotting (Tenney-Parker changes), and congestion by sickled erythrocytes.[72,78] Levels of von Willebrand factor and various cell adhesion molecules (eg, P-selectin and vascular endothelial growth factor) are increased within umbilical vein endothelial cells and smooth muscle cells, consistent with an activated response to hypoxemia. Few placental neutrophils are seen, indicating only a mild inflammatory reaction, in contrast to preeclampsia, in which neutrophils are a hallmark of placental hypoxemic injury.

For all women with sickle cell disease who are pregnant or contemplating pregnancy, a multidisciplinary team approach is essential, drawing on the expertise of obstetricians, nutritionists, primary care physicians, and hematologists. In the appropriate geographic locales, comprehensive prenatal care plans incorporating patient education, nutrition counseling, malaria prophylaxis, early detection of bacterial infections, and restricted use of blood transfusions may improve maternal mortality.[50] Following conception, routine chemical analysis; liver function tests; estimation of serum bilirubin, lactate dehydrogenase, and 24-hour urine protein levels; complete blood cell count; reticulocyte count; urinalysis and urine culture; blood type analysis; and antibody screens should be performed and repeated regularly. Fetal β-globin phenotyping should be performed early in pregnancy via chorionic villus sampling (at 9–12 weeks' gestation) or amniocentesis (at 16–18 weeks), with each procedure carrying a small risk of miscarriage (1%–2% or 0.5%–1%, respectively).[79] Fetal ultrasonography is recommended in the first and third trimesters. Maternal echocardiography may be performed to assess for pulmonary hypertension.[80]

Supportive care in sickle cell disease centers on pain management and red blood cell transfusions. Pain management in pregnant women with sickle cell disease can be challenging owing to concerns regarding fetal and neonatal narcotic dependence. Hydration should be encouraged throughout pregnancy and should be performed empirically during hospitalizations and throughout labor and delivery. A seminal randomized controlled trial demonstrated no benefit of prophylactic over restrictive transfusions, except in the reduction of maternal pain crises, at the expense of a marked increase in the number of blood products administered and the development of red cell alloantibodies.[70,72,81] A hemoglobin level of less than 5 g/dL, reduction in hemoglobin levels of 20% from baseline, acute chest syndrome, hypoxemia, preeclampsia, or other symptoms of anemia are all indications for transfusion in pregnant women with sickle cell disease. Simple transfusions may be used for a hemoglobin level of less than 5 g/dL and a reticulocyte count of less than 3%, whereas partial exchange transfusions with a target posttransfusion HbS level of less than 50% are preferred for a hemoglobin level of 8 to 10 g/dL.[76] Hydroxyurea has shown teratogenicity in animals and is excreted in breast milk; hence, the use of hydroxyurea is contraindicated during pregnancy and breastfeeding.

Thalassemias in Pregnancy

For pregnant and nonpregnant patients with α- or β-thalassemia, hemolytic anemia caused by ineffective erythropoiesis is the major complication.[82] Imbalanced nonstoichiometric production of α- and β-globin chains leads to disruptions in red cell physiology, causing intramedullary destruction of erythroid precursors and hemolysis of circulating red blood cells. Extramedullary hematopoiesis occurs when anemia is severe. In an attempt to maintain erythropoietic needs, iron use is increased through reduction in hepcidin levels, leading to hemochromatosis independent of transfusion therapy.[83] Splenectomy can be helpful in improving anemia but confers an increased risk of thrombosis, particularly in patients with HbE thalassemia.[66,67,69]

HbH disease

HbH is an unstable tetramer of β-chains (β_4) with high oxygen affinity and impaired oxygen delivery.[69,79,84] Precipitation of β_4 in erythrocytes disrupts red cell metabolism and impairs membrane deformability, leading to shortened erythrocyte survival. Clinical manifestations of HbH disease include microcytic anemia, hepatosplenomegaly, cholelithiasis, growth defects, thrombosis, and hemochromatosis; the last manifestation is associated with hepatic and cardiac dysfunction. Hemolytic crises occur in 10% of patients with HbH disease, sometimes in conjunction with parvovirus B19 infection.[85] In pregnant women with HbH disease, anemia can be profound with hemoglobin levels of less than 6 to 7 g/dL, particularly in the second and third trimesters. Pregnancy in HbH disease is associated with increased risks of preeclampsia, congestive heart failure, miscarriage, premature births, intrauterine growth restriction, low birth weight, and perinatal deaths compared with patients without thalassemia.[86] Rarely, fatal HbH hydrops fetalis can occur because of a specific α gene mutation.[87] Pregnant women with HbH disease may receive blood transfusions to maintain hemoglobin levels more than 7 g/dL. Recombinant human erythropoietin has been successfully used in a single case report of a pregnant patient with HbH disease and symptomatic anemia.[88]

Hemoglobin Bart's hydrops fetalis

Hemoglobin Bart's disease arises when all 4 α-globin genes are absent, leading to the accumulation and tetramerization of fetal γ-globin (γ_4) at 6 to 8 weeks' gestation, when α-globin expression would ordinarily begin.[89] Oxygen affinity of γ_4 is sufficiently high that oxygen cannot be delivered, leading to fetal ischemia, anemia, organomegaly (from extramedullary hematopoiesis), and intrauterine death. Pregnancies involving fetuses with hemoglobin Bart's disease carry several potential complications, including maternal anemia, preeclampsia, polyhydramnios, fetal malpresentation, antepartum hemorrhage, and preterm delivery.[90] For fetuses with hemoglobin Bart's disease, the severity of fetal anemia can be approximated by Doppler ultrasonographic assessment of middle cerebral artery peak velocity.[91] Intrauterine simple and exchange transfusions have been used with some success, although long-term sequelae including neurologic deficits, mild congenital malformations, hemochromatosis, and chronic transfusion dependence are of concern.[92,93] In utero and postnatal hematopoietic stem cell transplants have also been performed, the former relying on the immunologic naivete of fetal donor stem cell preparations and of fetal recipient immune responses; however, such techniques remain experimental.

β-Thalassemia intermedia and major

Hemolysis in β-thalassemia intermedia and β-thalassemia major is accompanied by hemochromatosis with multiorgan dysfunction, involving cardiac, hepatic, and endocrine tissues.[66,94] Hypogonadotropic hypogonadism may lead to infertility, with serum ferritin levels correlating inversely with the likelihood of pregnancy.[95] During pregnancy, as with the α-thalassemias, anemia in β-thalassemia can worsen and may require transfusion support, particularly in the second and third trimesters.[94] Pregnant women with β-thalassemia carry an increased risk of thrombosis, which may warrant consideration of empirical anticoagulation post partum and, in some cases, evaluation for associated thrombophilias.

APLASTIC ANEMIA AND PREGNANCY

Multiple cases of aplastic anemia associated with pregnancy and a few cases of pregnancy-induced aplastic anemia seen with or mimicking immune thrombocytopenia have been reported in patients presenting with petechiae or pallor during the second or third trimester of pregnancy.[96–99] Pathologically, pregnancy may induce aplastic anemia through erythropoietic inhibitory effects of estrogens and other hormones, although in some cases, pregnancy may uncover a preexisting aplastic anemia. Maternal death occurs in 20% to 50% of cases, usually from fatal hemorrhage or infection. Fetal complications include in utero death in up to one-third of cases and preterm labor from chorioamnionitis. Women with a preexisting diagnosis of aplastic anemia may have a more favorable prognosis than those with pregnancy-associated aplastic anemia, although prenatal management is the same and consists of blood transfusions to maintain a platelet count of more than 20×10^9/L and administration of growth factors (eg, granulocyte/monocyte colony stimulating factor) and, in select cases, cyclosporine. Hematopoietic cell transplant, the mainstay of treatment of aplastic anemia in nonpregnant patients, is contraindicated during pregnancy.[100] Among women who survive pregnancy-associated aplastic anemia, 50% to 70% achieve spontaneous remission, whereas the remainder require therapy with antithymocyte globulin, immunosuppression, and/or stem cell transplantation.

REFERENCES

1. Longo LD. Classic pages in obstetrics and gynecology. Notes on anhaemia, principally in its connections with the puerperal state, and with functional disease of the uterus; with cases: Walter Channing. The New England Quarterly Journal of Medicine and Surgery, vol. 1, pp. 157–188, 1842–1843. Am J Obstet Gynecol 1977;127(1):91.
2. George R. Minot - Nobel lecture. Nobelprize.org. Avaliable at: http://nobelprize.org/nobel_prizes/medicine/laureates/1934/minot-lecture.html. Accessed March 9, 2011.
3. UN Children's Fund, U, WHO. Iron deficiency anaemia. Assessment prevention, and control. A guide for programme managers. Geneva (Switzerland): World Health Organization; 2001.
4. Dieckmann WJ, Wegner CR. The blood in normal pregnancy. I: blood and plasma volumes. Arch Intern Med 1934;53(1):71–86.
5. Dillon RA. The anemias of pregnancy. N Engl J Med 1943;229(19):718–22.
6. Recommendations to prevent and control iron deficiency in the United States. Centers for Disease Control and Prevention. MMWR Recomm Rep 1998; 47(RR-3):1–29.
7. Healthy People 2010. US Government; 2000. Available at: http://www.healthypeople.gov/2020/default.aspx. Accessed February 17, 2011.
8. Weiss G, Goodnough LT. Anemia of chronic disease. N Engl J Med 2005; 352(10):1011–23.
9. Andrews NC. Forging a field: the golden age of iron biology. Blood 2008;112(2): 219–30.
10. Baker WF Jr. Iron deficiency in pregnancy, obstetrics, and gynecology. Hematol Oncol Clin North Am 2000;14(5):1061–77.
11. Milman N. Iron and pregnancy–a delicate balance. Ann Hematol 2006;85(9): 559–65.
12. Rehu M, Punnonen K, Ostland V, et al. Maternal serum hepcidin is low at term and independent of cord blood iron status. Eur J Haematol 2010;85(4):345–52.
13. Silversides CK, Colman JM. Physiological changes in pregnancy. In: Oakley C, Warnes CA, editors. Heart disease in pregnancy. 2nd edition. Malden (MA): Blackwell Publishing; 2007. p. 6.

14. Goodlin RC, Dobry CA, Anderson JC, et al. Clinical signs of normal plasma volume expansion during pregnancy. Am J Obstet Gynecol 1983;145(8):1001–9.

15. Frenkel EP, Yardley DA. Clinical and laboratory features and sequelae of deficiency of folic acid (folate) and vitamin B12 (cobalamin) in pregnancy and gynecology. Hematol Oncol Clin North Am 2000;14(5):1079–100, viii.

16. Rao R, Georgieff MK. Perinatal aspects of iron metabolism. Acta Paediatr Suppl 2002;438:124–9.

17. Killip S, Bennett JM, Chambers MD. Iron deficiency anemia. Am Fam Physician 2007;75(5):671–8.

18. Love AL, Billett HH. Obesity, bariatric surgery, and iron deficiency: true, true, true and related. Am J Hematol 2008;83(5):403–9.

19. Routine iron supplementation during pregnancy. Review article. US Preventive Services Task Force. JAMA 1993;270(23):2848–54.

20. Murray-Kolb LE, Beard JL. Iron deficiency and child and maternal health. Am J Clin Nutr 2009;89(3):946S–50S.

21. Reveiz L, Gyte GM, Cuervo LG. Treatments for iron-deficiency anaemia in pregnancy. Cochrane Database Syst Rev 2007;2:CD003094.

22. Rasmussen K. Is there a causal relationship between iron deficiency or iron-deficiency anemia and weight at birth, length of gestation and perinatal mortality? J Nutr 2001;131(2S–2):590S–601S [discussion: 601S–3S].

23. Kalaivani K. Prevalence & consequences of anaemia in pregnancy. Indian J Med Res 2009;130(5):627–33.

24. Breymann C, Honegger C, Holzgreve W, et al. Diagnosis and treatment of iron-deficiency anaemia during pregnancy and postpartum. Arch Gynecol Obstet 2010;282(5):577–80.

25. Akesson A, Bjellerup P, Bremme K, et al. Soluble transferrin receptor: longitudinal assessment from pregnancy to postlactation. Obstet Gynecol 2002; 99(2):260–6.

26. Makrides M, Crowther CA, Gibson RA, et al. Efficacy and tolerability of low-dose iron supplements during pregnancy: a randomized controlled trial. Am J Clin Nutr 2003;78(1):145–53.

27. al-Momen AK, al-Meshari A, al-Nuaim L, et al. Intravenous iron sucrose complex in the treatment of iron deficiency anemia during pregnancy. Eur J Obstet Gynecol Reprod Biol 1996;69(2):121–4.

28. Bayoumeu F, Subiran-Buisset C, Baka NE, et al. Iron therapy in iron deficiency anemia in pregnancy: intravenous route versus oral route. Am J Obstet Gynecol 2002;186(3):518–22.

29. Al RA, Unlubilgin E, Kandemir O, et al. Intravenous versus oral iron for treatment of anemia in pregnancy: a randomized trial. Obstet Gynecol 2005;106(6):1335–40.

30. Breymann C, Visca E, Huch R, et al. Efficacy and safety of intravenously administered iron sucrose with and without adjuvant recombinant human erythropoietin for the treatment of resistant iron-deficiency anemia during pregnancy. Am J Obstet Gynecol 2001;184(4):662–7.

31. Sifakis S, Angelakis E, Vardaki E, et al. Erythropoietin in the treatment of iron deficiency anemia during pregnancy. Gynecol Obstet Invest 2001;51(3):150–6.

32. Sobilo-Jarek L, Popowska-Drojecka J, Muszytowski M, et al. Anemia treatment with darbepoetin alpha in pregnant female with chronic renal failure: report of two cases. Adv Med Sci 2006;51:309–11.

33. Yusufji D, Mathan VI, Baker SJ. Iron, folate, and vitamin B12 nutrition in pregnancy: a study of 1000 women from southern India. Bull World Health Organ 1973; 48(1):15–22.

34. Açkurt F, Wetherilt H, Löker M, et al. Biochemical assessment of nutritional status in pre- and post-natal Turkish women and outcome of pregnancy. Eur J Clin Nutr 1995;49(8):613–22.
35. Msolla MJ, Kinabo JL. Prevalence of anaemia in pregnant women during the last trimester. Int J Food Sci Nutr 1997;48(4):265–70.
36. House JD, March SB, Ratnam S, et al. Folate and vitamin B12 status of women in Newfoundland at their first prenatal visit. CMAJ 2000;162(11):1557–9.
37. Garcia-Casal MN, Osorio C, Landaeta M, et al. High prevalence of folic acid and vitamin B12 deficiencies in infants, children, adolescents and pregnant women in Venezuela. Eur J Clin Nutr 2005;59(9):1064–70.
38. Karaoglu L, Pehlivan E, Egri M, et al. The prevalence of nutritional anemia in pregnancy in an east Anatolian province, Turkey. BMC Public Health 2010;10:329.
39. Metz J, McGrath K, Bennett M, et al. Biochemical indices of vitamin B12 nutrition in pregnant patients with subnormal serum vitamin B12 levels. Am J Hematol 1995;48(4):251–5.
40. Pardo J, Gindes L, Orvieto R. Cobalamin (vitamin B12) metabolism during pregnancy. Int J Gynaecol Obstet 2004;84(1):77–8.
41. Ladipo OA. Nutrition in pregnancy: mineral and vitamin supplements. Am J Clin Nutr 2000;72(Suppl 1):280S–90S.
42. Christian P, Shrestha J, LeClerq SC, et al. Supplementation with micronutrients in addition to iron and folic acid does not further improve the hematologic status of pregnant women in rural Nepal. J Nutr 2003;133(11):3492–8.
43. Haider BA, Bhutta ZA. Multiple-micronutrient supplementation for women during pregnancy. Cochrane Database Syst Rev 2006;4:CD004905.
44. Fawzi WW, Msamanga GI, Urassa W, et al. Vitamins and perinatal outcomes among HIV-negative women in Tanzania. N Engl J Med 2007;356(14):1423–31.
45. Boel M, Carrara VI, Rijken M, et al. Complex interactions between soil-transmitted helminths and malaria in pregnant women on the Thai-Burmese border. PLoS Negl Trop Dis 2010;4(11):e887.
46. Dreyfuss ML, Stoltzfus RJ, Shrestha JB, et al. Hookworms, malaria and vitamin A deficiency contribute to anemia and iron deficiency among pregnant women in the plains of Nepal. J Nutr 2000;130(10):2527–36.
47. Shulman CE, Graham WJ, Jilo H, et al. Malaria is an important cause of anaemia in primigravidae: evidence from a district hospital in coastal Kenya. Trans R Soc Trop Med Hyg 1996;90(5):535–9.
48. Brooker S, Hotez PJ, Bundy DA. Hookworm-related anaemia among pregnant women: a systematic review. PLoS Negl Trop Dis 2008;2(9):e291.
49. Ndibazza J, Muhangi L, Akishule D, et al. Effects of deworming during pregnancy on maternal and perinatal outcomes in Entebbe, Uganda: a randomized controlled trial. Clin Infect Dis 2010;50(4):531–40.
50. Rahimy MC, Gangbo A, Adjou R, et al. Effect of active prenatal management on pregnancy outcome in sickle cell disease in an African setting. Blood 2000;96(5):1685–9.
51. Brabin BJ, Hakimi M, Pelletier D. An analysis of anemia and pregnancy-related maternal mortality. J Nutr 2001;131(2S–2):604S–14S [discussion: 614S–5S].
52. Menendez C, D'Alessandro U, ter Kuile FO. Reducing the burden of malaria in pregnancy by preventive strategies. Lancet Infect Dis 2007;7(2):126–35.
53. Shulman CE, Dorman EK, Cutts F, et al. Intermittent sulphadoxine-pyrimethamine to prevent severe anaemia secondary to malaria in pregnancy: a randomised placebo-controlled trial. Lancet 1999;353(9153):632–6.

54. ter Kuile FO, van Eijk AM, Filler SJ. Effect of sulfadoxine-pyrimethamine resistance on the efficacy of intermittent preventive therapy for malaria control during pregnancy: a systematic review. JAMA 2007;297(23):2603–16.

55. Brabin BJ, Warsame M, Uddenfeldt-Wort U, et al. Monitoring and evaluation of malaria in pregnancy - developing a rational basis for control. Malar J 2008; 7(Suppl 1):S6.

56. Volberding PA, Baker KR, Levine AM. Human immunodeficiency virus hematology. Hematology Am Soc Hematol Educ Program 2003;294–313.

57. Dairo MD, Lawoyin TO, Onadeko MO, et al. HIV as an additional risk factors for anaemia in pregnancy: evidence from primary care level in Ibadan, Southwestern Nigeria. Afr J Med Med Sci 2005;34(3):275–9.

58. Fawzi WW, Msamanga GI, Spiegelman D, et al. A randomized trial of multivitamin supplements and HIV disease progression and mortality. N Engl J Med 2004;351(1):23–32.

59. Angastiniotis M, Modell B. Global epidemiology of hemoglobin disorders. Ann N Y Acad Sci 1998;850:251–69.

60. Langlois S, Ford JC, Chitayat D, et al. Carrier screening for thalassemia and hemoglobinopathies in Canada. J Obstet Gynaecol Can 2008;30(10):950–71.

61. Ryan K, Bain BJ, Worthington D, et al. Significant haemoglobinopathies: guidelines for screening and diagnosis. Br J Haematol 2010;149(1):35–49.

62. Benson JM, Therrell BL Jr. History and current status of newborn screening for hemoglobinopathies. Semin Perinatol 2010;34(2):134–44.

63. Schechter AN. Hemoglobin research and the origins of molecular medicine. Blood 2008;112(10):3927–38.

64. Bunn HF. Pathogenesis and treatment of sickle cell disease. N Engl J Med 1997; 337(11):762–9.

65. Nagel RL, Fabry ME, Steinberg MH. The paradox of hemoglobin SC disease. Blood Rev 2003;17(3):167–78.

66. Rund D, Rachmilewitz E. Beta-thalassemia. N Engl J Med 2005;353(11): 1135–46.

67. Vichinsky E. Hemoglobin e syndromes. Hematology Am Soc Hematol Educ Program 2007;79–83.

68. Higgs DR, Weatherall DJ. The alpha thalassaemias. Cell Mol Life Sci 2009;66(7): 1154–62.

69. Vichinsky E. Complexity of alpha thalassemia: growing health problem with new approaches to screening, diagnosis, and therapy. Ann N Y Acad Sci 2010;1202: 180–7.

70. Howard RJ, Tuck SM, Pearson TC. Pregnancy in sickle cell disease in the UK: results of a multicentre survey of the effect of prophylactic blood transfusion on maternal and fetal outcome. Br J Obstet Gynaecol 1995;102(12):947–51.

71. Villers MS, Jamison MG, De Castro LM, et al. Morbidity associated with sickle cell disease in pregnancy. Am J Obstet Gynecol 2008;199(2):125.e1–5.

72. Koshy M, Burd L, Wallace D, et al. Prophylactic red-cell transfusions in pregnant patients with sickle cell disease. A randomized cooperative study. N Engl J Med 1988;319(22):1447–52.

73. Seoud MA, Cantwell C, Nobles G, et al. Outcome of pregnancies complicated by sickle cell and sickle-C hemoglobinopathies. Am J Perinatol 1994;11(3): 187–91.

74. Smith JA, Espeland M, Bellevue R, et al. Pregnancy in sickle cell disease: experience of the Cooperative Study of Sickle Cell Disease. Obstet Gynecol 1996; 87(2):199–204.

75. Serjeant GR, Loy LL, Crowther M, et al. Outcome of pregnancy in homozygous sickle cell disease. Obstet Gynecol 2004;103(6):1278–85.
76. Koshy M. Sickle cell disease and pregnancy. Blood Rev 1995;9(3):157–64.
77. Rogers DT, Molokie R. Sickle cell disease in pregnancy. Obstet Gynecol Clin North Am 2010;37(2):223–37.
78. Trampont P, Roudier M, Andrea AM, et al. The placental-umbilical unit in sickle cell disease pregnancy: a model for studying in vivo functional adjustments to hypoxia in humans. Hum Pathol 2004;35(11):1353–9.
79. Chui DH, Fucharoen S, Chan V. Hemoglobin H disease: not necessarily a benign disorder. Blood 2003;101(3):791–800.
80. Castro O, Gladwin MT. Pulmonary hypertension in sickle cell disease: mechanisms, diagnosis, and management. Hematol Oncol Clin North Am 2005;19(5):881–96, vii.
81. Ngô C, Kayem G, Habibi A, et al. Pregnancy in sickle cell disease: maternal and fetal outcomes in a population receiving prophylactic partial exchange transfusions. Eur J Obstet Gynecol Reprod Biol 2010;152(2):138–42.
82. Rivella S. Ineffective erythropoiesis and thalassemias. Curr Opin Hematol 2009;16(3):187–94.
83. Gardenghi S, Grady RW, Rivella S. Anemia, ineffective erythropoiesis, and hepcidin: interacting factors in abnormal iron metabolism leading to iron overload in beta-thalassemia. Hematol Oncol Clin North Am 2010;24(6):1089–107.
84. Nathan DG, Stossel TB, Gunn RB, et al. Influence of hemoglobin precipitation on erythrocyte metabolism in alpha and beta thalassemia. J Clin Invest 1969;48(1):33–41.
85. Origa R, Sollaino MC, Giagu N, et al. Clinical and molecular analysis of haemoglobin H disease in Sardinia: haematological, obstetric and cardiac aspects in patients with different genotypes. Br J Haematol 2007;136(2):326–32.
86. Tongsong T, Srisupundit K, Luewan S. Outcomes of pregnancies affected by hemoglobin H disease. Int J Gynaecol Obstet 2009;104(3):206–8.
87. Lorey F, Charoenkwan P, Witkowska HE, et al. Hb H hydrops foetalis syndrome: a case report and review of literature. Br J Haematol 2001;115(1):72–8.
88. Macciò A, Madeddu C, Chessa P, et al. Use of erythropoiesis stimulating agents for the treatment of anaemia and related fatigue in a pregnant woman with HbH disease. Br J Haematol 2009;146(3):335–7.
89. Chui DH, Waye JS. Hydrops fetalis caused by alpha-thalassemia: an emerging health care problem. Blood 1998;91(7):2213–22.
90. Liang ST, Wong VC, So WW, et al. Homozygous alpha-thalassaemia: clinical presentation, diagnosis and management. A review of 46 cases. Br J Obstet Gynaecol 1985;92(7):680–4.
91. Oepkes D, Seaward PG, Vandenbussche FP, et al. Doppler ultrasonography versus amniocentesis to predict fetal anemia. N Engl J Med 2006;355(2):156–64.
92. Lucke T, Pfister S, Durken M. Neurodevelopmental outcome and haematological course of a long-time survivor with homozygous alpha-thalassaemia: case report and review of the literature. Acta Paediatr 2005;94(9):1330–3.
93. Yi JS, Moertel CL, Baker KS. Homozygous alpha-thalassemia treated with intra-uterine transfusions and unrelated donor hematopoietic cell transplantation. J Pediatr 2009;154(5):766–8.
94. Borgna-Pignatti C, Marsella M, Zanforlin N. The natural history of thalassemia intermedia. Ann N Y Acad Sci 2010;1202:214–20.

95. Cohen AR, Galanello R, Pennell DJ, et al. Thalassemia. Hematology Am Soc Hematol Educ Program 2004;14–34.
96. Deka D, Banerjee N, Roy KK, et al. Aplastic anaemia during pregnancy: variable clinical course and outcome. Eur J Obstet Gynecol Reprod Biol 2001;94(1): 152–4.
97. Choudhry VP, Gupta S, Gupta M, et al. Pregnancy associated aplastic anemia– a series of 10 cases with review of literature. Hematology 2002;7(4):233–8.
98. Aboujaoude R, Alvarez J, Alvarez M, et al. Pregnancy-induced bone marrow aplasia mimicking idiopathic thrombocytopenia: a case report. J Reprod Med 2007;52(6):526–8.
99. Kwon JY, Lee Y, Shin JC, et al. Supportive management of pregnancy-associated aplastic anemia. Int J Gynaecol Obstet 2006;95(2):115–20.
100. Marsh JC, Ball SE, Cavenagh J, et al. Guidelines for the diagnosis and management of aplastic anaemia. Br J Haematol 2009;147(1):43–70.

Myeloproliferative Disorders in Pregnancy

Claire N. Harrison, DM, FRCP, FRCPath*,
Susan E. Robinson, MSc, MRCP, FRCPath

KEYWORDS

• Myeloproliferative • Pregnancy • MPN

The myeloproliferative neoplasms (MPNs), previously known as the myeloproliferative disorders, are generally indolent stem cell malignancies, characterized by a propensity to thrombotic or hemorrhagic events and, less frequently, transformation to myelofibrosis or acute myeloid leukemia. The MPNs defined by the World Health Organization (WHO)[1] encompass the more commonly encountered essential thrombocythemia (ET), polycythemia vera (PV), and primary myelofibrosis (PMF), and the rarer entities MPN unclassified, MPN syndromes overlapping with myelodysplasia, mast cell disorders, chronic neutrophilic leukemia, and hypereosinophilic syndrome. The combined incidence of ET, PV, and PMF is approximately 6 in 100,000 to 9 in 100,000, with a peak frequency between 50 and 70 years. However, for ET in particular there is a second peak in women of reproductive age, and 15% of patients with PV are younger than 40 years at the time of diagnosis. Thus these diseases are encountered in women of reproductive potential, and may indeed be diagnosed in pregnancy or during investigation of recurrent pregnancy loss or infertility. Historical case reports of pregnancy and retrospective case series, albeit likely to be subject to reporting bias, suggest significant maternal morbidity and poor fetal outcome. Pregnancy in these conditions is clearly complicated, and a proportion of women with MPN will require disease-specific intervention in pregnancy.

PATHOGENESIS OF MPN

MPNs result from the transformation of a hemopoietic progenitor cell, characterized by overproduction of mature blood cells. In 2005, 4 groups simultaneously reported the discovery of a point mutation in exon 14 of Janus Kinase 2 (JAK2V617F), where phenylalanine is substituted by valine, which enables constitutive activation of JAK 2.[2–5] Both wild-type and mutant JAK2 bind to the intracytoplasmic tail of many

Department of Haematology, Guy's and St Thomas' NHS Foundation Trust, Guy's Hospital, Great Maze Pond, London, SE1 9RT, UK
* Corresponding author.
E-mail address: Claire.Harrison@gstt.nhs.uk

Hematol Oncol Clin N Am 25 (2011) 261–275
doi:10.1016/j.hoc.2011.01.008
0889-8588/11/$ – see front matter © 2011 Elsevier Inc. All rights reserved.

common hemopoietic cytokine receptors, which include those cognate receptors for erythropoietin, thrombopoietin (TPO), and granulocyte colony stimulating factor. When the ligand binds to one of these receptors, phosphorylation of JAK2 and the receptor itself occurs, initiating signaling via the JAK-STAT, MAPK, and PI3K pathways. This process is independent of the presence of ligand receptor interaction in the presence of JAK2V617F (**Fig. 1**). The JAK2V617F mutation is present in 95% of patients with PV and 50% of patients with ET or myelofibrosis. Many of the remaining patients with JAK2V617F-negative PV have a mutation in exon 12.[6] A proportion of patients with ET or myelofibrosis have one of several mutations of the transmembrane domain of the TPO receptor cMPL, which also causes constitutive activation.[7] All these mutations have been shown to produce an MPN-like phenotype in murine models.

PREGNANCY OUTCOME DATA AND RISK FACTORS FOR MPN

ET is the commonest MPN in women of childbearing age, and a significant number of cases of pregnancy have been reported in the literature, but these data are insufficient to devise evidence-based management guidelines. A meta-analysis reported the outcome of 461 pregnancies in women diagnosed with ET.[8] The live birth rate was 50% to 70%; first trimester loss occurred in 25% to 40% and late pregnancy losses in 10%. Rates of placental abruption (3.6%) and intrauterine growth restriction (IUGR) (4.5%) were higher than in the general population. Postpartum thrombotic episodes were reported in 5.2% of pregnancies and pre-/postpartum hemorrhage in 5.2%. A summary of 208 historical cases of ET collated from case series that included greater than 6 pregnancies produced comparable data (**Table 1**). The literature for pregnancies affected by PV is sparse; pregnancy outcome in the authors' own case series of 18 pregnancies in PV combined with 20 historical reports was concordant with the pregnancy outcomes in ET, and is summarized in **Table 2**. In PV first trimester loss was the most frequent complication (21%), followed by late pregnancy loss (18%), IUGR (15%), and premature delivery (13%), which included 3 neonatal deaths resulting in a 50% survival rate. Maternal morbidity was also significant including 3 thromboses, 1 large postpartum hemorrhage, 4 cases of preeclampsia, and 1 maternal death associated with evidence of a deep vein thrombosis, pulmonary emboli, sagittal sinus thrombosis, and disseminated intravascular coagulation. The literature regarding PMF is more limited. A report of 4 pregnancies in PMF combined with 4 historical cases suggested a 50% risk of fetal loss; no maternal complications of thrombosis or disease progression were noted, but the numbers are probably too small to draw any firm conclusions (**Table 3**).

PATHOPHYSIOLOGY OF PREGNANCY LOSS IN MPN, AND RISK FACTORS

Thrombosis is consistently reported as the number one direct cause of maternal mortality.[9] In addition, thrombotic occlusion of the placental circulation may be a late manifestation of placental dysfunction. In MPN pregnancies the prothrombotic state may affect the remodeling of maternal spiral arteries essential for adequate blood volume delivery to the placenta. In pregnancy the placental circulation changes from a low-flow high-resistance system to a high-flow low-resistance system: if remodeling of the maternal spiral arteries is impaired by microthrombi leading to impaired blood delivery, the resultant placental hypoperfusion may form the basis of the abnormal fetal-maternal interaction and increase the risk of preeclampsia and growth restriction in MPN pregnancies. However, this would not account for recurrent early pregnancy loss. Further work is required to look at the pathogenesis of recurrent first trimester loss in these diseases. Multiple factors are likely to contribute to the

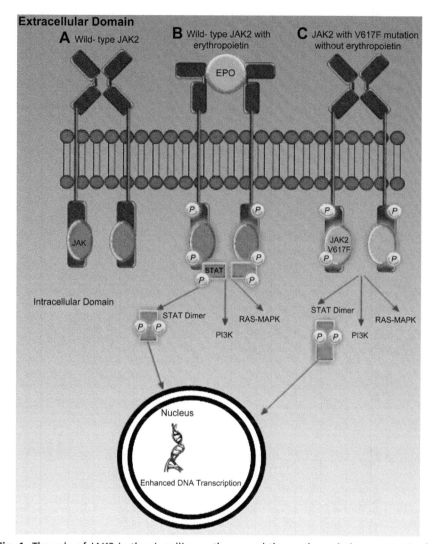

Fig. 1. The role of JAK2 in the signalling pathway and the erythropoietin receptor. In the absence of erythropoietin, the erythropoietin receptor binds JAK2 as an inactive dimer (*A*). The binding of erythropoietin induces conformational change in the erythropoietin receptor and phosphorylation of JAK2 and the cytoplasmic tail of the receptor (*B*) leading to signalling through the Janus kinases and signal transducers and activators of transcription (JAK-STAT), phosphatidylinositol 3 kinase (PI3K) and RAS and mitogen activated protein kinase (RAS-MAPK). In cells with JAK2 V617F the signalling pathways are constitutively increased even in the absence of erythropoietin (*C*). (*Adapted from* Campbell PJ, Green A. The mechanisms of disease. The Myeloproliferative Disorders. The New England Journal of Medicine 2006;355:2452–66.)

pathogenesis of thrombosis in MPN, including degree of thrombocytosis, leukocytosis, raised hematocrit, activation of platelets and leukocytes, the formation of platelet leukocyte aggregates, circulating prothrombotic and endothelial factors, and their interactions.[10]

Table 1
Summary of the literature regarding ET in pregnancy

Author[Ref.]	Patients, n	Pregnancies, n	Maternal Outcome	Live Birth Total	Pregnancy Loss Total	Loss <12/40	Loss >12/40	IUGR	Placental Abruption	Live Birth Premature Delivery <37/40	Live Birth FTD
Belluci et al[42]	3	11	Detail not available	4	7	6	1	Detail not available	1	2	2
Beard et al[43]	6	9	1 phlebitis, 1 leg ulcer, 1 PPH	8	1	1	0	0	0	1	7
Leone et al[44]	8	10	Detail not available	7	3	0	3	Detail not available	0	0	7
Pagliaro et al[45]	9	15	2 VTE, 2 TIA, 1 hemorrhage	9	6	4 including 1 TOP	2	2	0	4	5
Randi et al[46]	13	16	3 VTE	13	3	3	0	0	0	3	10
Cincotta et al[47]	12	30	1 PE	17	13	5 including 1 ectopic	8	2	5	5	12
Bangerter et al[48]	9	17	1 TIA, 2 acquired vWD, 3 vaginal bleeds, 2 epistaxis	11	6	6	0	0	0	3	8
Niittyvuopio et al[49]	16	40	1 eclampsia, 2 PET, 1 vaginal bleed	26 (1 twin)	15	13	2	1	0	2	23
Gangat et al[16]	36	63	1 PET, 2 hematoma, 1 PPH	38	25	22 including 1 ectopic, 1 TOP	3	Detail not available	1	1	37
Melillo et al[15]	92	122	5 DVT, 3 PET, 1 PPH	92	30	23	7	2	1	12	80
Passamonti et al[50]	78	113	5 PET	44	34	Detail not available	Detail not available	7	Detail not available	Detail not available	Detail not available
Palandri et al[51]	13	24	Detail not available	15	9	Detail not available	Detail not available	0	1	0	Detail not available
Total	295	470	—	284/470 (60%)	152/470 (32%)	83/333 (25%)	26/333 (8%)	14/386 (4%)	9/357 (3%)	33/357 (9%)	191/333 (57%)

Abbreviations: DVT, deep vein thrombosis; FTD, full-term delivery; IUGR, intrauterine growth restriction; PE, pulmonary embolism; PET, preeclampsia/toxemia; PPH, postpartum hemorrhage; TIA, transient ischemic attack; TOP, termination of pregnancy; VTE, venous thromboembolism; vWD, von Willebrand disease.

Table 2
Summary of the literature regarding PV in pregnancy

Author[Ref.]	Patients, n	Pregnancies, n	Treatment During Pregnancy	High Risk	Maternal Outcome	Live Births, n	Pregnancy Loss, n	First Trimester Miscarriage	Stillbirth (Gestation)	IUGR	Placental Abruption	Live Birth <37/40	Live Birth FTD
Crowley et al[52]	1	1	Aspirin + dipyridamole	No	Death	0	1	1 TOP	0	0	0	0	0
Centrone et al[53]	1	3	Nil	No	Alive	1	2	2	0	0	0	0	1
Ferguson et al[54]	1	2	Nil	No	Alive, PET	2	0	0	0	0	0	0	2 PET
Ruch and Klein[55]	1	2	None	No	Alive, PET	1	1	0	1 (35/40) PET	1	0	0	1
Subtil et al[56]	1	3	Aspirin, heparin, venesection	No	Alive, PE postpartum	1	2	0	2 (24/40 and 28/40)	2	0	1 (32/40)	0
Hochman and Stein[57]	1	4	Nil	Yes	Alive, PET	2	2	0	2 (5 & 7 months) PET	0	0	1 (7 months, PET), 1 (8 months)	0
Harris and Conrad[58]	2	2	Nil	No	Alive, PPH	2	0	0	0	0	0	0	2
Ruggeri et al[59]	1	2	Heparin 3/52 postpartum	No	Alive, PE 24/7 postpartum	1	1	1	0	0	0	0	1
Pata et al[60]	1	1	Hydroxyurea 9/40 then nil	No	Alive	1	0	0	0	0	0	0	1
Robinson et al[61]	8	18 (1 twin)	Varied: venesection, aspirin, interferon LMWH, vitamin C+E	No	Alive, 1 PET	11	7	4	2	3	0	1 (34/40, IUGR), 1 (36/40), 1 (26/40) (NND)	9
Total	18	38	—	1 yes	1 death, 4 PET, 2 PE, 1 PPH	22, 3 neonatal deaths	16	8	7	6	0	6	17

Abbreviations: LMWH, low molecular weight heparin; NND, neonatal death.
Data from Robinson S, Bewley S, Hunt BJ, et al. The management and outcome of 18 pregnancies in women with polycythemia vera. Haematologica 2005;90:1477–83.

Table 3
Summary of the literature regarding PMF in pregnancy

Author[Ref.]	Patients, n	Pregnancy, n	Treatment Prepregnancy	Treatment During Pregnancy	Maternal Outcome	First Trimester Miscarriage	Stillbirth (Gestation)	IUGR	Placental Abruption	Live Birth Premature Delivery <37 wk
Taylor et al[62]	1	1	Supportive	Supportive	No complications	0	0	0	0	1 elective induction at 36 wk
Gotic et al[63]	1	1	None	None	No complications	0	30 (placental infarctions)	0	0	0
		2	None	None	No complications	0	27 (placental infarctions)	0	0	0
		3	Interferon-α	Interferon-α	No complications	0	0	1	0	1 elective delivery at 34 wk due to IUGR, birth weight 2000 g
Tulpule[64]	A	3 (2 preceding diagnosis PMF)	Aspirin	Aspirin	Disseminated TB	0	0	0	0	1 FTND
	B	1	Aspirin	Aspirin, LMWH	Postpartum hemorrhage	0	0	0	0	1 FTND
	B	2	Aspirin	Aspirin, LMWH	No complications	0	24/40 cardiac malformation	0	0	0
	B	3	Aspirin	Aspirin, LMWH	No complications	1	0	0	0	0
Total	4	8	3	3		0	3	1	0	4

Abbreviation: FTND, full-term normal delivery.
Data from Tulpule S, Bewley S, Robinson SE, et al. The management and outcome of four pregnancies in women with idiopathic myelofibrosis. Br J Haematol 2008; 142:480–2.

A history of thrombosis, hemorrhage, and extreme thrombocytosis in pregnant women with ET are considered risk factors for fetal/maternal complications.[11–13] However, there are no validated predictors of pregnancy outcome. Age, parity, thrombophilia, platelet count, leukocyte count, and hemoglobin level have not been found to be predictive of pregnancy outcome in ET.[14–16] It is currently unclear whether the presence of JAK2V617F and MPLW515L/K increase the risk of poor pregnancy outcome in MPN. In 2007, Passamonti and colleagues[14] reported an analysis of 103 pregnancies in 63 women with ET. The JAK2V617F-positive women had an odds ratio (OR) of 2.02 (95% confidence interval [CI]: 1.1–3.8, $P = .05$) of developing complications in pregnancy compared with JAK2V617F-negative women, indicating a possible relationship between JAK2V617F and fetal loss. The Mayo Clinic study data suggested the rate of pregnancy loss was similar between JAK2V617F-positive and JAKV617F-negative pregnancies[16]; however, the Italian registry found the JAK2V617F mutation was associated with a poorer outcome (fetal losses JAK2V617F-positive 9/25, 36% vs wild-type 2/24, 8.3%; $P = .037$).[15] Prospective data collection of MPN pregnancies as opposed to historical case reports would be informative regarding current epidemiology of MPN in pregnancy and risk factors related to pregnancy outcomes.

There are also data regarding JAK2V617F screening in women with pregnancy loss without a diagnosis of a MPN. A total of 3496 pairs of women in a first-pregnancy case-control study of first unexplained pregnancy loss were screened for JAK2V617F. The mutation was detected more frequently in women with pregnancy loss (1.06%) than in control subjects (OR 5.33, 95% CI 2.37–11.90.)[17] This result led to the hypothesis that JAK2V617F may be further enriched in women who had multiple miscarriages. Three hundred and eighty-nine women with a history of recurrent miscarriage were screened for JAK2V617F. The mutation was not detected in any case, yielding a 95% CI for the prevalence of the mutation ranging from 0 to 0.009 ($P = .038$), excluding a 1% prevalence in this population.[18]

DIAGNOSIS

The diagnosis of MPN in pregnancy requires an increased awareness that these conditions may occur in women with reproductive potential. Consideration of a new diagnosis of MPN in pregnancy may be prompted by an abnormal full blood count, a thrombotic or hemorrhagic event, or adverse pregnancy outcome. Awareness that plasma expansion in pregnancy may mask the typical full blood count findings in MPN is required to remain vigilant and to consider diagnosis in women who present in pregnancy with thrombosis, hemorrhage, or adverse pregnancy outcome, for whom there is no alternative explanation.

DIAGNOSIS AND MANAGEMENT OF MPN IN WOMEN OF REPRODUCTIVE POTENTIAL

Following a diagnosis of an MPN in a woman of reproductive age, it is imperative to discuss and provide written information regarding contraceptive advice, fertility treatment, and the management of future pregnancies. Ideally, prior to pregnancy this discussion should be revisited in a preconceptual meeting to enable an up to date risk assessment and to formulate an individualized management plan according to perceived risk for the woman and potential fetus. The key goal is to improve outcome and avoid fetal and maternal morbidity and mortality.

Contraception and Fertility Treatment

There is currently insufficient evidence to either support or refute an association between estrogen-based hormonal treatment and thrombosis in MPNs. A retrospective review of thrombotic events in 305 women with ET, median follow-up 133 months, suggested estrogen-based hormone therapy may be safe in ET outside the setting of combined oral contraceptive pill use, and that use of the combined oral contraceptive may be associated with an increased risk of deep vein thrombosis.[19] Hence the use of estrogen-based contraceptives is avoided in women with MPN and alternative contraceptives are considered. If women require treatment with a cytoreductive drug or indeed any drug of teratogenic potential, it is imperative in the consent process to inform them regarding the implications of unplanned pregnancy whilst taking these agents, coupled with contraceptive advice. If women with MPN present with fertility issues, optimal disease management needs to be addressed alongside referral for standard fertility investigations. In the event that reproductive therapy is considered, this requires a multidisciplinary approach. There are no data regarding ovarian stimulation therapy in MPN. Ovarian hyperstimulation is known to be associated with an increased risk of thrombosis. Each case would need to be assessed on an individual basis and thromboprophylaxis considered.

Preconceptual Meeting

From preconceptual planning to the postpartum period, access to joint care from an obstetrician with experience of high-risk pregnancies and a hematologist in a multidisciplinary setting is paramount. The preconceptual meeting should encompass:

- A discussion of up to date pregnancy outcome in MPNs
- An individual risk assessment
- A discussion of therapeutic options
- Information regarding the multidisciplinary approach
- Information regarding follow-up in pregnancy and additional monitoring
- A comprehensive delivery and postpartum plan
- Discussion around breast feeding.

Following this meeting, a written summary of the information discussed and the proposed individualized management plan for future pregnancies should be made available to the woman and health professional in the multidisciplinary team.

Risk Assessment

Standard management of patients with a diagnosis of an MPN outside of pregnancy is to offer treatment according to an assessment of thrombotic or hemorrhagic potential. Likewise, before embarking on a pregnancy or during pregnancy a risk assessment according to disease status, concomitant illness, and prior obstetric history forms the basis of the individual woman's risks and benefits of therapeutic options in pregnancy. Box 1 lists factors to consider during the risk assessment, which may suggest an increased risk of fetal or maternal complications. Dependent on perceived risks, women may be offered a standard or increased risk management strategy. Treatment options include aspirin, heparin, venesection, cytoreductive agents, and thromboembolic deterrent stockings. If one or more of the listed risk factors are present, local practice is to consider cytoreductive therapy and low molecular weight heparin (LMWH).

MANAGEMENT STRATEGY FOR STANDARD-RISK PREGNANCY IN MPN
Aspirin

The use of aspirin in nonpregnant patients with PV is supported by the European Collaborative Low-dose Aspirin in Polycythemia vera (ECLAP) study,[20] which

---

Box 1
High-risk MPN pregnancy criteria

- Previous venous or arterial thrombosis, regardless of whether associated with a previous pregnancy

- Previous hemorrhage attributed to MPN, regardless of whether associated with a previous pregnancy[a]

- Previous pregnancy complication toward which MPN may have contributed:

  Three pregnancy losses less than 12 weeks since last menstrual period (LMP)

  One or more pregnancy loss greater than 12 weeks since LMP

  Intrauterine growth restriction, preeclampsia, or other evidence of placental dysfunction

  Intrauterine death or still birth with no other cause identified

  Antepartum or major postpartum hemorrhage requiring red cell transfusion

- Platelet count rising to >1500 × 10^9/L before or during pregnancy[a]

- Diabetes or hypertension requiring treatment[a]

[a] These criteria would be an indication for cytoreductive treatment but not LMWH.

---

demonstrated a reduction in risk of thrombosis in PV patients. Hydroxyurea and low-dose aspirin is the treatment of choice in high-risk ET in nonpregnant patients,[21] resulting in a significant reduction in thrombotic events. These studies fostered the widespread use of aspirin in low-risk ET, despite the lack of evidence-based data. Recently a retrospective review of observation versus aspirin as primary prophylaxis for thrombosis in 300 low-risk ET patients concluded that antiplatelet agents reduce the risk of venous thrombosis in JAK2V617F-positive ET patients and the rate of arterial events in patients with cardiovascular risk factors. In the remaining low-risk ET patients aspirin was not effective as primary prophylaxis of thrombosis, and observation may be an option.[22] No prospective data are available regarding aspirin versus observation in low-risk MPN in pregnancy, but as pregnancy itself is prothrombotic, low-dose aspirin would certainly be recommended in this situation. These findings, combined with the support of the Collaborative Low-dose Aspirin in Pregnancy study (CLASP),[23] which suggested aspirin is safe in pregnancy, and the use of aspirin in antiphospholipid syndrome associated with poor pregnancy outcome, have led to the widespread continuation of aspirin in women with a diagnosis of MPN in pregnancy. In the absence of clear contraindication, that is, asthma, peptic ulceration, or hemorrhage, local practice is to continue with low-dose aspirin. In the event of a platelet count greater than 1000 × 10^9/L, an acquired von Willebrand disease should be excluded before commencing aspirin.

Control of Platelet Count and Packed Cell Volume

In nonpregnant patients with MPN in whom a standardized risk assessment suggests they are at high risk of thrombosis, key treatment aims include maintaining a platelet count of less than 400 × 10^9/L and a packed cell volume (PCV) of less than 0.45 and possibly less than 0.42 in women who remain symptomatic. In pregnancy the increase in plasma volume reduces both the platelet count and PCV, altering blood rheology. An understanding of the physiologic dilution in pregnancy and brisk return to prepregnancy levels in the postpartum period is important when considering optimal intervals between monitoring women and suitable treatment targets. The target PCV in pregnant women with MPN has been the subject of debate[24,25]; certainly the PCV should be maintained below 0.45 and maintenance of gestational appropriate target ranges considered.

Venesection/Therapeutic Phlebotomy

Although the natural decrease in PCV may obviate the need to venesect, it is an option in resistant cases. If venesection fails to control the PCV then cytoreductive therapy may be considered. Venesection may be associated with syncope in the third trimester, due to reduced venous return, in which case formal intravenous fluid replacement may be required.

MANAGEMENT STRATEGY FOR HIGH-RISK PREGNANCY IN MPN

In addition to the standard measures described, cytoreductive therapy and LMWH may be considered in women with additional risk factors (see **Box 1**).

Cytoreductive Therapy

None of the cytoreductive drugs discussed in this review have a product license for use in pregnancy. If a woman is taking hydroxyurea or anagrelide prior to pregnancy this should be gradually withdrawn, followed by a 3- to 6-month washout period prior to conception. Patients with a clear indication for cytoreductive therapy prior to pregnancy should be converted to interferon-α. A few pregnancies have been reported in women treated with hydroxyurea, mostly without fetal complication.[12,26] However, the use of hydroxyurea is probably contraindicated at the time of conception in both men and women and during pregnancy, due to the risk of teratogenicity. The use of anagrelide is also not recommended; there are only 6 case reports of anagrelide in pregnancy.[27] The molecule is small enough to cross the placenta, and there is a theoretical possibility of thrombocytopenia in the fetus. Following the cessation of hydroxyurea or anagrelide, the platelet count and PCV will need to be closely monitored. In PV, venesection should be commenced once the PCV rises above the appropriate gestational range.

Several case reports in the past have suggested the relative safety of interferon-α during pregnancy, with little or no effect on the fetus, and there are no reports of teratogenic effects in animals. However, there is one report of a young woman who became pregnant while receiving interferon-α for ET.[28] She delivered a small-for-gestational-age baby girl at 33 weeks' gestation. The infant displayed a facial rash characteristic of neonatal lupus and transient thrombocytopenia; maternal and neonatal serology were typical for drug-induced lupus. There is also some evidence to suggest interferon-α may decrease fertility, so it is best avoided in women who experience difficulty conceiving.[29] The introduction of interferon-α should also be considered if the raised PCV is resistant to venesection or there is a persistent thrombocytosis following cessation of cytoreductive therapy. Treatment should be guided by monitoring the full blood count as standard practice. Cytoreduction with interferon-α should also be considered if any of the risk factors in **Box 1** are present, or develop in pregnancy. The benefits of interferon in pregnancy are supported by the study of Melillo and colleagues.[15]

Low Molecular Weight Heparin

LMWH is safe in pregnancy. Heparin-induced thrombocytopenia has not been described in pregnancy, and the risk of osteopenia is extremely low.[30] LMWH has been used anecdotally in women with MPN and previous pregnancy morbidity in addition to cytoreductive therapy. There are no prospective trial data of heparin use in

MPN pregnancies to support its use. In antiphospholipid syndrome, treatment with aspirin and LMWH is associated with improved outcomes for women with previous late fetal loss or early delivery due to placental dysfunction[31]; however, a recent controlled study of women with antiphospholipid antibodies, thrombophilia, or positive antinuclear antibody and recurrent pregnancy loss found live birth rates in the group receiving aspirin to be similar to the group receiving aspirin and LMWH.[32] In women with a history of pregnancy morbidity, it is the authors' practice to offer a weight-adjusted prophylactic dose of LMWH once daily on an empirical basis. In women with a previous history of venous thrombosis, the same weight-adjusted prophylactic dose is commenced in the first trimester and is increased to twice daily from 16 weeks. Women with a history of recurrent venous thrombosis, venous thrombosis in pregnancy, or arterial thrombosis require a higher dose of LMWH assessed on an individual basis.

GRADUATED ELASTIC COMPRESSION STOCKINGS

The guidance from the Royal College of Obstetricians and Gynecologists (RCOG) recommends the use of properly applied graduated compression stockings of appropriate strength in pregnancy and the puerperium for women who are hospitalized and have a contraindication to LMWH, women who are hospitalized post-cesarean section (combined with LMWH) and considered to be at particularly high risk of venous thromboembolism (VTE) (such as previous VTE, more than 3 risk factors), women who are outpatients with prior VTE (usually combined with LMWH), and women traveling a long distance for more than 4 hours.[33] In the context of women with MPN in pregnancy, all of these criteria would be applicable.

MATERNAL AND FETAL MONITORING

The authors' practice is to monitor the full blood count on a monthly basis until 24 weeks, then fortnightly. The local protocol for fetal monitoring includes a booking scan at 12 weeks and a detailed anomaly scan at 20 weeks. Uterine artery Dopplers are performed at 20 weeks and, if abnormal, repeated at 24 weeks. Regular growth scans are performed from 20 weeks onward. The presence of persistent bilateral notching on uterine artery Dopplers at 24 weeks indicates resistance to flow, and possible placental dysfunction would prompt escalation from a standard to a high-risk protocol. In the postpartum phase the platelet count and PCV may increase dramatically, but can usually be controlled with cytoreductive therapy or venesection.

LABOR

It is important to discuss the implications of the use of thromboprophylaxis with the obstetrician and anesthetist, and to plan for eventualities including instrumental delivery and epidural or spinal anesthesia. Local protocols regarding the interruption of LMWH should be adhered to during labor. The third stage of labor should be actively managed, and adequate hydration maintained throughout labor and the postpartum phase.

POSTPARTUM THROMBOPROPHYLAXIS

The recent RCOG guideline (reducing risk of thrombosis and embolism during pregnancy and the puerperium, Guideline 37) for thromboprophylaxis in pregnancy[33] suggests constant reassessment for venous thrombotic risk during pregnancy. Once adequate hemostasis is achieved postpartum, all women with MPN are offered 6 weeks of LMWH prophylaxis in the absence of a history of a significant hemorrhagic event.

BREAST FEEDING

Breast feeding is safe with heparin or warfarin provided the baby receives adequate vitamin K, but is traditionally contraindicated with cytoreductive agents. However, the recommendation to avoid breast feeding with interferon-α is based on reports that this agent is variably excreted in breast milk and may be active orally.[34,35] There is an absence of safety data, rather than evidence of harm to the neonate. The benefits of breast feeding are well described, including a reduction in risk of infection and gastroenteritis. The authors' practice is that any decision about breast feeding should be made on an individual basis after explanation of the potential risks and benefits.

THE POTENTIAL FOR GENETIC SUSCEPTIBILITY TO MPN

"What is the chance of my children being affected by MPN?" is a frequent question posed by young pregnant women with an MPN. In the 1990s studies of large kindreds with a predisposition to an MPN phenotype (thrombocytosis) led to the identification of mutations in the 5′ untranslated region of the TPO gene[36] and in *cMpl*, the cognate receptor for TPO.[37] With the discovery of the JAK2V617F mutation in 2005, interest in the potential genetic predisposition to MPN was reignited. The JAK2V617F mutation has not been reported in constitutional DNA, and families have been reported in which members affected with MPN may be discordant for the JAK2V617F mutation. Recent epidemiology studies suggest inherited risk factors may contribute to the development of MPNs. The largest study comprising 24,577 first-degree relatives of 11,039 MPN patients reported a relative risk of 5.7 and 7.4 of developing an MPN for first-degree relatives of patients with PV and ET, respectively.[38] Three groups have also described a common haplotype, 46/1, which confers a susceptibility to developing an MPN.[39–41] At present, routine testing of offspring is not recommended and the women should be counseled accordingly.

SUMMARY

Clinically it is necessary to establish how MPN pregnancies are managed currently and to provide relevant up to date outcome data through prospective data collection. This strategy would enable a stronger evidence base to inform future development of guidelines and, in principle, potential study protocols regarding areas of practice where the evidence base for practice is lacking. Potential research projects include looking further into the pathogenesis of poor pregnancy outcome in MPN, and the effect of MPN-associated gene mutations and biomarkers in predicting poor pregnancy outcome. Women with reproductive potential and a diagnosis of an MPN should be offered a multidisciplinary clinical pathway, encompassing preconceptual planning and an individual risk assessment and management strategy.

REFERENCES

1. Swerdlow SH. WHO classification of tumours of haemopoietic and lymphoid tissues. WHO classification of tumours version 2. 2. Lyon (France): IARC; 2008.
2. Baxter EJ, Scott LM, Campbell PJ, et al. Acquired mutation of the tyrosine kinase JAK2 in human myeloproliferative disorders. Lancet 2005;365(9464):1054–61.
3. James C, Ugo V, Le Couedic JP, et al. A unique clonal JAK2 mutation leading to constitutive signalling causes polycythaemia vera. Nature 2005;434(7037):1144–8.
4. Kralovics R, Passamonti F, Buser AS, et al. A gain-of-function mutation of JAK2 in myeloproliferative disorders. N Engl J Med 2005;352(17):1779–90.

5. Levine RL, Wadleigh M, Cools J, et al. Activating mutation in the tyrosine kinase JAK2 in polycythemia vera, essential thrombocythemia, and myeloid metaplasia with myelofibrosis. Cancer Cell 2005;7(4):387–97.
6. Scott LM, Tong W, Levine RL, et al. JAK2 exon 12 mutations in polycythemia vera and idiopathic erythrocytosis. N Engl J Med 2007;356(5):459–68.
7. Pikman Y, Lee BH, Mercher T, et al. MPLW515L is a novel somatic activating mutation in myelofibrosis with myeloid metaplasia. PLoS Med 2006;3(7):e270.
8. Barbui T, Finazzi G. Myeloproliferative disease in pregnancy and other management issues. Hematology 2006;2006(1):246–52.
9. Confidential Enquiry into Maternal and Child Health. Saving mothers' lives: reviewing maternal deaths to make motherhood safer—2003–2005. London (UK): Centre for Maternal and Child Enquiries; 2007.
10. Harrison CN. Platelets and thrombosis in myeloproliferative diseases. Hematology 2005;2005(1):409–15.
11. Barbui T, Barosi G, Grossi A, et al. Practice guidelines for the therapy of essential thrombocythemia. A statement from the Italian Society of Hematology, the Italian Society of Experimental Hematology and the Italian Group for Bone Marrow Transplantation. Haematologica 2004;89(2):215–32.
12. Harrison C. Pregnancy and its management in the Philadelphia negative myeloproliferative diseases. Br J Haematol 2005;129(3):293–306.
13. Griesshammer M, Struve S, Barbui T. Management of Philadelphia negative chronic myeloproliferative disorders in pregnancy. Blood Rev 2008;22(5):235–45.
14. Passamonti F, Randi ML, Rumi E, et al. Increased risk of pregnancy complications in patients with essential thrombocythemia carrying the JAK2 (617V>F) mutation. Blood 2007;110(2):485–9.
15. Melillo L, Tieghi A, Candoni A, et al. Outcome of 122 pregnancies in essential thrombocythemia patients: a report from the Italian registry. Am J Hematol 2009;84(10):636–40.
16. Gangat N, Wolanskyj AP, Schwager S, et al. Predictors of pregnancy outcome in essential thrombocythemia: a single institution study of 63 pregnancies. Eur J Haematol 2009;82(5):350–3.
17. Mercier E, Lissalde-Lavigne G, Gris JC. JAK2 V617F mutation in unexplained loss of first pregnancy. N Engl J Med 2007;357(19):1984–5.
18. Dahabreh IJ, Jones AV, Voulgarelis M, et al. No evidence for increased prevalence of JAK2 V617F in women with a history of recurrent miscarriage. Br J Haematol 2009;144(5):802–3.
19. Gangat N, Wolanskyj AP, Schwager SM, et al. Estrogen-based hormone therapy and thrombosis risk in women with essential thrombocythemia. Cancer 2006; 106(11):2406–11.
20. Landolfi R, Marchioli R. European Collaboration on Low-dose Aspirin in Polycythemia Vera (ECLAP): a randomized trial. Semin Thromb Hemost 1997;23(5): 473–8.
21. Harrison CN, Campbell PJ, Buck G, et al. Hydroxyurea compared with anagrelide in high-risk essential thrombocythemia. N Engl J Med 2005;353(1):33–45.
22. varez-Larran A, Cervantes F, Pereira A, et al. Observation versus antiplatelet therapy as primary prophylaxis for thrombosis in low-risk essential thrombocythemia. Blood 2010;116(8):1205–10.
23. CLASP: a randomised trial of low-dose aspirin for the prevention and treatment of pre-eclampsia among 9364 pregnant women. CLASP (Collaborative Low-dose Aspirin Study in Pregnancy) Collaborative Group. Lancet 1994;343(8898): 619–29.

24. Spivak JL. The optimal management of polycythaemia vera. Br J Haematol 2002; 116(2):243–54.

25. McMullin MF, Bareford D, Craig J, et al. The optimal management of polycythaemia vera. Br J Haematol 2003;120(3):543–4.

26. Liebelt EL, Balk SJ, Faber W, et al. NTP-CERHR expert panel report on the reproductive and developmental toxicity of hydroxyurea. Birth Defects Res B Dev Reprod Toxicol 2007;80(4):259–366.

27. Sobas MA, Perez Encinas MM, Rabunal Martinez MJ, et al. Anagrelide treatment in early pregnancy in a patient with JAK2V617F-positive essential thrombocythemia: case report and literature review. Acta Haematol 2009;122(4):221–2.

28. Fritz M, Vats K, Goyal RK. Neonatal lupus and IUGR following alpha-interferon therapy during pregnancy. J Perinatol 2005;25(8):552–4.

29. Griesshammer M, Bergmann L, Pearson T. Fertility, pregnancy and the management of myeloproliferative disorders. Baillieres Clin Haematol 1998;11(4):859–74.

30. Greer IA, Nelson-Piercy C. Low-molecular-weight heparins for thromboprophylaxis and treatment of venous thromboembolism in pregnancy: a systematic review of safety and efficacy. Blood 2005;106(2):401–7.

31. Bramham K, Hunt BJ, Germain S, et al. Pregnancy outcome in different clinical phenotypes of antiphospholipid syndrome. Lupus 2010;19(1):58–64.

32. Laskin CA, Spitzer KA, Clark CA, et al. Low molecular weight heparin and aspirin for recurrent pregnancy loss: results from the randomized, controlled HepASA trial. J Rheumatol 2009;36(2):279–87.

33. Royal College of Obstetricians and Gynaecologists. Green Top Guideline no. 37. Reducing the risk of thrombosis and embolism during pregnancy and the puerperium. London (UK): Royal College of Obstetricians and Gynaecologists; 2009.

34. Bayley D, Temple C, Clay V, et al. The transmucosal absorption of recombinant human interferon-alpha B/D hybrid in the rat and rabbit. J Pharm Pharmacol 1995;47(9):721–4.

35. Kumar AR, Hale TW, Mock RE. Transfer of interferon alfa into human breast milk. J Hum Lact 2000;16(3):226–8.

36. Wiestner A, Schlemper RJ, van der Maas AP, et al. An activating splice donor mutation in the thrombopoietin gene causes hereditary thrombocythaemia. Nat Genet 1998;18(1):49–52.

37. Ding J, Komatsu H, Wakita A, et al. Familial essential thrombocythemia associated with a dominant-positive activating mutation of the c-MPL gene, which encodes for the receptor for thrombopoietin. Blood 2004;103(11):4198–200.

38. Landgren O, Goldin LR, Kristinsson SY, et al. Increased risks of polycythemia vera, essential thrombocythemia, and myelofibrosis among 24,577 first-degree relatives of 11,039 patients with myeloproliferative neoplasms in Sweden. Blood 2008;112(6):2199–204.

39. Jones AV, Campbell PJ, Beer PA, et al. The JAK2 46/1 haplotype predisposes to MPL-mutated myeloproliferative neoplasms. Blood 2010;115(22):4517–23.

40. Olcaydu D, Harutyunyan A, Jager R, et al. A common JAK2 haplotype confers susceptibility to myeloproliferative neoplasms. Nat Genet 2009;41(4):450–4.

41. Kilpivaara O, Mukherjee S, Schram AM, et al. A germline JAK2 SNP is associated with predisposition to the development of JAK2(V617F)-positive myeloproliferative neoplasms. Nat Genet 2009;41(4):455–9.

42. Bellucci S, Janvier M, Tobelem G, et al. Essential thrombocythemias. Clinical evolutionary and biological data. Cancer 1986;58(11):2440–7.

43. Beard J, Hillmen P, Anderson CC, et al. Primary thrombocythaemia in pregnancy. Br J Haematol 1991;77(3):371–4.

44. Leone G, De Stefano V, D'Addosio A. Essential thrombocythemia: pregnancy. Haematologica 1991;76(Suppl 3):365–7 [in Italian].
45. Pagliaro P, Arrigoni L, Muggiasca ML, et al. Primary thrombocythemia and pregnancy: treatment and outcome in fifteen cases. Am J Hematol 1996;53(1):6–10.
46. Randi ML, Rossi C, Fabris F, et al. Essential thrombocythemia in young adults: treatment and outcome of 16 pregnancies. J Intern Med 1999;246(5):517–8.
47. Cincotta R, Higgins JR, Tippett C, et al. Management of essential thrombocythaemia during pregnancy. Aust N Z J Obstet Gynaecol 2000;40(1):33–7.
48. Bangerter M, Guthner C, Beneke H, et al. Pregnancy in essential thrombocythaemia: treatment and outcome of 17 pregnancies. Eur J Haematol 2000;65(3): 165–9.
49. Niittyvuopio R, Juvonen E, Kaaja R, et al. Pregnancy in essential thrombocythaemia: experience with 40 pregnancies. Eur J Haematol 2004;73(6):431–6.
50. Passamonti F, Rumi E, Randi ML, et al. Aspirin in pregnant patients with essential thrombocythemia: a retrospective analysis of 129 pregnancies. J Thromb Haemost 2010;8(2):411–3.
51. Palandri F, Polverelli N, Ottaviani E, et al. Long-term follow-up of essential thrombocythemia in young adults: treatment strategies, major thrombotic complications and pregnancy outcomes. A study of 76 patients. Haematologica 2010; 95(6):1038–40.
52. Crowley JP, Barcohana Y, Sturner WQ. Disseminated intravascular coagulation following first trimester abortion in polycythemia vera. Increased platelet count apparently contributed to fatal outcome. R I Med J 1987;70(3):109–12.
53. Centrone AL, Freda RN, McGowan L. Polycythemia rubra vera in pregnancy. Obstet Gynecol 1967;30(5):657–9.
54. Ferguson JE, Ueland K, Aronson WJ. Polycythemia rubra vera and pregnancy. Obstet Gynecol 1983;62(3 Suppl):16s–20s.
55. Ruch WA, Klein RL. Polycythemia vera and pregnancy: report of a case. Obstet Gynecol 1964;23:107–11.
56. Subtil D, Deruelle P, Trillot N, et al. Preclinical phase of polycythemia vera in pregnancy. Obstet Gynecol 2001;98(5 Pt 2):945–7.
57. Hochman A, Stein JA. Polycythemia and pregnancy. Report of a case. Obstet Gynecol 1961;18:230–5.
58. Harris RE, Conrad FG. Polycythemia vera in the childbearing age. Arch Intern Med 1967;120(6):697–700.
59. Ruggeri M, Tosetto A, Castaman G, et al. Pulmonary embolism after pregnancy in a patient with polycythemia vera. Am J Hematol 2001;67(3):216–7.
60. Pata O, Tok CE, Yazici G, et al. Polycythemia vera and pregnancy: a case report with the use of hydroxyurea in the first trimester. Am J Perinatol 2004;21(3):135–7.
61. Robinson S, Bewley S, Hunt BJ, et al. The management and outcome of 18 pregnancies in women with polycythemia vera. Haematologica 2005;90(11):1477–83.
62. Taylor UB, Bardeguez AD, Iglesias N, et al. Idiopathic myelofibrosis in pregnancy: a case report and review of the literature. Am J Obstet Gynecol 1992; 167(1):38–9.
63. Gotic M, Cvetkovic M, Bozanovic T, et al. Successful treatment of primary myelofibrosis with thrombocytosis during pregnancy with alfa-interferon. Srp Arh Celok Lek 2001;129(11–12):304–8 [in Serbian].
64. Tulpule S, Bewley S, Robinson SE, et al. The management and outcome of four pregnancies in women with idiopathic myelofibrosis. Br J Haematol 2008; 142(3):480–2.

Leukemia and Lymphoma in Pregnancy

Uri Abadi, MD[a], Gideon Koren, MD[b,c],*, Michael Lishner, MD[d,e]

KEYWORDS

- Pregnancy • Leukemia • Lymphoma • Chemotherapy
- Malformations • Fetus

The diagnosis of cancer during pregnancy is a traumatic event, posing a challenge for patients, their family, and the medical team. The need to treat the patient for a potentially lethal disease and concerns about adverse fetal outcomes raise therapeutic, ethical, moral, and social dilemmas. This "maternal-fetal conflict" must include close attention to the cultural attitudes and beliefs of patients and their family. Lymphoma is the fourth most common malignancy in pregnancy, with an estimated prevalence of 1 in 6000 pregnancies.[1–3] Leukemia is estimated to occur in 1 in 100,000 pregnancies.[1–3] Because of the increasing age of pregnancy in the western world, the incidence of malignancy during pregnancy is expected to increase.

Over the past few years, significant progress has been made in the treatment of patients with hematologic malignancies, including new imaging techniques and the addition of innovative drugs that increase therapeutic efficacy. Incorporation of these new tools during pregnancy is questionable in some instances and contraindicated in others due to concerns of fetal harm and the lack of safety data in human pregnancies.

The low incidence of hematologic malignancies during pregnancy precludes large prospective controlled trials, and information in this area is limited to retrospective series and case reports, which further complicates decision making. This article reviews the different therapeutic options for pregnant women with hematologic malignancy and discusses optimization of therapy for the mother, while minimizing risks to the fetus.

The authors have nothing to disclose.

[a] Department of Medicine, Hematology Institute, Meir Medical Center, Tcheirnechovsky Street, Kfar Saba, Israel

[b] Department of Pediatrics, University of Toronto, 555 University Avenue, Toronto, ON M5G 1X8, Canada

[c] Hospital for Sick Children, 555 University Avenue, Toronto, ON M5G 1X8, Canada

[d] Sackler Faculty of Medicine, Tel Aviv University, Ramat Aviv, Tel Aviv 69978, Israel

[e] Meir Medical Center, Tcheirnechovsky Street, Kfar Saba, Israel

* Corresponding author. Hospital for Sick Children, 555 University Avenue, Toronto, ON M5G 1X8, Canada.

E-mail address: gidiup_2000@yahoo.com

DIAGNOSIS AND EVALUATION OF PREGNANT WOMEN WITH HEMATOLOGIC MALIGNANCY

The presenting signs and symptoms of lymphoma and leukemia during pregnancy are similar to those occurring in nonpregnant women. However, some common symptoms normally reported during pregnancy, such as fatigue and shortness of breath, or physiologic changes, such as pregnancy-associated anemia and thrombocytopenia, might delay the diagnostic workup. Avoiding imaging studies because of fetal exposure to radiation may further delay the initial diagnosis. The diagnosis of lymphoma is usually established by performing lymph node biopsy. The surgical procedure of lymph node biopsy, done under local or general anesthesia, does not seem to pose a risk to the fetus when using modern anesthetic techniques, and the rate of miscarriage is not different from that of healthy pregnant women.[4]

Staging of a patient with lymphoma requires imaging studies, usually computed tomographic (CT) scan or positron emission tomography (PET) combined with CT scan (PET-CT). These studies are often associated with considerable doses of radiation, and although the dose is well below the teratogenic threshold, it is advisable to minimize exposing the fetus to radiation if possible. Ultrasonography and magnetic resonance imaging can be used safely, whereas reassessment with CT scan or PET-CT can be performed after delivery. Chest radiography can be safely performed using abdominal shielding. Bone marrow biopsy and aspiration, which are part of lymphoma staging and the key procedures in diagnosing leukemia, can be performed safely in pregnant women.

CHEMOTHERAPY IN PREGNANCY

Pregnancy is associated with physiologic changes that may affect the pharmacokinetics of chemotherapeutic agents. Such changes include increased plasma volume, third spacing in the amniotic fluid, and increased renal clearance and hepatic metabolism of drugs.[5–7] Because pharmacokinetic studies in pregnant women are lacking, it is unknown whether dose modification may be needed.

Teratogenicity is the main concern when treating pregnant women. Most cytotoxic agents have a molecular weight less than 400 kDa and can thus freely cross the placenta and reach the fetus.[7] However, information regarding drug concentrations in the placenta, amniotic fluid, and fetus is limited to small studies with conflicting results. Although the information regarding the teratogenicity of specific chemotherapeutic drugs is limited, almost all cytotoxic drugs have been found to be teratogenic in animal studies[2,5,6]; however, doses used to treat humans are usually less than the teratogenic limit documented in animals, making it difficult to extrapolate human teratogenic thresholds from animal data. Most information regarding chemotherapy in pregnancy is from series that used multiagent protocols, and it is therefore difficult to separate the fetal effects of individual drugs.

Genetic variability probably explains some of the heterogeneity in pregnancy outcome after chemotherapy; for example, severe effects of doxorubicin (Adriamycin) were documented on a male fetus, whereas his female twin was unaffected.[8]

The fetus is most vulnerable to teratogenic effects during organogenesis, which occurs during weeks 2 to 8 of pregnancy.[5–7] Several organs, including the eyes and genitalia, as well as the hematopoietic and nervous systems, remain vulnerable after the first trimester.[6,7] Treatment with combination chemotherapy during the first trimester has an estimated teratogenicity rate of 10% and 20%. This risk was found to be lower with single agent than combination therapy[9,10] and decreased when antimetabolites were omitted.[9] In addition to fetal malformations, chemotherapy during the first trimester increased the risk for spontaneous abortion and fetal death.[11,12]

Chemotherapy during the second and third trimesters has been associated with increased risk of intrauterine growth retardation (IUGR), fetal death, preterm delivery, and low birth weight[6,7]; however, it is impossible to discern the direct effects of the drugs from those of maternal morbidity. Most of the available data do not show increased risk of fetal malformations during the later stages of pregnancy.[6,7]

LONG-TERM EFFECTS OF FETAL EXPOSURE TO CHEMOTHERAPY

Fetal exposure to chemotherapy has raised concerns regarding more subtle and late-onset adverse effects. Concerns regarding late effects include adverse neurodevelopmental outcomes, compromised fertility, and childhood malignancy. Information regarding long-term outcomes of fetal exposure to chemotherapy is very limited. A series by Aviles and Neri[13] assessing outcomes in 84 children exposed to chemotherapy in utero, with an average follow-up period of 18.7 years, showed apparent normal neurologic development, school performance, and sexual development. And 12 of the children later became parents to normal children. The apparent risk of childhood malignancies was not increased. Another series with 111 children exposed to chemotherapy during pregnancy and followed up for 1 to 19 years showed favorable long-term outcomes.[14] It seems that after the first trimester, exposure of the fetus to chemotherapy does not increase the risk of adverse neurodevelopment, infertility, or childhood malignancies, although this is based on limited information.

RADIOTHERAPY IN PREGNANCY

Fetal exposure to radiotherapy during the first trimester may be teratogenic and may increase the risk of childhood malignancy. Concerns regarding long-term neurodevelopmental outcomes exist as well.[15,16] The dose of fetal exposure to radiation depends on field size and the distance from the radiation field margins to the uterus. An exposure of 0.1 to 0.2 Gy during the first trimester is considered the threshold for severe fetal malformations.[16] For these reasons, radiotherapy during pregnancy should be limited to highly specific situations when the radiation field is far from the fetus, such as lymphoma with disease confined to the neck region, using abdominal shielding. Radiotherapy should be executed after consultation with an expert medical physicist.

HODGKIN LYMPHOMA

Although Hodgkin lymphoma (HD) represents less then 1% of all malignancies, its first peak occurs in the third decade of life, during the reproductive age. Thus, it is the most common lymphoma diagnosed during pregnancy.[2,3]

The current treatment consists of the ABVD protocol (Adriamycin, bleomycin, vinblastine, and dacarbazine) for most patients, with or without radiotherapy. More aggressive protocols such as escalated BEACOPP (bleomycin, etoposide, Adriamycin, cyclophosphamide, vincristine, prednisone, and procarbazine) are used for high-risk patients with advanced disease.

Most information regarding HD during pregnancy is derived from case reports and small series. Data regarding the use of ABVD are limited, but the available information, including a few reports of treatment during the first trimester, suggests that this protocol may be safe for use in pregnancy.[6,7,13,17,18] However, because chemotherapy is generally considered teratogenic during the first trimester, it is recommended to defer treatment to later in pregnancy whenever possible.

In a patient with advanced disease diagnosed during the first trimester, delaying therapy may adversely affect maternal survival,[19] and thus, treatment with combination chemotherapy is initiated, advising the family to consider pregnancy termination. In a patient diagnosed during the second or the third trimester, initiation of treatment with combination chemotherapy is commonly recommended.

Alternative approaches for the management of HD during pregnancy may include

- In women with early stage disease limited to the neck region, radiotherapy has been suggested, using proper shielding to the abdomen. However, such an option must be considered carefully because of the potentially severe adverse effects of radiotherapy to the fetus.[20]
- Another alternative to multiagent chemotherapy is therapy with single-agent vinblastine, which is effective for HD with modest toxicity and lower likelihood of fetal adverse outcome. In a series described by Connors,[21] 6 women were treated with single-agent vinblastine, delaying combination chemotherapy until after delivery, with favorable fetal outcome.

The prognosis of pregnant women with HD seems to be similar to that in nonpregnant women. A case-control study of 48 women with HD during pregnancy showed a 20-year survival rate comparable to that of matched control subjects.[19]

A suggested algorithm for the management of HD in pregnancy is presented in **Fig. 1**.

NON-HODGKIN LYMPHOMA

Non-Hodgkin lymphoma (NHL) is a heterogeneous group of malignancies. The authors have divided the treatment of NHL during pregnancy according to the indolent, aggressive, and very aggressive types of NHL.

Indolent NHL

Indolent NHL, including follicular lymphoma, small lymphocytic lymphoma/chronic lymphocytic leukemia, and marginal zone lymphoma, is usually diagnosed at an older age, with a median age of 60 years for the diagnosis of follicular lymphoma, and is thus very uncommon during pregnancy. Consequently, there is a lack of evidence regarding optimal treatment of these malignancies.

Indolent NHL tends to progress slowly, causes few symptoms, and is considered incurable. Hence, the approach to its management is watchful waiting until symptomatic progression (**Fig. 2**). For this reason, most women with indolent lymphoma diagnosed during pregnancy can be followed up closely without treatment, unless symptoms occur. When therapy is needed, single agent (chlorambucil) or combination chemotherapy such as CVP (cyclophosphamide, vincristine, and prednisone) or CHOP (cyclophosphamide, doxorubicin, vincristine, and prednisone) is used. A few case reports of women with NHL treated with these protocols during pregnancy are available in the literature, although none reported congenital anomalies, including 4 cases treated during the first trimester.[2,6,13,17,18,22] Neonatal leukopenia and colitis were reported in an infant whose mother was exposed to chemotherapy in the third trimester.[23]

An alternative approach is the use of single-agent rituximab without chemotherapy. The use of rituximab was not associated with fetal morbidity or mortality in several

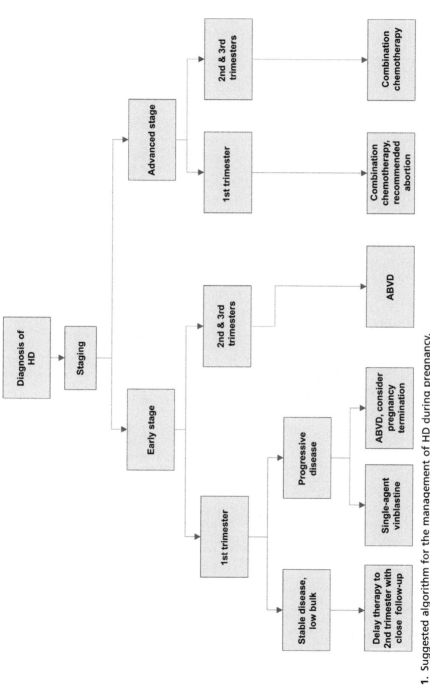

Fig. 1. Suggested algorithm for the management of HD during pregnancy.

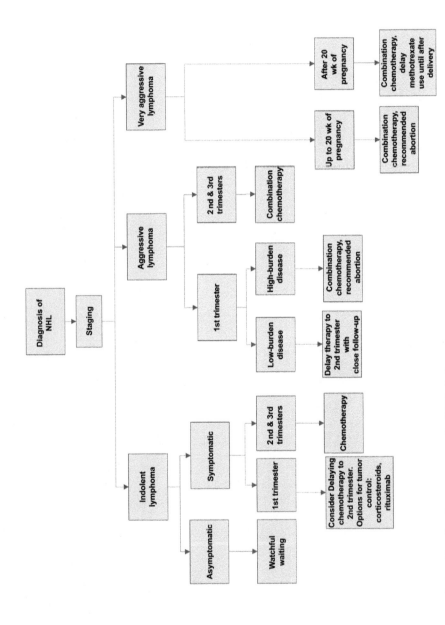

Fig. 2. Suggested algorithm for the management of NHL during pregnancy.

case reports.[17,18,24,25] A neonate with transient B-cell depletion and otherwise normal development was reported.[26]

Fludarabine is a purine analogue often used for the treatment of indolent NHL, but data regarding its effect on fetal development are lacking. In general, antimetabolites tend to be more teratogenic than other antineoplastic agents, and thus, fludarabine is not generally recommended during pregnancy.[17,18]

Radiolabeled monoclonal antibodies are contraindicated during pregnancy because of the teratogenic risks from radiation exposure.

The use of amoxicillin, clarithromycin, and omeprazole for the eradication of *Helicobacter pylori* in patients with gastric mucosa-associated lymphoid tissue lymphoma is considered safe during pregnancy, and they may be administered without delay.[27,28]

Aggressive NHL

It is the most frequently encountered group of NHL and includes diffuse large B-cell lymphoma (DLBCL), mantle cell lymphoma, and mature T- and natural killer–cell lymphomas.

The most common regimen used for these malignancies is CHOP, with the addition of rituximab in CD20[+] tumors. As noted earlier, information regarding treatment with CHOP during pregnancy is limited to a few case reports and small series. Although no congenital anomalies have been noted using this protocol, including 4 cases of women treated during the first trimester,[13,17,18,22,29] the numbers are too small to render an estimate of safety. Other reports describe treatment with different regimens containing alkylating agents and anthracyclines in patients with NHL, and although no fetal anomalies have been reported, there were a few cases of preterm delivery and intrauterine fetal death.[12,17,18,22] The fetal safety of late trimester use of cyclophosphamide and doxorubicin is suggested by reports of pregnant women with breast cancer treated with protocols containing these agents. In 2 series of 53 pregnant women with breast cancer treated with these agents during the second and third trimesters, no fetal complications were noted.[6,30]

Because of the rapidly progressive nature of aggressive NHL, treatment of pregnant women should not be delayed, and multiagent chemotherapy should be initiated promptly with CHOP, adding rituximab in DLBCL. When the disease is diagnosed during the first trimester, appropriate treatment with multiagent chemotherapy should be begun promptly, and pregnancy termination should be considered by the family because of the increased risk of fetal malformation (see **Fig. 2**). Treatment delay with close follow-up should be considered for women approaching the end of the first trimester with limited disease and low bulk. It seems safe to administer combination chemotherapy with CHOP and rituximab in the second and third trimesters, and treatment should begin soon after diagnosis.

Very Aggressive NHL

This group of diseases includes Burkitt lymphoma (BL) and precursor B- and T-cell lymphoblastic lymphoma/leukemia. These malignancies are characterized by very rapid tumor growth, high risk for central nervous system (CNS) involvement or relapse, and high risk for tumor lysis syndrome. Treatment should include intensive combination chemotherapy, with the addition of CNS prophylaxis. The information regarding treatment of BL during pregnancy is limited to only several case reports. Recent publications suggest that women treated with effective intensive modern combination chemotherapy can be cured.[31,32] Information regarding fetal outcome with these intensive protocols is extremely limited. One case report described fetal death in a patient treated from the beginning of the second trimester, whereas in another patient treated during the third trimester with early planned delivery by cesarean delivery, the fetal outcome was uneventful.[32] High-dose methotrexate, which is an essential part of the protocols for BL, is highly teratogenic and should not be used in the first trimester. Several reports regarding the use of this drug in pregnancy described fetal anomalies, as well as fetal myelosuppression.[2,5,13,17,18] In the few case reports of BL during pregnancy, treatment with methotrexate was postponed until after delivery.

Because patients with aggressive lymphomas must be treated immediately and because of concerns for fetal harm using appropriate protocols, pregnancy termination should be discussed with the family when therapy has to commence during the first trimester (see **Fig. 2**). Because of the high toxicity of these protocols, extending the recommendation for pregnancy termination up to 20 weeks of pregnancy should be considered. When possible, early delivery should be recommended at later stages of pregnancy.

ACUTE LEUKEMIA

Leukemia in pregnancy has an estimated incidence of 1 in 100,000, with acute myeloid leukemia (AML) representing most cases.[33] These malignancies are characterized by a rapidly progressive clinical course and are fatal unless treated promptly with aggressive combination chemotherapy.

The potential risk to the fetus induced by this treatment and the necessity for immediate treatment pose a serious dilemma to the patient and the physician. As with other malignancies during pregnancy, the published information is limited to small retrospective series and case reports.

AML

Treatment of AML consists of remission induction with cytarabine and an anthracycline, usually daunorubicin or idarubicin, and postremission therapy with consolidation using high-dose cytarabine or with allogeneic stem cell transplantation.

Several series and case reports of treatment of AML in pregnancy exist.[18,33–36] In most cases described, patients diagnosed during the first trimester underwent planned abortion and subsequently were treated with induction chemotherapy.[35,36] In the few cases treated with chemotherapy during the first trimester, poor pregnancy outcomes were reported with congenital anomalies and spontaneous abortions.[34–37] In 1 series, it was suggested that delaying therapy is associated with poor maternal outcome.[35] Thus, for patients diagnosed with AML during the first trimester, termination of pregnancy and immediate induction chemotherapy should be considered.

Several retrospective series reported on patients diagnosed and treated during the second and third trimesters of pregnancy. Preterm delivery, IUGR, spontaneous abortions, and stillbirths were noted but without congenital anomalies.[34,35]

Considering the need for prompt treatment and fetal outcome, patients in the second and third trimesters should be treated with immediate induction of chemotherapy. Once recovery of bone marrow is achieved in near-term pregnancies, cesarean delivery should be considered to enable continuation of chemotherapy without risk to the fetus. Concerns have been raised regarding the potential fetal cardiotoxicity of anthracyclines because cardiac damage has been described in some cases.[38,39] However, anthracyclines are an important component of AML chemotherapy and should be used cautiously, with close neonatal follow-up. Idarubicin, which is more lipophilic, has increased placental transfer and potential toxicity, and thus, daunorubicin has been preferred.

Induction with cytarabine and anthracycline is associated with considerable maternal toxicity, including mucositis and prolonged neutropenia accompanied by bacterial and sometimes invasive fungal infections that require systemic therapy.

Penicillin, cephalosporins, metronidazole, and aminoglycosides seem to be safe during pregnancy.[28] Amphotericin B is the antifungal drug with the widest experience during pregnancy, with no reports of teratogenicity.[40,41] Fluconazole has dose-dependent teratogenic effects in animals. Voriconazole might be teratogenic as well, and evidence regarding the use of caspofungin and posaconazole is lacking. Hence, it seems that the antifungal drug of choice during pregnancy for invasive fungal infections should be amphotericin B.

Based on the available data, it seems that if treated with appropriate regimens, pregnant women with AML have outcomes similar to those of nonpregnant woman.[36]

Acute Promyelocytic Leukemia

Acute promyelocytic leukemia (APL) is a specific subtype of AML (AML M3), with unique clinical, laboratory, and therapeutic characteristics. APL is an uncommon malignancy representing about 13% of AML cases, but it tends to be more common in young patients of reproductive age. Patients usually present with bleeding diathesis caused by disseminated intravascular coagulation (DIC), which may be life threatening. However, an excellent long-term outcome with modern protocols combining all-trans retinoic acid (ATRA) with chemotherapy can be achieved.

APL presenting with DIC is a medical emergency, and treatment with blood products and ATRA must begin immediately to reverse the coagulopathy. Concurrent treatment is initiated with anthracyclines, usually daunorubicin or idarubicin, as part of remission induction.

ATRA and other retinoids are associated with considerable teratogenicity when used in the first trimester, including CNS defects and cardiovascular malformations (retinoid embryopathy).[5,33] Because patients diagnosed with APL during the first trimester should begin treatment with ATRA and chemotherapy immediately, pregnancy termination must be considered, and if executed, reversal of the coagulopathy must be awaited (**Fig. 3**). Recently published recommendations by the European LeukemiaNet also advise against first trimester use of ATRA.[42] For women who insist on pregnancy preservation, an option of using daunorubicin as a single drug has been suggested. Choosing this option will likely increase the risk of bleeding.

Case reports describing treatment of patients with APL during the second and third trimesters suggest normal pregnancy outcomes for most cases.[35,36] There have been reports of preterm delivery,[18] and treatment with daunorubicin is preferred because of idarubicin's increased transfer through the placenta.

Treatment of patients presenting with APL during the second or third trimester should be initiated immediately, using ATRA and daunorubicin for induction therapy, with delivery planned according to the stage of pregnancy and after recovery of bone marrow suppression and resolution of the coagulopathy. Recommendations by the European LeukemiaNet suggest an alternative option for treatment, initially using only ATRA, and waiting to use chemotherapy after delivery. Using this approach may increase the risk of APL differentiation syndrome and possibly ATRA resistance. In patients treated with ATRA with or without chemotherapy, it is recommended to apply close neonatal follow-up with special emphasis on cardiac function.[42]

Arsenic trioxide, which is an effective first line treatment agent for relapsed APL, is considered teratogenic based on animal models and a few series describing environmental poisoning.[43] Its use during pregnancy is contraindicated.[42]

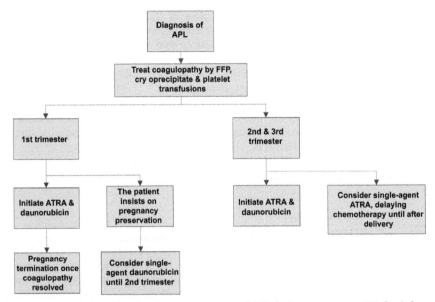

Fig. 3. Suggested algorithm for the management of APL during pregnancy. FFP, fresh frozen plasma.

ACUTE LYMPHOBLASTIC LEUKEMIA

Acute lymphoblastic leukemia (ALL) is rare among adults, and information regarding treatment of pregnant women with ALL is very limited. ALL is an aggressive malignancy, which necessitates prompt initiation of polychemotherapy, usually based on cyclophosphamide, corticosteroids, anthracyclines, vincristine, cytarabine, and asparaginase. Because of the high risk of CNS involvement or relapse, treatment with intrathecal and systemic high-dose methotrexate is part of most modern protocols. Additional courses of consolidation chemotherapy and maintenance therapy are also used. Patients at high risk for relapse are treated with allogeneic stem cell transplantation. Philadelphia chromosome positive ALL is treated with tyrosine kinase inhibitors (TKIs) as well.

In the few available case reports, spontaneous abortions and premature labor were reported during all stages of pregnancy after treatment initiation.[34–36] Teratogenicity is a major concern during the first trimester.[5,33] According to available data, pregnancy termination in patients with ALL diagnosed before 20 weeks of pregnancy should be considered with the family while treatment with multiagent chemotherapy is initiated. When ALL is diagnosed after 20 weeks of pregnancy, treatment should be initiated promptly. When the woman is near term, labor should be planned for a period without bone marrow suppression.

Imatinib mesylate, which is part of the treatment of Philadelphia chromosome positive ALL, is considered teratogenic, with reports of spontaneous abortions and fetal malformations.[44] Second line TKIs are considered teratogenic as well, although specific information regarding their effect on the fetus is unavailable.

CHRONIC MYELOID LEUKEMIA

Chronic myeloid leukemia (CML) has an annual incidence of 1 to 2 in 100,000 cases and represents about 15% to 20% of leukemia in adults. The median age at diagnosis is 50 years, and about 10% of patients are at childbearing age.[33] The disease is characterized by the presence of translocation,[21,45] with the formation of the bcr-abl chimeric protein, which acts as a constitutively active tyrosine kinase. Imatinib is a TKI that has dramatically changed disease outcome from a fatal disease with a median survival of 7 years to a chronic disease with long-term survival.

Several case reports and series on patients taking imatinib during pregnancy exist.[44,46,47] The most comprehensive report regarding the use of imatinib during pregnancy is a retrospective study that reported on 180 women.[44] Most of the women had CML; 103 of them were administered imatinib during the first trimester, and 35 women underwent planned abortion, of them 3 was because of fetal malformations. Spontaneous abortions occurred in 18 cases, and there was 1 stillbirth. Fetal malformations were reported in 12 pregnancies, including skeletal abnormalities, exomphalos, renal abnormalities, hydrocephalus, cardiac defects, pyloric stenosis, and hypospadias. Skeletal abnormalities and exomphalos were noted in 3 different cases, and also in animal studies, thus they probably represent a specific teratogenic effect of imatinib.[48]

According to these data, imatinib is teratogenic and should not be used during pregnancy. An asymptomatic woman diagnosed with chronic phase CML during pregnancy, without excessive leukocytosis, can probably be watched closely during pregnancy, delaying imatinib therapy initiation until after delivery. If therapy is needed, interferon α, which appears to be safe during pregnancy, should be administered until after delivery. Hydroxyurea may be used during the second or third trimester for patients who do not tolerate interferon side effects. Hydroxyurea is contraindicated during the first trimester due to teratogenicity. Leukapheresis is another therapeutic option, which is rarely used.

Another clinical dilemma is raised in women treated with imatinib due to chronic phase CML who wish to become pregnant. Because imatinib therapy must be discontinued during pregnancy for prolonged periods, concerns regarding disease progression and evolution of drug resistance have been raised. Several small studies have attempted to address the issue of safety of imatinib therapy cessation: Ault and colleagues[49] reported on 9 women who have interrupted imatinib treatment because of pregnancy. Of these 9 patients, only 1 was in complete cytogenetic response, 3 were in partial cytogenetic response, and 2 were in minor cytogenetic response. After stopping imatinib use, 6 of 9 patients progressed with regard to cytogenetic response, and 5 lost their complete hematologic response. After the end of pregnancy, imatinib treatment was reinitiated in all the women with repeated response to therapy. Rousselot and colleagues[50] have published a series of 12 patients who have stopped treatment for various reasons. All these patients had an excellent response to imatinib before therapy withdrawal, with complete molecular response. Six patients had a molecular relapse, which was retreated later with return to complete molecular response. The remaining 6 patients continued to be in complete molecular response at a median period of 18 months. In another study by Burchert and colleagues,[51] imatinib use was stopped in 20 patients who were previously treated with a combination of imatinib and interferon, and maintenance therapy with pegylated interferon was initiated with a median follow-up period of 2.4 years, with 75% of patients remaining in remission. The patients with relapses were retreated with imatinib and achieved molecular response again.

According to this limited information, imatinib therapy discontinuation could be offered to a woman with chronic phase CML and a prolonged major or complete molecular response after discussing the potential risks associated with therapy interruption. A regular and frequent hematologic and molecular follow-up is warranted.

Women with lesser degrees of response are at risk of relapse if imatinib therapy is discontinued, and this risk should be clearly explained to patients and their family.

If a decision to become pregnant and discontinue imatinib use has been made, treatment with interferon during pregnancy should be considered, with reinitiation of imatinib therapy after delivery. Disease monitoring by blood cell counts and real-time quantitative polymerase chain reaction should take place during pregnancy, maintaining the option to reinitiate treatment if disease progression occurs.

For patients with chronic phase CML treated with imatinib, with an unplanned pregnancy, the same considerations and recommendations regarding imatinib therapy discontinuation are appropriate as for planned pregnancy. For these patients, it has been suggested to continue imatinib use with close ultrasonographic pregnancy follow-up and to consider pregnancy termination if fetal malformations appear.[48] However, evidence supporting such an approach is limited.

In patients with first-trimester pregnancy and concomitant accelerated phase CML, TKI therapy should probably be initiated with consideration of pregnancy termination. Pregnant women diagnosed with blast crisis should undergo combination chemotherapy together with TKI therapy, and pregnancy termination should be considered. As previously noted, second-generation TKIs are considered teratogenic as well, although specific information of their effect on the human fetus is lacking.

SUMMARY

When treating a pregnant woman diagnosed with a hematologic malignancy, 2 factors must be considered: optimizing the mother's chances for cure and the safety of the fetus. The patient must be counseled on all available therapeutic options and presented with the pros and cons of each.

It is critical for the hematologist to remember that we live in a very heterogeneous society with a wide range of religions and beliefs. It is important for the hematologist not to display a paternalistic approach, telling the pregnant patient "what to do" but rather ensure that she, her family, and others she may choose to bring in (eg, religious and spiritual leaders) be optimally informed in terms and language understandable to them.

In general, when a hematologic malignancy is diagnosed during the first trimester, treatment should be postponed to the second trimester if the patient's chances of recovery are not compromised. When treatment delay poses a risk to the patient, immediate treatment should be offered after informing the family of the attendant fetal risks. When the diagnosis is made during the second or third trimester, standard treatment should usually be promptly initiated.

REFERENCES

1. Pentheroudakis G, Pavlidis N. Cancer and pregnancy: poena magna, not anymore. Eur J Cancer 2006;42:126–40.
2. Koren G, Lishner M, Santiago S, editors. The Motherisk guide to cancer in pregnancy and lactation. 2nd edition. Toronto: Motherisk Program; 2005.
3. Pavlidis NA. Coexistence of pregnancy and malignancy. Oncologist 2002;7:279–87.
4. Cohen-Kerem R, Railton C, Oren D, et al. Pregnancy outcome following non-obstetric surgical intervention. Am J Surg 2005;190:467–73.
5. Pereg D, Lishner M. Maternal and fetal effects of systemic therapy in the pregnant woman with cancer. In: Surbone A, Peccatori F, Pavilidis N, editors. Cancer and pregnancy. 1st edition. Berlin: Springer; 2008. p. 21–38.

6. Cardonick E, Iacobucci A. Use of chemotherapy during human pregnancy. Lancet Oncol 2004;5:283–91.
7. Weisz B, Meirow D, Schiff E, et al. Impact and treatment of cancer during pregnancy. Expert Rev Anticancer Ther 2004;4:889–902.
8. Zemlickis D, Lishner M, Erlich R, et al. Teratogenicity and carcinogenicity in a twin exposed in utero to cyclophosphamide. Teratog Carcinog Mutagen 1993;13: 139–43.
9. Doll DC, Ringenberg QS, Yarbro JW. Management of cancer during pregnancy. Arch Intern Med 1998;148:2058–64.
10. Randall T. National registry seeks scarce data on pregnancy outcomes during chemotherapy. JAMA 1993;269:323.
11. Leslie KK, Koil C, Rayburn WF. Chemotherapeutic drugs in pregnancy. Obstet Gynecol Clin North Am 2005;32:627–40.
12. Zemlickis D, Lishner M, Degendorfer P, et al. Fetal outcome after in utero exposure to cancer chemotherapy. Arch Intern Med 1992;152:573–6.
13. Aviles A, Neri N. Hematological malignancies and pregnancy: a final report of 84 children who received chemotherapy in utero. Clin Lymphoma 2001;2:173–7.
14. Nulman I, Laslo D, Fried S, et al. Neurodevelopment of children exposed in utero to treatment of maternal malignancy. Br J Cancer 2001;85:1611–8.
15. Streffer C, Shore R, Konermann G, et al. Biological effects after prenatal irradiation (embryo and fetus). A report of the International Commission on Radiological Protection. Ann ICRP 2003;33:205–6.
16. Otake M, Schull WJ. Radiation-related brain damage and growth retardation among the prenatally exposed atomic bomb survivors. Int J Radiat Biol 1998; 74:159–71.
17. Pereg D, Koren G, Lishner M. The treatment of Hodgkin's and non-Hodgkin's lymphoma in pregnancy. Hematologica 2007;92:1230–7.
18. Azim HA, Pavlidis N, Peccatori FA. Treatment of the pregnant mother with cancer: a systematic review on the use of cytotoxic, endocrine, targeted agents and immunotherapy during pregnancy. Part II: hematological tumors. Cancer Treat Rev 2010;36:110–21.
19. Lishner M, Zemlickis D, Degendorfer P, et al. Maternal and foetal outcome following Hodgkin's disease in pregnancy. Br J Cancer 1992;65:114–7.
20. Fenig E, Mishaeli M, Kalish Y, et al. Pregnancy and radiation. Cancer Treat Rev 2001;27:1–7.
21. Connors JM. Hodgkin's lymphoma clinical challenges. Challenging problems: coincident pregnancy, HIV Infection, and older age. Hematology Am Soc Hematol Educ Program 2008;334–9.
22. Lambert J, Wijermans PW, Dekker GA, et al. Chemotherapy in non-Hodgkin's lymphoma during pregnancy. Neth J Med 1991;38:80–5.
23. Garcia L, Valcarcel M, Santiago-Borrero PJ. Chemotherapy during pregnancy and its effects on the fetus-neonatal myelosuppression: two case reports. J Perinatol 1999;19:230–3.
24. Ojeda-Uribe M, Gilliot C, Jung G, et al. Administration of rituximab during the first trimester of pregnancy without consequences for the newborn. J Perinatol 2006; 26:252–5.
25. Kimby E, Sverrisdottir A, Elinder G. Safety of rituximab therapy during the first trimester of pregnancy: a case history. Eur J Haematol 2004;72:292–5.
26. Decker M, Rothermundt C, Hollander G, et al. Rituximab plus CHOP for treatment of diffuse large B-cell lymphoma during second trimester of pregnancy. Lancet Oncol 2006;7:693–4.

27. Diav-Citrin O, Arnon J, Shechtman S, et al. The safety of proton pump inhibitors in pregnancy: a multicentre prospective controlled study. Aliment Pharmacol Ther 2005;21:269–75.

28. Einarson A, Shuhaiber S, Koren G. Effects of antibacterials on the unborn child: what is known and how should this influence prescribing. Paediatr Drugs 2001;3: 803–16.

29. Lishner M, Zemlickis D, Sutcliffe SB, et al. Non-Hodgkin's lymphoma and pregnancy. Leuk Lymphoma 1994;14:411–3.

30. Berry DL, Theriault RL, Holmes FA, et al. Management of breast cancer during pregnancy using a standardized protocol. J Clin Oncol 1999;17:855–61.

31. Peterson C, Darrell RL, Sanger W. Burkitt's lymphoma in early pregnancy. J Clin Oncol 2010;28:e136–8.

32. Lam MS. Treatment of Burkitt's lymphoma during pregnancy. Ann Pharmacother 2006;40:2048–52.

33. Shapira T, Pereg D, Lishner M. How I treat acute and chronic leukemia in pregnancy. Blood Rev 2008;22:247–59.

34. Reynoso EE, Shepherd FA, Messner HA, et al. Acute leukemia during pregnancy: the Toronto Leukemia Study Group experience with long-term follow-up of children exposed in utero to chemotherapeutic agents. J Clin Oncol 1987;5: 1098–106.

35. Greenlund LJ, Letendre L, Tefferi A. Acute leukemia during pregnancy. A single institutional experience with 17 cases. Leuk Lymphoma 2001;41:571–7.

36. Chelghoum Y, Vey N, Raffoux E, et al. Acute leukemia during pregnancy: a report on 37 patients and a review of the literature. Cancer 2005;104:110–7.

37. Schafer AI. Teratogenic effects of antileukemic chemotherapy. Arch Intern Med 1981;141:514–5.

38. Aviles A, Neri N, Nambo MJ. Long term evaluation of cardiac function in children who received anthracyclines during pregnancy. Ann Oncol 2006;17:286–8.

39. Germann N, Goffiner F, Godwasser F. Anthracyclines during pregnancy: embryo-fetal outcome in 160 patients. Ann Oncol 2004;15:146–50.

40. King CT, Rogers PD, Cleary JD, et al. Antifungal therapy during pregnancy. Clin Infect Dis 1998;27:1151–60.

41. Sobel JD. Use of antifungal drugs in pregnancy: a focus on safety. Drug Saf 2000; 23:77–85.

42. Sanz MA, Grimwade D, Tallman MS, et al. Management of acute promyelocytic leukemia: recommendations from an expert panel on behalf of the European LeukemiaNet. Blood 2009;113:1875–91.

43. Golub MS, Macintosh MS, Baumrind N. Developmental and reproductive toxicity of inorganic arsenic: animal studies and human concerns. J Toxicol Environ Health B Crit Rev 1998;1:199–241.

44. Pye SM, Cortes J, Ault P, et al. The effects of imatinib on pregnancy outcome. Blood 2008;111:5505–8.

45. Pacifici GM, Nottoli R. Placental transfer of drugs administered to the mother. Clin Pharmacokinet 1995;28:235–69.

46. Ault P, Kantarjian H, O'Brien S, et al. Pregnancy among patients with CML treated with imatinib. J Clin Oncol 2006;24:1204–8.

47. Prabash K, Sastry PS, Biswas G, et al. Pregnancy outcome of two patients treated with imatinib. Ann Oncol 2005;16:1983–4.

48. Apperley J. CML in pregnancy and childhood. Best Pract Res Clin Haematol 2009;22:455–74.

49. Ault P, Kantarjian H, O'Brien S, et al. Pregnancy among patients with chronic myeloid leukemia treated with imatinib. J Clin Oncol 2006;24:1204–8.
50. Rousselot P, Huguet F, Rea D, et al. Imatinib mesylate discontinuation in patients with chronic myelogenous leukemia in complete molecular remission for more than 2 years. Blood 2007;109:58–60.
51. Burchert A, Muller MC, Kostrewa P, et al. Sustained molecular response with interferon alfa maintenance after induction therapy with imatinib plus interferon alfa in patients with chronic myeloid leukemia. J Clin Oncol 2010;28:1429–35.

Thrombocytopenia in Pregnancy

Paula L. Bockenstedt, MD

KEYWORDS

- Thrombocytopenia • Pregnancy • Immune thrombocytopenia
- Preeclampsia • Microangiopathic hemolysis

Thrombocytopenia affects up to 10% of all pregnancies. Thrombocytopenia in pregnancy may be related to preexisting conditions commonly seen in women of childbearing age, such as systemic lupus erythematosus (SLE) and immune thrombocytopenia (ITP), or it may be attributable to disorders intrinsic to pregnancy, such as gestational thrombocytopenia or HELLP syndrome. Occasionally, a previously undiagnosed congenital platelet disorder may be recognized for the first time during evaluation of the thrombocytopenic obstetric patient. Fortunately, most thrombocytopenia in pregnancy is physiologic. Although women with severe thrombocytopenia or platelet functional defects are generally able to maintain a normal pregnancy, it is at delivery that the hemostatic consequences of more significant thrombocytopenia in pregnancy become life-threateningly apparent. At delivery, placental separation occurs at a time when the normal maternal blood flow is approximately 700 mL/minute through the placental vessels. This flow is dampened by uterine contraction leading to placental/myometrial extravascular compression and simultaneous occlusion by physiologic thrombosis of the open maternal vessels. Defects in either mechanism to arrest uterine bleeding can lead to significant and potentially lethal hemorrhage. Careful analysis of the time of onset of thrombocytopenia, associated clinical manifestations, and specific laboratory testing is critical to provide timely diagnosis and appropriate maternal and fetal care in preparation for this hemostatic challenge.

The platelet count decreases by approximately 10% during normal pregnancy, most apparent in the third trimester.[1–4] In addition, platelet counts may be slightly lower in women with twin or multiple fetus pregnancies. There is no clear numerical definition of thrombocytopenia in pregnancy. A count below 115,000 to 120,000/μL in pregnancy is a suggested threshold and it is recommended that all pregnant women with a platelet count below 100,000/μL undergo evaluation. Of women presenting with mild thrombocytopenia during pregnancy, defined as platelet count greater than 70,000/μL, 65% will not be associated with any definable pathology. Statistically,

The author has nothing to disclose.

Division of Hematology/Oncology, University of Michigan Medical Center, University of Michigan, C344 Med Inn Building, 1500 East Medical Center Drive, Ann Arbor, MI 48105, USA

E-mail address: pbockens@umich.edu

Hematol Oncol Clin N Am 25 (2011) 293–310

doi:10.1016/j.hoc.2011.01.004

the most common causes of thrombocytopenia are gestational thrombocytopenia (70%), preeclampsia (21%), immune thrombocytopenia (3%), and other causes (6%).[4,5]

GESTATIONAL THROMBOCYTOPENIA

Gestational thrombocytopenia is a benign disorder that occurs in about 5% of pregnancies. Platelet counts are typically greater than 70,000/μL with about 70% of platelet counts being between 130,000 and 150,000/μL. The etiology of gestational thrombocytopenia may be related to increased activation and peripheral consumption of platelets, but an immune clearance mechanism may also be present during pregnancy. Evidence for an immune-based destruction is the transient, reversible nature of the thrombocytopenia following pregnancy and the presence of platelet-associated antibody levels indistinguishable from levels found in women with ITP.[6] Thus, gestational thrombocytopenia is not easily differentiated from mild immune thrombocytopenia.[7]

Diagnosis

Diagnostic features of gestational thrombocytopenia include a mild, asymptomatic thrombocytopenia with platelet count of greater than 70,000/μL, typically occurring in the third trimester of pregnancy. There is no prior history of thrombocytopenia in the nongravid state and resolution of the thrombocytopenia follows delivery by 7 days.[4,5] Recurrent thrombocytopenia in subsequent pregnancies is observed in 20% of women with gestational thrombocytopenia. The peripheral blood smear shows no red blood cell morphologic changes other than those associated with a possible coincidental microcytic, hypochromic anemia of iron deficiency commonly seen in young women and during pregnancy.

Management

There is no indication for therapy in the patient with gestational thrombocytopenia. Epidural anesthesia is safe at platelet counts above 100,000/μL and some studies indicate that epidural can be performed even at counts of 50,000 to 80,000/μL.[3,8] However, individual anesthesiology practice policies will necessarily dictate the absolute platelet count required. Some physicians recommend preterm anesthesia consultation about the risks and benefits of intravenous analgesics versus a brief course of corticosteroids (<1–2 weeks) to increase the platelet count above the required threshold for epidural anesthesia. Vaginal delivery is the preferred method of delivery unless other obstetric concerns arise.

The risk of neonatal thrombocytopenia in infants born to mothers with gestational thrombocytopenia is considered to be negligible.[9,10] Nevertheless, all infants born to mothers with thrombocytopenia should be evaluated by a neonatologist.

IMMUNE THROMBOCYTOPENIA

Chronic immune thrombocytopenia (ITP) is a disorder of both increased platelet destruction and insufficient compensatory bone marrow production of new platelets.[11–13] In chronic ITP, most autoantibodies are directed against platelet glycoprotein receptors GPIIb–IIIa or GPIb-IX-V and are formed in the white pulp of the spleen. The stimulus for autoantibody production in ITP is probably attributable to abnormal T-cell activity.[11,14] Antibody-coated platelets are then susceptible to opsonization and Fc receptor-mediated phagocytosis by mononuclear macrophages, primarily but not exclusively in the spleen.[14,15] The IgG autoantibodies are also thought to damage megakaryocytes.[16,17] ITP may be idiopathic or secondary to medications, lymphoid malignancies, viral processes, such as HIV and hepatitis C, or autoimmune diseases such as SLE or autoimmune thyroiditis. ITP occurs in 1 to 2 of every 1000 pregnancies and accounts for 5% of cases of pregnancy-associated thrombocytopenia.[18] Distinction between ITP and gestational thrombocytopenia, the most frequent cause of maternal thrombocytopenia, is important because pregnancies in women with ITP are complicated by severe neonatal thrombocytopenia in 9% to 15% of all cases with a risk of neonatal intracranial hemorrhage of 1% to 2%.[19,20]

Diagnosis

ITP is a diagnosis of exclusion. Women with ITP complicating pregnancy generally report a history of thrombocytopenia in the nonpregnant state. Evidence for preexisting thrombocytopenia includes a history of easy bruisability, epistaxis, petechiae, and menorrhagia before pregnancy, generally when platelet count is less than 50,000/μL. Splenomegaly is absent in ITP. The peripheral blood smear shows thrombocytopenia with an increased mean platelet volume and normal red blood cell morphology. Laboratory testing for liver enzymes, prothrombin time (PT), activated partial thromboplastin time (aPTT), and urinalysis are normal. Testing for HIV or hepatitis C should also be considered. Bone marrow aspirate and biopsy are generally performed only if there are abnormalities in other blood cell lines or if splenectomy is entertained. Platelet antibody testing is not recommended as a routine procedure in clinical decision making because of the poor sensitivity and specificity, and low positive predictive value of results.[16] Women with a history of previous miscarriage and thrombocytopenia should be carefully evaluated for other clinical features of antiphospholipid syndrome or SLE because additional management considerations are necessary in those disorders. Inquiry should be made as to whether prior pregnancies were complicated by thrombocytopenia and whether the newborn had thrombocytopenia or bleeding complications. When ITP is diagnosed for the first time during pregnancy, the platelet count is typically abnormal early in pregnancy with mean platelet count below 70,000/μL.[21] This contrasts with gestational thrombocytopenia where the thrombocytopenia is noted for the first time late in pregnancy and platelet counts are above 70,000/μL. In one study of 92 women during 119 pregnancies over 11 years, women with a diagnosis of ITP before pregnancy were less likely to require therapy of ITP than those pregnant patients with newly diagnosed ITP.[22] There are variable reports of exacerbation of ITP during pregnancy or in the postpartum period, however. Approximately half of patients with a prior diagnosis of ITP experience a mild decline in platelet count progressively during pregnancy.[7]

Management

The clinical management of the pregnant patient with ITP requires close consultation between the obstetrician and the hematologist. Pregnant women with ITP should be evaluated once a month in the first and second trimesters, once every 2 weeks after the seventh month, and once a week after 36 weeks with routine obstetric care and assessment of blood pressure, urinalysis for protein, and serial platelet count.[23] Fetal assessment with ultrasounds can be performed as indicated and if there is concern for fetal hemorrhage, Doppler assessment of peak systolic velocity in the fetal middle cerebral artery can be performed.

Decisions to treat thrombocytopenia are determined by the patient's bleeding symptoms. As term approaches, more aggressive therapy may be required to improve platelet count as the potential need for surgery or epidural anesthesia is considered.

The American Society of Hematology (ASH) and the British Committee for Standards in Hematology General Hematology Task Force Guidelines consider treatment to be appropriate for severe thrombocytopenia or thrombocytopenia with bleeding.[21,24] Treatment is recommended for women with a platelet count below 10,000/μL at any time during pregnancy.[7] Because of the increasing potential for imminent delivery, treatment is also recommended for platelet counts of less than 30,000/μL in the second and third trimesters. There is no consensus in treatment of the asymptomatic patient in the first trimester with platelet counts between 10,000 and 30,000/μL.[24] Therapies for ITP in pregnancy are similar to initial therapy for ITP in the nonpregnant state. Platelet transfusion is generally not indicated except in cases of severe hemorrhage or immediately before surgery or delivery owing to the very short period of response in platelet count.[7]

Glucocorticoids, such as prednisone, are generally the first line of treatment. The mechanism of action of glucocorticoid is to block antibody production and to reduce phagocytosis of antibody-coated platelets by the reticuloendothelial system in the spleen. A typical starting dose is 1 mg/kg of prednisone based on the prepregnancy weight with taper once a response has been achieved. Unfortunately, the adverse effects of steroids are increased in pregnancy and include gestational diabetes, weight gain, bone loss, hypertension, placental abruption, and premature labor.

Intravenous immunoglobulin (IVIg) may also be used in steroid-resistant patients or as a first-line agent, sparing the adverse side effects of prednisone. IVIg can be administered for platelets less than 10,000/μL during the third trimester or less than 30,000/μL in presence of acute hemorrhage, or for improvement of platelet count several days before delivery.[21] The therapeutic response to IVIg is attributable to several different immunologic mechanisms including blockade of splenic macrophages.[25] High-dose IVIg of 2 g/kg over 2 to 5 days is effective in raising the platelet count rapidly over several days but the effects are transient, generally lasting 1 to 4 weeks. The disadvantages of IVIg are that it is more costly than prednisone and IVIg is a blood product with a theoretic risk of blood-borne infections. IVIg is also helpful in patients with secondary immune thrombocytopenia as seen in SLE and HIV.

In pregnant patients with ITP beyond the optimal second trimester for splenectomy, who fail steroids, and for whom IVIg has been ineffective or is not an option, intravenous anti-RhD may be considered.[26] Anti-RhD is a pooled IgG product taken from the plasma of RhD-negative donors who have been immunized to the D antigen. Experience with its use in pregnancy is limited, however. Use of anti-RhD in the second and third trimesters in 6 of 8 patients resulted in a partial response with no major maternal or fetal complications noted.[27] Anti-RhD immunoglobulin binds to maternal red blood cells. Presentation of antibody-bound red cells to Fc receptors in the spleen results in preferential splenic phagocytosis of the red cells rather than platelets. Response occurs in 75% of patients within 1 to 2 days with peak effect in 7 to 14 days and duration up to 4 weeks.[28] Use of anti-RhD results in mild anemia. In a series reported by Michel and colleagues,[27] there was only one instance in which the hemoglobin fell greater than 2 gm/dL. The direct antiglobulin test was positive in 3 of the 7 newborns but none were anemic or jaundiced. In a series of 120 patients treated with anti-RhD during pregnancy in 2009, only one infant had jaundice, which resolved on phototherapy.[26] Anti-RhD therapy in ITP has been associated with acute hemoglobinemia or hemoglobinuria and subsequent acute renal insufficiency with 5 deaths reported of 121,389 nonpregnant patients treated.[29,30]

Rituxan is classified as a category C drug in pregnancy and its use has been limited to pregnant patients with lymphoma. No fetal malformations have been reported, nor any immune deficits described, but information is limited.[12]

Other agents used in the treatment of the nonpregnant patient with ITP, such as cytotoxic and immunsuppressive agents with potential teratogenic effects, are discouraged in pregnancy. Interpretation of the hazards in using these agents in pregnancy is complicated by the fact that they have been generally used in situations unrelated to ITP and in which multiple agents including radiation were also used. Use of cyclophosphamide (Category D), an alkylating agent, during pregnancy has resulted in birth defects. In humans, exposure during the first trimester is associated with multiple defects of the calvaria and craniofacial and eye malformations. Use after the first trimester is associated with less risk of congenital malformations but growth retardation, impaired hematopoiesis, and developmental delay are reported.[31] Low-dose cyclosporin A has been used in pregnant patients with no documented defects in the infant immune system and with nonsignificant increases reported in congenital malformations, rate of prematurity, and low birth weight.[32,33] Azathioprine (category D) has been used safely in female renal transplant patients who are pregnant. The human fetal liver lacks the enzyme inosinate pyrophosphorylase, which converts azathioprine to its active form and it is therefore protected from the drug even though it crosses the placenta.[34] Neonatal hematologic and immune impairment have been reported in some exposed infants, however.[23]

Splenectomy during pregnancy is reserved for severe refractory ITP and is generally performed in the second trimester owing to risks of inducing premature labor in the first trimester and obstruction of the surgical field by the gravid uterus in the third trimester.[2] Remission is achieved in 75% of women initially. Splenectomy does not affect the incidence of neonatal thrombocytopenia or the transplacental passage of circulating maternal antiplatelet antibodies.[35–37]

There is little information on the effects of the thrombopoietin mimetics, romiplostim and eltrombopag, in pregnancy or the developing fetal bone marrow.[38] A pregnancy registry has been developed for patients who become pregnant while on either of these agents.

Delivery

Vaginal delivery is the preferred method of delivery.[7] Epidural anesthesia during labor in thrombocytopenic patients is controversial because of concern for epidural hematoma. There are several reports of successful use of regional anesthesia in patients with ITP who have platelet counts of less than 100,000/μL without bleeding complications.[3,23] Current guidelines state that there is no contraindication to regional anesthesia in patients with platelet counts of greater than 100,000/μL. Individuals with platelet counts between 50,000 and 100,000/μL require careful individual assessment. Regional anesthesia is contraindicated in those pregnant patients with platelet counts below 50,000/μL.[21,24]

Fetal platelet counts do not correlate with maternal platelet counts.[37] Fortunately, 90% of fetuses of mothers with ITP do not have thrombocytopenia. Determination of fetal platelet count requires an invasive procedure such as fetal scalp vein sampling or cordocentesis.[39] The safety of these procedures needs to be weighed against the likelihoods of significant thrombocytopenia and subsequent birth process–related intracranial hemorrhage. Fetal scalp vein monitoring is technically difficult and requires ruptured membranes and cervical dilatation to at least 3 cm. Contamination of the fetal blood sample with amniotic fluid frequently results in fetal platelet clumping and spurious lab results.[39] Cordocentesis has a 1% to 2% complication rate with risk of cord hematoma and pregnancy loss.[5,10,40,41] Several studies comparing vaginal delivery to cesarean section found no increased risk in intracranial hemorrhage after vaginal delivery even in infants with severe thrombocytopenia.[7,13] Monitoring for neonatal thrombocytopenia is required for several days following delivery, as fetal platelet counts continue to drop after delivery with nadir 1 to 2 days after delivery in pregnancies complicated by ITP.[42]

PREECLAMPSIA

Preeclampsia is the second most frequent cause of thrombocytopenia in pregnancy, accounting for 21% of cases. Preeclampsia affects 3% to 14% of pregnancies and is the most common medical disorder of pregnancy.[43] Thrombocytopenia develops in 50% of patients with preeclampsia, generally in the third trimester, and correlates with the severity of the disorder. Preeclampsia is a syndrome characterized by the onset of hypertension and proteinuria after 20 weeks of gestation in a previously normotensive woman. The diagnostic criteria for preeclampsia include hypertension (systolic blood pressure [BP] greater than or equal to 140 mm Hg and diastolic BP 90 mm Hg) and proteinuria (300 mg protein/24 hours).[44,45] Preeclampsia is defined as either mild or severe. Preeclampsia may be of early onset (<34 weeks) or late onset (≥34 weeks) and may also occur during labor or in the postpartum state.[45] The pathophysiologic mechanisms in preeclampsia are not fully understood but the placentation process appears to be abnormal (for review see Sankaralingam and colleagues[46]). Trophoblastic cells have been shown to have defects in expression of adhesion molecules, vascular endothelial growth factors, and their receptors.[46–48] High levels of P-selectin and CD63 expression and increased levels of CD40 ligand are found in preeclamptic pregnancies.[49] Feto-placental ischemia develops, leading to impaired prostaglandin synthesis and release. This contributes to the development of hypertension, reduced placental flow, vascular damage, and platelet activation clinically manifested by a decrease in platelet number and increased new fibrin generation.[50] Angiogenic factors, such as vascular endothelial growth factor 1 (VEGF1), placental growth factor (PlGF), and soluble fms-like tyrosine kinase-1 (sFlt-1), are elevated in preeclampsia above normal pregnancy ranges, often before preeclampsia is recognized clinically. Measurement of these factors is currently limited to research settings.[51] Risk factors for preeclampsia include nongestational diabetes, family history of preeclampsia, maternal age older than 40 years, and antiphospholipid sydrome.[52] The recurrence rate of early severe preeclampsia is 25% to 65% and for mild preeclampsia is 5% to 7% in subsequent pregnancies.[52]

Diagnosis

Preeclampsia is suspected with new-onset hypertension with systolic blood pressure greater than or equal to 140 mm Hg and diastolic blood pressure 90 mm Hg. Laboratory studies useful in the diagnosis of thrombocytopenia related to preeclampsia include a complete blood count, peripheral blood smear, serum creatinine, uric acid, and 24-hour urine protein collection if urine dipstick indicates greater than 1+ protein. Coagulation studies are generally normal and disseminated intravascular coagulation is absent unless the disorder is severe.[44]

Management

Most cases of late-onset preeclampsia are handled entirely by the obstetrician. The management of the pregnant patient is directed at stabilization of blood pressure followed by delivery of the fetus. Because most cases of preeclampsia occur late in pregnancy after 34 weeks, at a time when the fetal lung is mature, immediate delivery of the infant is the optimal treatment.[53] Decisions for delivery are otherwise based on the balance of maternal and fetal risks of which platelet count less than 100,000/μL is one criterion.[44] Platelet transfusion may be necessary to support hemostasis for procedures or active bleeding but platelet survival is shortened. Some studies report that mild preeclampsia may respond to aspirin therapy, but this has not been confirmed.[51,54] Neonatal thrombocytopenia is reported in preeclamptic deliveries;

however, all reported infants were preterm deliveries of which 2 had intracranial hemorrhage despite cesarean section delivery.[4,5,10]

HELLP SYNDROME

HELLP syndrome is a poorly understood disorder of pregnancy characterized by microangiopathic hemolysis (H), elevated liver enzymes (EL), and low platelet count (LP). HELLP syndrome occurs in 0.5% to 0.9% of pregnancies. In preeclampsia/ HELLP, the hypoxic placenta releases soluble extravascular domains of at least 2 receptors for angiogenic factors that play a role in the pathogenesis of HELLP. One factor is soluble VEGF receptor-1, which inactivates VEGF. The second factor, soluble endoglin, inactivates transforming growth factor (TGF) β-1 and TGF β-3. These pro-angiogenic factors are inhibited from binding to their physiologic receptors in cell membranes and contribute to the progressive renal dysfunction/ hypertension and hepatic necrosis in HELLP syndrome.[46]

HELLP accounts for 12% of thrombocytopenia cases in pregnancy.[55] HELLP syndrome may represent advanced preeclampsia, although 15% to 20% of patients presenting with HELLP syndrome do not have antecedent hypertension or proteinuria which is a requirement for diagnosis of preeclampsia. HELLP syndrome complicates 10% to 20% of severe preeclamptic or eclamptic pregnancies and occurs predominantly in the third trimester between 28 and 36 weeks of gestation, although a very small percentage of cases do occur at less than 27 weeks of gestation.[56–58] HELLP syndrome, like preeclampsia, may also occur postpartum with 30% of patients presenting within 48 hours of delivery but may occur up to 1 week later. The mean age of women with HELLP syndrome is older than that seen with preeclampsia and most White women with HELLP are multiparous.

Diagnosis

Patients present with abdominal pain and tenderness in the epigastrium and right upper quadrant, which may be accompanied by nausea, vomiting, and malaise. Headache is reported in 30% to 60% of women and visual symptoms in 20%. The syndrome appears to be exacerbated during the night and symptoms improve during the day. Hypertension and proteinuria are present in 85% of cases. Generalized edema precedes the syndrome in more than half the cases.[58] The thrombocytopenia in HELLP syndrome is attributable to platelet activation and adherence to damaged vascular endothelium resulting in microangiopathy. The diagnostic laboratory features are microangiopathic hemolytic anemia, serum aspartate aminotransferase (AST) greater than 70 IU/dL, lactate dehydrogenase (LDH) greater than 600 IU/dL, and total bilirubin greater than 1.2 mg/dL with predominance of indirect bilirubin and low serum haptoglobin. The platelet count is generally less than 100,000/μL. Twenty-one percent of women with HELLP syndrome develop disseminated intravascular coagulation (DIC). Other serious morbidities include 1% incidence of subcapsular liver hematoma with 1% to 2% risk of hepatic rupture, 1% incidence of retinal detachment, 6% incidence of pulmonary edema, 8% incidence of renal failure, and 16% incidence of placental abruption.[58,59] Although thrombocytopenia is present, bleeding attributable solely to a low platelet count is not typical. The PT and aPTT are prolonged and factors

V, VIII, and fibrinogen are decreased, helping to distinguish the microangiopathic and coagulopathic changes in HELLP syndrome from those related to thrombotic thrombocytopenic purpura/hemolytic uremic syndrome (TTP/HUS).[60]

Management

The central management of HELLP syndrome is delivery of the fetus.[58] Delivery is indicated if the pregnancy is greater than 34 weeks' gestation, there are signs of fetal distress, or there are signs of maternal multiorgan damage including DIC, liver infarction, capsular hemorrhage, renal failure, or placental abruption. More than half of women will require transfusion support for platelet count less than 20,000/μL or if bleeding is present. The platelet count should be maintained at greater than 40,000 to 50,000/μL for cesarean section delivery.[61] HELLP syndrome usually peaks 24 to 48 hours following delivery with peak rise in LDH and platelet nadir at 24 to 48 hours postpartum. In the absence of other complications such as severe DIC, renal dysfunction, and ascites, the platelet count should begin to rise by the fourth day postpartum and rise to 100,000/μL by the sixth postpartum day. Plasma exchange may be used if the bilirubin and creatinine continue to rise for more than 72 hours.[62]

Urgent delivery is recommended to stop progression of HELLP. For pregnancies of fewer than 34 weeks' gestation and in which the maternal and fetal status is reassuring, glucocorticoids are recommended to accelerate fetal pulmonary maturity followed by delivery in 48 hours and may have some beneficial effect on maternal HELLP syndrome with a shorter length of hospital stay and a greater platelet count increase over 48 hours. However, there is no measurable effect on the maternal morbidity or transfusion requirement of HELLP syndrome.[55] Observation alone without plan for delivery is not generally recommended because HELLP syndrome features rarely reverse until delivery of the infant.

ANTIPHOSPHOLIPID SYNDROME

Antiphospholipid syndrome (APS) is characterized by vascular thrombosis and or pregnancy complications in association with laboratory evidence of antiphospholipid antibodies (aPL) and/or lupus anticoagulant.[63] Although no longer included in the revised Sapporo diagnostic criteria for APS, thrombocytopenia is a manifestation of primary APS with prevalence in 30% to 46% of patients.[64] The pathogenesis of the thrombocytopenia related to aPL is not entirely clear, but one mechanism is the binding of aPL to activated platelets via beta 2 glycoprotein I. Antibodies also binding to specific platelet glycoprotein receptors have been identified in 40% of patients with APS.[65,66] The presence of moderate to high titers of aPL in a patient with ITP may indicate pro-thrombotic risk. Sixty percent of nonpregnant patients diagnosed with ITP with positive aPL developed thrombosis in a 5-year follow-up study.[67] High titers of IgG anticardiolipin have a 78% and 77% predictive value for thrombosis and thrombocytopenia respectively, and only 44% for recurrent fetal loss.[68] In 742 patients with ITP from 9 published series, the frequency of aPL varied from 25% to 67% with mean of 43%.[69] Among some 623 patients with ITP reported in a total of 4 series, 33 of 48 ITP patients with aPL experienced thrombosis. In a study by Diz-Küçükkaya and colleagues,[67] 5 patients had recurrent spontaneous abortions or third trimester stillbirths. There was no discriminating difference in initial platelet count, type of aPL antibody, or platelet response to therapy between the aPL-positive ITP patient with subsequent thrombosis compared with those without subsequent thrombosis. Immunosuppressive therapy of ITP in patients with APS increased the platelet count and reduced the titers of antibodies directed to specific platelet glycoproteins but had no effect on the titers of aPL.[70] Notably, most thrombotic episodes occurred after the platelet count reached greater than 100,000/μL following glucocorticoid therapy or splenectomy in the ITP patients with aPL reactivity. None of these studies were designed to specifically address treatment of pregnant aPL-positive ITP patients with APS features.

Diagnosis

Symptoms of APS include a history of recurrent miscarriage, stillbirths, eclampsia or preeclampsia, premature delivery at less than 34 weeks, migraine headaches, Raynaud phenomena, livedo reticularis, transient ischemic attack, seizures, and prior history of venous or arterial thrombosis. Secondary APS occurs in the setting of autoimmune diseases such as SLE or rheumatoid arthritis. Symptoms and clinical signs of these disorders when evaluating the thrombocytopenic patient should prompt a referral for rheumatologic consultation because additional obstetric and neonatal concerns may arise with those disorders. The laboratory diagnosis requires the presence of a lupus anticoagulant, anticardiolipin antibodies in medium or high titer, or anti beta 2 glycoprotein I antibodies in high titer present on 2 or more occasions 12 weeks apart (for review see Baker and Bick[71,72] and Miyakis and colleagues[72]).

Management

Thrombocytopenia in association with APS is generally less severe than that seen with ITP. When platelet counts are less than 50,000/μL and symptomatic bleeding is present, treatment follows decision making similar to that in ITP, with steroids, IVIg, and occasionally splenectomy. Treatment of thrombocytopenia in APS must be balanced with the risk of thrombosis, as the disorder is characterized by venous and arterial thrombosis even in the setting of thrombocytopenia. Data are lacking about thrombotic risk and possible benefits of antithrombotic therapy in pregnant women with thrombocytopenia and positive APL but no prior history of thrombosis. Guidelines recommend combination of low-dose aspirin and heparin or low molecular weight heparin but drug therapy may be individualized with low-dose aspirin alone in young women with recurrent early miscarriage alone and no history of stillbirths or personal history of thrombosis.[63,66,73,74] There is no reduction in risk of preeclampsia, intrauterine growth retardation, and prematurity with aspirin alone. All women with APS require adequate 6- to 8- week minimum postpartum thromboprophylaxis.[63]

LIVER DISEASE

Thrombocytopenia may be related to liver disease and hypersplenism in pregnancy. Abnormal liver tests occur in 3% to 5% of pregnancies with a wide variety of causes.[75] Most liver disease in pregnancy is attributable to 1 of the 5 liver diseases unique to pregnancy: hyperemesis gravidarum, intrahepatic cholestasis of pregnancy, preeclampsia, HELLP syndrome, and acute fatty liver of pregnancy. Of these disorders, only HELLP, preeclampsia, and acute fatty liver of pregnancy are associated with thrombocytopenia. Acute fatty liver of pregnancy (AFLP) has an incidence of 1 in 10,000 to 15,000 pregnancies with a maternal mortality rate of 18% and fetal mortality of 23%.[76–78] Patients with AFLP are commonly nulliparous and the disorder has an increased incidence in twin pregnancies. In some cases, the etiology of AFLP is related to abnormalities in intramitochondrial fatty acid beta-oxidation (FAO).[79] Maternal heterozygosity for long-chain 3-hydroxyacyl-CoA dehydrogenase deficiency (LCHAD) reduces the maternal capacity to oxidize long-chain fatty acids both in the liver and placenta. In addition to dietary and other factors that exacerbate the defect, when a heterozygous woman carries a fetus that is homozygous, fetal hepatotoxic fatty acids accumulate and return to the maternal circulation causing maternal liver and vascular damage.[79]

Diagnosis

Acute fatty liver occurs exclusively in the third trimester from 28 to 40 weeks and rarely in later second trimester.[80] Symptoms include 1- to 2-week history of anorexia, nausea, vomiting, headache, and right upper quadrant pain. Physical signs include jaundice, hypertension, edema, ascites, and hepatic encephalopathy. Half of these patients will have criteria for preeclampsia and some may have features that overlap with HELLP syndrome. DIC is the hallmark for AFLP, whereas only 7% of patients with preeclampsia and 20% to 40% of patients with HELLP have DIC. The liver aminotransferase levels will be elevated usually to the 300- to 500-IU/dL range but may be as high as 1000 IU/dL and bilirubin less than 5 mg/dL. A normochromic normocytic anemia, elevated white blood cell count, and normal to low platelet count is usually present. On liver biopsy, there is evidence of microvesicular infiltration of free fatty acids in hepatocytes with lobular disarray and mild portal inflammation with cholestasis. AFLP is more likely to be associated with liver and renal failure and concomitant coagulopathy, hypoglycemia, and encephalopathy than HELLP syndrome.

Management

The management of AFLP is immediate termination of pregnancy, because there are no reports of spontaneous recovery during pregnancy. Vaginal delivery is associated with a reduced incidence of major intra-abdominal bleeding in women with coagulopathy owing to reduced clotting factor synthesis or consumptive DIC. Coagulation studies should be optimized by transfusion to maintain international normalized ratio (INR) less than 1.5 and platelet count greater than 50,000/μL for delivery. Although antithrombin III (ATIII) levels are markedly low at 11%, administration of ATIII concentrates has not been shown to be of benefit.[78] Recovery usually begins within 2 to 3 days after delivery. Overall improvement does not occur until 1 to 4 weeks later and, surprisingly, with no signs of residual chronic liver disease. Infants of mothers with AFLP should be screened for LCHAD deficiency, which has been found in 20% of infants born to mothers with AFLP but not in pregnancies with HELLP syndrome.

Chronic liver disease in pregnancy may be associated with various degrees of thrombocytopenia depending on the underlying etiology of the liver disease and degree of hypersplenism present. The disease activity of viral hepatitis C may increase with increased viral RNA load during pregnancy with a subsequent fall postpartum.[75] Autoimmune hepatitis may be associated with a flare of activity, most frequently noted in the postpartum state.[76,81] Flares are treated with an increase in steroids and azathioprine, both of which are likely to have beneficial effects on the platelet count in these disorders.

In pregnancies in which there is liver cirrhosis and portal hypertension, increased fetal and maternal complications are noted in 50% of the cases, including increased risk of fetal loss. The main risk is maternal variceal bleeding, which is observed in 20% to 25% of cirrhotic pregnancies especially during the second trimester and during labor. Vaginal delivery is the preferred method of delivery to avoid abdominal surgery and risk of hemorrhage. If the patient has known large varices, labor is to be avoided and surgical delivery is preferred. Patients with significant coagulation defects and platelet counts less than 30,000 to 50,000/μL will benefit from transfusion to avoid significant bleeding.

OTHER RARE THROMBOCYTOPENIC DISORDERS
Type IIB von Willebrand Disease

Type IIB von Willebrand disease (vWD) is an autosomal dominant subtype of vWD characterized by gain of function mutations in the A1 domain of von Willebrand factor (vWF), resulting in increased affinity of vWF binding to platelet GpIb.[82–84] Platelets bind to the mutant vWF and form complexes that are sequestered in the microcirculation and that are proteolyzed by the metalloproteinase ADAMTS13, resulting in increased platelet clearance and thrombocytopenia. Women with type IIB vWD typically experience worsening of thrombocytopenia owing to estrogen-related increased production of the mutant vWF during pregnancy and may be mistaken to have ITP.[85,86] Previous history of bleeding symptoms dating from early childhood, family history of a bleeding disorder associated with mild thrombocytopenia, and lack of response of the thrombocytopenia to steroids or IVIg should prompt consideration of this disorder.

Diagnosis

Assessment of vWF levels is complicated by the normal rise in factor VIII and vWF levels throughout pregnancy.[83] In some instances, these values will fall within the normal range at term explaining the low incidence of bleeding complications antenatally for most pregnant type I vWD patients. However, in type IIB vWD, the multimer analysis is abnormal and becomes increasingly so during pregnancy.[86] The vWF levels seldom normalize entirely in type IIB disease. Unlike other subtypes of vWD, the platelet count is abnormal. Diagnostic laboratory studies include factor VIII level, vWF antigen, vWF ristocetin cofactor activity, and vWF multimer analysis and platelet count. Ristocetin-induced platelet agglutination typically demonstrates heightened response to low-dose ristocetin, unlike in healthy individuals and in other forms of vWD in which there is no aggregation response at low dose.

Management

It is recommend that factor VIII, vWF antigen, and activity levels be checked late in the third trimester.[83] Factor VIII and vWF levels greater than 50 IU/dL are considered safe for regional anesthesia. Pregnancy-related increases in vWF fall to baseline within 7 to 21 days, which may explain the high incidence of delayed postpartum hemorrhage in 29% of pregnant patients with vWD. Patients with factor VIII levels of less than 50 IU/dL should be treated immediately before delivery and whenever bleeding is anticipated. Desmopressin (DDAVP) and plasma-derived vWF concentrates are the primary therapies in vWD, but the use of DDAVP in pregnancy is controversial.[87,88] Fibrinolytic inhibitors may be used as adjunctive therapy postpartum to decrease bleeding. DDAVP was formerly contraindicated in type IIB vWD because of the spontaneous platelet agglutination leading to exacerbation of thrombocytopenia. It has been used despite this in some instances in type IIB vWD without noted increased bleeding.[89] However, in the pregnant patient with type IIB vWD in whom the platelet count may dip as low as 20,000/μL at term, vWF concentrates are the preferred therapy. Moreover, in situations where more protracted therapy is required, such as in prophylaxis for cesarean section, the tachyphylaxis of factor VIII/vWF response observed after sequential dosing of DDAVP limits utility of this agent in type IIB vWD. Platelet transfusion is generally not necessary in type IIB vWD. Vaginal delivery is the preferred method of delivery without use of forceps or vacuum suction assistance because the infant has a 50% chance of inheriting type IIB vWD from the affected mother.[84]

Thrombotic Thrombocytopenic Purpura

Thrombotic thrombocytopenic purpura (TTP) and hemolytic uremic syndrome (HUS) are rare related hematologic disorders that affect 4 to 11 per 1 million in the United States. TTP is caused by an acquired deficiency of ADAMTS13, a disintegrin that specifically cleaves the highly adhesive long VWF strings as they are normally secreted from endothelial cells. TTP is characterized by systemic platelet adhesion/ aggregation, organ ischemia, profound thrombocytopenia, and fragmentation of erythrocytes. The red cell fragmentation occurs as blood flows through turbulent areas of the microcirculation partially occluded by platelet clumps. A microangiopathic hemolytic anemia occurs and serum levels of LDH are extremely elevated owing to hemolysis and tissue ischemia.[90] Pregnancy is associated with 13% of TTP/HUS cases in women. TTP is of rapid onset in the late second or early third trimester or postpartum. Symptoms of bruising occur at a median of 8.5 days before diagnosis.[91] Features of TTP may overlap with the more common HELLP syndrome with both disorders characteristically exhibiting microangiopathic hemolysis, thrombocyto- penia, and renal insufficiency. ADAMTS13 levels are also lower than normal pregnancy levels in HELLP syndrome and ADAMTS13 levels may not distinguish this from TTP. Maternal mortality has been declining from a peak of 80% pre-1980 to a present rate of 9% owing to the use of plasma infusion and plasmapheresis early in this disorder in addition to steroids. Stillbirth rate is high at 32% to 44% because of placental infarction.[90,92]

Congenital Thrombocytopenic Defects

Although rare, congenital thrombocytopenic defects such as gray platelet syndrome, Bernard Soulier syndrome (BSS), Fechtner syndrome, and the May Heggelin anomaly are rare hereditary platelet disorders that may complicate pregnancy.[93–95] Congenital thrombocytopenia should be considered in pregnant individuals who have bleeding symptoms that date to early childhood. A review of the peripheral blood smear platelet morphology is helpful to exclude many of these disorders. There are only 100 reported cases of gray platelet syndrome worldwide. Bleeding symptoms are relatively mild and patients may not be recognized early in life. It is associated with mild to moderate thrombocytopenia with absence of platelet granules resulting in a pale gray color on Wright Giemsa stain of peripheral blood. Diagnosis is made by electron microscopy. May Heggelin anomaly, Sebastian syndrome, Fechtner syndrome, and Epstein syndrome are all related macrothrombocytopenic disorders associated with the non–muscle myosin heavy-chain IIA (MYH9) gene. May Heggelin anomaly is charac- terized by giant platelets, thrombocytopenia, and Dohle bodies in the cytoplasm of granulocytes. Sebastian, Fechtner, and Epstein have associated deafness, nephritis, and cataracts in addition to macrothrombocytopenia. Bleeding symptoms in the affected May Heggelin individual are generally mild, as platelet function tends to be preserved although absolute number of platelets is decreased. There are a few reports of bleeding at delivery in individuals with May Heggelin anomaly.[94]

Bernard Soulier syndrome (BSS) is present in 1 in 1 million individuals and is char- acterized by macrothrombocytopenia and absent or reduced platelet GPIb-IX-V, important in vWF-mediated platelet adhesion.[95] Because the disorder generally presents in infancy with purpura, epistaxis, or gingival bleeding, and later menor- rhagia and urinary bleeding, BSS is generally diagnosed before pregnancy. On platelet aggregation there is absent or decreased platelet aggregation with ristocetin despite normal vWF levels. Confirmation can be obtained by specific genetic analysis of genes for GPIb-IX-V complex. Therapy for bleeding in BSS requires judicious use of platelet transfusion, as alloimmunization is frequent. Significant bleeding requires platelet transfusion with leuko-poor or leuko-depleted, preferably HLA-matched platelet transfusion to reduce formation of antibodies to normal platelet or HLA class I antigens. Mean platelet count varies from 10,000 to 150,000/μL with mean count of 58,300/μL. Mean blood loss following delivery is 1.2 L with 33% of women experiencing early hemorrhage and 40% experiencing postpartum hemorrhage 28 hours to 6 weeks later.[96] Alloimmunization is of concern because an antibody may be directed against a functionally important region of the GpIb receptor making subsequent transfusion ineffective. IVIg, plasmapheresis, and corticosteroids have also been tried in an attempt to improve response to platelet transfusion in pregnancy and to prevent alloimmune neonatal thrombocytopenia. Additional options for hemostatic agents include recombinant VIIa, DDAVP, and tranexamic acid. Neonatal alloimmune thrombocytopenia (NAIT) has been reported in 6 infants of mothers with BSS who were positive for maternal antiplatelet antibodies with 2 deaths from hemorrhage.

SUMMARY

In conclusion, thrombocytopenia in pregnancy is most frequently a benign process that does not require intervention. However, 35% of cases of thrombocytopenia in pregnancy are related to disease processes that may have serious bleeding consequences at delivery or for which thrombocytopenia may be an indicator of a more severe systemic disorder requiring emergent maternal and fetal care. Thus, all pregnant women with platelet counts less than 100,000/μL require careful hematological and obstetric consultation to exclude more serious disorders.

REFERENCES

1. Matthews JH, Benjamin S, Gill DS, et al. Pregnancy-associated thrombocytopenia: definition, incidence and natural history. Acta Haematol 1990;84(1):24–9.
2. Verdy E, Bessous V, Dreyfus M, et al. Longitudinal analysis of platelet count and volume in normal pregnancy. Thromb Haemost 1997;77(4):806–7.
3. Beilin Y, Zahn J, Comerford M. Safe epidural analgesia in thirty parturients with platelet counts between 69,000 and 98,000 mm(−3). Anesth Analg 1997;85(2):385–8.
4. Burrows RF, Kelton JG. Thrombocytopenia at delivery: a prospective survey of 6715 deliveries. Obstet Gynecol 1990;162(3):731–4.
5. Burrows RF, Kelton JG. Fetal thrombocytopenia and its relation to maternal thrombocytopenia. N Engl J Med 1993;329(20):1463–6.
6. Lescale KB, Eddleman KA, Cines DB, et al. Antiplatelet antibody testing in thrombocytopenic pregnant women. Obstet Gynecol 1996;174(3):1014–8.
7. Kelton J. Idiopathic thrombocytopenic purpura complicating pregnancy. Blood Rev 2002;16(1):43–6.
8. Tanaka M, Balki M, McLeod A, et al. Regional anesthesia and non-preeclamptic thrombocytopenia: time to re-think the safe platelet count. Rev Bras Anestesiol 2009;59(2):142–53.
9. Anteby E, Shalev O. Clinical relevance of gestational thrombocytopenia of <100,000/microliters. Am J Hematol 1994;47(2):118–22.
10. Burrows RF, Kelton JG. Pregnancy in patients with idiopathic thrombocytopenic purpura: assessing the risks for the infant at delivery. Obstet Gynecol Surv 1993;48(12):781–8.

11. Cines D, Bussel J, Liebman H, et al. The ITP syndrome: pathogenic and clinical diversity. Blood 2009;113(26):6511–21.
12. Cines D, Bussel J. How I treat idiopathic thrombocytopenic purpura (ITP). Blood 2005;106(7):2244–51.
13. McMillan R, Nugent D. The effect of antiplatelet autoantibodies on megakaryocytopoiesis. Int J Hematol 2005;81(2):94–9.
14. Stasi R, Cooper N, Del Poeta G, et al. Analysis of regulatory T-cell changes in patients with idiopathic thrombocytopenic purpura receiving B cell-depleting therapy with rituximab. Blood 2008;112(4):1147–50.
15. Grozovsky R, Hoffmeister K, Falet H. Novel clearance mechanisms of platelets. Curr Opin Hematol 2010;17(6):585–9.
16. Cines D, Blanchette V. Immune thrombocytopenic purpura. N Engl J Med 2002; 346(13):995–1008.
17. Cooper N, Bussel J. The pathogenesis of immune thrombocytopaenic purpura. Br J Haematol 2006;133(4):364–74.
18. Stavrou E, McCrae K. Immune thrombocytopenia in pregnancy. Hematol Oncol Clin North Am 2009;23(6):1299–316.
19. Ajzenberg N, Dreyfus M, Kaplan C, et al. Pregnancy-associated thrombocytopenia revisited: assessment and follow-up of 50 cases. Blood 1998;92(12): 4573–80.
20. Gill KK, Kelton JG. Management of idiopathic thrombocytopenic purpura in pregnancy. Semin Hematol 2000;37(3):275–89.
21. George JN, Woolf SH, Raskob GE, et al. Idiopathic thrombocytopenic purpura: a practice guideline developed by explicit methods for the American Society of Hematology. Blood 1996;88(1):3–40.
22. Webert K, Mittal R, Sigouin C, et al. A retrospective 11-year analysis of obstetric patients with idiopathic thrombocytopenic purpura. Blood 2003;102(13): 4306–11.
23. Sukenik-Halevy R, Ellis MH, Fejgin MD. Management of immune thrombocytopenic purpura in pregnancy. Obstet Gynecol Surv 2008;63:182–8.
24. British Committee for Standards in Haematology General Haematology Task Force. Guidelines for the investigation and management of idiopathic thrombocytopenic purpura in adults, children and in pregnancy. Br J Haematol 2003;120(4): 574–96.
25. Baerenwaldt A, Biburger M, Nimmerjahn F. Mechanisms of action of intravenous immunoglobulins. Expert Rev Clin Immunol 2010;6(3):425–34.
26. Cromwell C, Tarantino M, Aledort L. Safety of anti-D during pregnancy. Am J Hematol 2009;84(4):261–2.
27. Michel M, Novoa M, Bussel J. Intravenous anti-D as a treatment for immune thrombocytopenic purpura (ITP) during pregnancy. Br J Haematol 2003;123(1):142–6.
28. Cooper N. Intravenous immunoglobulin and anti-RhD therapy in the management of immune thrombocytopenia. Hematol Oncol Clin North Am 2009;23(6):1317–27.
29. Gaines AR. Disseminated intravascular coagulation associated with acute hemoglobinemia or hemoglobinuria following Rh(0)(D) immune globulin intravenous administration for immune thrombocytopenic purpura. Blood 2005;106(5): 1532–7.
30. Gaines AR. Acute onset hemoglobinemia and/or hemoglobinuria and sequelae following Rh(o)(D) immune globulin intravenous administration in immune thrombocytopenic purpura patients. Blood 2000;95(8):2523–9.
31. Temprano K, Bandlamudi R, Moore T. Antirheumatic drugs in pregnancy and lactation. Semin Arthritis Rheum 2005;35(2):112–21.

32. Oz BB, Hackman R, Einarson T, et al. Pregnancy outcome after cyclosporine therapy during pregnancy: a meta-analysis. Transplantation 2001;71(8):1051–5.
33. Di Paolo S, Schena A, Morrone LF, et al. Immunologic evaluation during the first year of life of infants born to cyclosporine-treated female kidney transplant recipients: analysis of lymphocyte subpopulations and immunoglobulin serum levels. Transplantation 2000;69(10):2049–54.
34. Erkman J, Blythe JG. Azathioprine therapy complicated by pregnancy. Obstet Gynecol 1972;40(5):708–10.
35. Payne SD, Resnik R, Moore TR, et al. Maternal characteristics and risk of severe neonatal thrombocytopenia and intracranial hemorrhage in pregnancies complicated by autoimmune thrombocytopenia. Obstet Gynecol 1997;177(1):149–55.
36. Samuels P, Bussel JB, Braitman LE, et al. Estimation of the risk of thrombocytopenia in the offspring of pregnant women with presumed immune thrombocytopenic purpura. N Engl J Med 1990;323(4):229–35.
37. Fujimura K, Harada Y, Fujimoto T, et al. Nationwide study of idiopathic thrombocytopenic purpura in pregnant women and the clinical influence on neonates. Int J Hematol 2002;75(4):426–33.
38. Chouhan J, Herrington J. Treatment options for chronic refractory idiopathic thrombocytopenic purpura in adults: focus on romiplostim and eltrombopag. Pharmacotherapy 2010;30(7):666–83.
39. Adams DM, Bussel JB, Druzin ML. Accurate intrapartum estimation of fetal platelet count by fetal scalp samples smear. Am J Perinatol 1994;11(1):42–5.
40. Christiaens G. Immune thrombocytopenic purpura in pregnancy. Baillieres Clin Haematol 1998;11(2):373–80.
41. Garmel SH, Craigo SD, Morin LM, et al. The role of percutaneous umbilical blood sampling in the management of immune thrombocytopenic purpura. Prenat Diagn 1995;15(5):439–45.
42. Kelton JG. Management of the pregnant patient with idiopathic thrombocytopenic purpura. Ann Intern Med 1983;99(6):796–800.
43. Cunningham FG, Lindheimer MD. Hypertension in pregnancy. N Engl J Med 1992;326(14):927–32.
44. Sibai B. Diagnosis and management of gestational hypertension and preeclampsia. Obstet Gynecol 2003;102(1):181–92.
45. Report of the National High Blood Pressure Education Program Working Group on High Blood Pressure in Pregnancy. Am J Obstet Gynecol 2000;183:S1–22.
46. Sankaralingam S, Arenas I, Lalu M, et al. Preeclampsia: current understanding of the molecular basis of vascular dysfunction. Expert Rev Mol Med 2006;8(3):1–20.
47. Redman C. Current topic: pre-eclampsia and the placenta. Placenta 1991;12(4):301–8.
48. McCrae KR, Samuels P, Schreiber AD. Pregnancy-associated thrombocytopenia: pathogenesis and management. Blood 1992;80(11):2697–714.
49. Oron G, Ben-Haroush A, Hod M, et al. Serum-soluble CD40 ligand in normal pregnancy and in preeclampsia. Obstet Gynecol 2006;107(4):896–900.
50. Kobayashi T, Tokunaga N, Sugimura M, et al. Coagulation/fibrinolysis disorder in patients with severe preeclampsia. Semin Thromb Hemost 1999;25(5):451–4.
51. Pereira T, Rudnicki M, Soler JM, et al. Meta-analysis of aspirin for the prevention of preeclampsia: do the main randomized controlled trials support an association between low-dose aspirin and a reduced risk of developing preeclampsia? Clinics (Sao Paulo) 2006;61(2):179–82.
52. Barton J, Sibai B. Prediction and prevention of recurrent preeclampsia. Obstet Gynecol 2008;112(2):359–72.

53. Stubbs TM, Lazarchick J, Van Dorsten J, et al. Evidence of accelerated platelet production and consumption in nonthrombocytopenic preeclampsia. Obstet Gynecol 1986;155:263–5.
54. Gauer R, Atlas M, Hill J. Clinical inquiries. Does low-dose aspirin reduce preeclampsia and other maternal-fetal complications? J Fam Pract 2008;57(1):54–6.
55. Sibai BM. Diagnosis, controversies, and management of the syndrome of hemolysis, elevated liver enzymes, and low platelet count. Obstet Gynecol 2004;103:981–91.
56. Haram K, Softeland E, Hervig T, et al. [Thrombocytopenia in pregnancy]. Tidsskr Nor Laegeforen 2003;123:2250–2 [in Norwegian].
57. Haeger M, Unander M, Norder-Hansson B, et al. Complement, neutrophil, and macrophage activation in women with severe preeclampsia and the syndrome of hemolysis, elevated liver enzymes, and low platelet count. Obstet Gynecol 1992;79:19–26.
58. Haram K, Svendsen E, Abildgaard U. The HELLP syndrome: clinical issues and management. A review. BMC Pregnancy Childbirth 2009;9(1):8.
59. Hupuczi P, Rigo B, Sziller I, et al. Follow-up analysis of pregnancies complicated by HELLP syndrome. Fetal Diagn Ther 2006;21:519–22.
60. Sibai BM. Imitators of severe pre-eclampsia/eclampsia. Clin Perinatol 2004;31: 835–52.
61. Baxter JK, Weinstein L. HELLP syndrome: the state of the art. Obstet Gynecol Surv 2004;59:838–45.
62. Eser B, Guven M, Unal A, et al. The role of plasma exchange in HELLP syndrome. Clin Appl Thromb Hemost 2005;11:211–7.
63. Abrahams VM. Mechanisms of antiphospholipid antibody-associated pregnancy complications. Thromb Res 2009;124(5):521–5.
64. Krause I, Blank M, Fraser A, et al. The association of thrombocytopenia with systemic manifestations in the antiphospholipid syndrome. Immunobiology 2005;210(10):749–54.
65. Espinosa G, Cervera R, Font J, et al. Antiphospholipid syndrome: pathogenic mechanisms. Autoimmun Rev 2003;2(2):86–93.
66. Meroni P, Gerosa M, Raschi E, et al. Updating on the pathogenic mechanisms 5 of the antiphospholipid antibodies-associated pregnancy loss. Clin Rev Allergy Immunol 2008;34(3):332–7.
67. Diz-Küçükkaya R, Hacihanefioğlu A, Yenerel M, et al. Antiphospholipid antibodies and antiphospholipid syndrome in patients presenting with immune thrombocytopenic purpura: a prospective cohort study. Blood 2001;98(6):1760–4.
68. Harris EN, Chan JK, Asherson RA, et al. Thrombosis, recurrent fetal loss, and thrombocytopenia. Predictive value of the anticardiolipin antibody test. Arch Intern Med 1986;146(11):2153–6.
69. Comellas-Kirkerup L, Hernndez-Molina G, Cabral A. Antiphospholipid-associated thrombocytopenia or autoimmune hemolytic anemia in patients with or without definite primary antiphospholipid syndrome according to the Sapporo revised classification criteria: a 6-year follow-up study. Blood 2010;116(16):3058–63.
70. Leuzzi RA, Davis GH, Cowchock FS, et al. Management of immune thrombocytopenic purpura associated with the antiphospholipid antibody syndrome. Clin Exp Rheumatol 1997;15(2):197–200.
71. Baker W, Bick R. The clinical spectrum of antiphospholipid syndrome. Hematol Oncol Clin North Am 2008;22(1):33–52, v.
72. Miyakis S, Lockshin MD, Atsumi T, et al. International consensus statement on an update of the classification criteria for definite antiphospholipid syndrome (APS). J Thromb Haemost 2006;4(2):295–306.

73. Shehata HA, Nelson-Piercy C, Khamashta MA. Management of pregnancy in anti-phospholipid syndrome. Rheum Dis Clin North Am 2001;27(3):643–59.
74. Derksen RH, Khamashta MA, Branch DW. Management of the obstetric antiphos-pholipid syndrome. Arthritis Rheum 2004;50(4):1028–39.
75. Hay JE. Liver disease in pregnancy. Hepatology 2008;47(3):1067–76.
76. Lee N, Brady C. Liver disease in pregnancy. World J Gastroenterol 2009;15(8):897–906.
77. Knox TA, Olans LB. Liver disease in pregnancy. N Engl J Med 1996;335(8):569–76.
78. Castro MA, Fassett MJ, Reynolds TB, et al. Reversible peripartum liver failure: a new perspective on the diagnosis, treatment, and cause of acute fatty liver of pregnancy, based on 28 consecutive cases. Obstet Gynecol 1999;181(2):389–95.
79. Ibdah JA, Bennett MJ, Rinaldo P, et al. A fetal fatty-acid oxidation disorder as a cause of liver disease in pregnant women. N Engl J Med 1999;340:1723–31.
80. Ramasamy I. Inherited bleeding disorders: disorders of platelet adhesion and aggregation. Crit Rev Oncol Hematol 2004;49(1):1–35.
81. Heneghan MA, Norris SM, O'Grady JG, et al. Management and outcome of preg-nancy in autoimmune hepatitis. Gut 2001;48(1):97–102.
82. Gadisseur A, Hermans C, Berneman Z, et al. Laboratory diagnosis and molecular classification of von Willebrand disease. Acta Haematol 2009;121(2–3):71–84.
83. James A, Manco-Johnson M, Yawn B, et al. Von Willebrand disease: key points from the 2008 National Heart, Lung, and Blood Institute guidelines. Obstet Gyne-col 2009;114(3):674–8.
84. Zeitler P, von Stockhausen HB. Type IIB von Willebrand Jürgens syndrome as the cause of neonatal thrombocytopenia. Klin Padiatr 1998;210(2):85–8 [in German].
85. Rick ME, Williams SB, Sacher RA, et al. Thrombocytopenia associated with preg-nancy in a patient with type IIB von Willebrand's disease. Blood 1987;69(3):786–9.
86. Casonato A, Sartori MT, Bertomoro A, et al. Pregnancy-induced worsening of thrombocytopenia in a patient with type IIB von Willebrand's disease. Blood Coa-gul Fibrinolysis 1991;2(1):33–40.
87. Pacheco L, Costantine M, Saade G, et al. von Willebrand disease and preg-nancy: a practical approach for the diagnosis and treatment. Obstet Gynecol 2010;203(3):194–200.
88. Lee CA, Chi C, Pavord SR, et al. The obstetric and gynaecological management of women with inherited bleeding disorders—review with guidelines produced by a taskforce of UK Haemophilia Centre Doctors' Organization. Haemophilia 2006;12(4):301–36.
89. Casonato A, Pontara E, Dannhaeuser D, et al. Re-evaluation of the therapeutic efficacy of DDAVP in type IIB von Willebrand's disease. Blood Coagul Fibrinolysis 1994;5(6):959–64.
90. Moake J. Thrombotic microangiopathies: multimers, metalloprotease, and beyond. Clin Transl Sci 2009;2(5):366–73.
91. Martin J, Bailey A, Rehberg J, et al. Thrombotic thrombocytopenic purpura in 166 pregnancies: 1955–2006. Obstet Gynecol 2008;199(2):98–104.
92. Myers L. Postpartum plasma exchange in a woman with suspected thrombotic thrombocytopenic purpura (TTP) vs. hemolysis, elevated liver enzymes, and low platelet syndrome (HELLP): a case study. Nephrol Nurs J 2010;37(4):399–402.
93. Chatwani A, Bruder N, Shapiro T, et al. May-Hegglin anomaly: a rare case of maternal thrombocytopenia in pregnancy. Obstet Gynecol 1992;166(1):143–4.

94. Ishii A, Honnma T, Ishida M, et al. Pregnancy complicated by the May-Hegglin anomaly. J Perinat Med 1993;21(3):247–52.
95. Nurden P, Nurden A. Congenital disorders associated with platelet dysfunctions. Thromb Haemost 2008;99(2):253–63.
96. Peitsidis P, Datta T, Pafilis I, et al. Bernard Soulier syndrome in pregnancy: a systematic review. Haemophilia 2010;16(4):584–91.

Microangiopathic Disorders in Pregnancy

Salley G. Pels, MD[a,*], Michael J. Paidas, MD[b,c]

KEYWORDS

• Microangiopathic disorders • TTP • HUS
• Preeclampsia • HELLP

Microangiopathic disorders in pregnancy present a challenge both diagnostically and therapeutically. Although these conditions are rare, they can lead to devastating maternal and fetal outcomes if misdiagnosed and treated improperly.

The microangiopathic disorders present with thrombocytopenia, hemolytic anemia, and multiorgan damage. The diagnosis of thrombotic thrombocytopenic purpura (TTP) has long been based on the clinical pentad of neurologic abnormalities, thrombocytopenia, microangiopathic hemolytic anemia, fever, and renal dysfunction. Hemolytic uremic syndrome (HUS) is often manifested by acute renal failure and hypertension, as well as microangiopathic anemia and thrombocytopenia. Renal dysfunction in HUS is often more severe than that in TTP, whereas neurologic abnormalities are more prevalent in TTP. HUS is more frequently observed in children who have had a preceding gastrointestinal infection; however, this condition has also been reported in adults and pregnant women. Patients with these diagnoses may or may not have hypertension, a hallmark of the disorders of preeclampsia.

Preeclampsia and hypertension, elevated liver enzymes, and low platelets (HELLP) are thought of as a spectrum of disorders, with HELLP being the most severe manifestation. Preeclampsia is defined as new onset of hypertension and proteinuria after 20 weeks' gestation in its mildest form. Patients may progress and develop eclampsia, with neurologic abnormalities that are often attributed to the hypertension, such as headache, blurry vision, and seizures.[1] Leaky cerebral vasculature also leads to

---

The authors have nothing to disclose.
[a] Section of Hematology Oncology, Department of Pediatrics, Yale University School of Medicine, 333 Cedar Street, LMP2073, New Haven, CT 06520-8063, USA
[b] Division of Maternal Fetal Medicine, Department of Obstetrics, Gynecology and Reproductive Sciences, Yale University School of Medicine, 333 Cedar Street, FMB339B, New Haven, CT 06520-8063, USA
[c] Section of Hematology Oncology, Department of Pediatrics, Yale University School of Medicine, 333 Cedar Street, LMP2073, New Haven, CT 06520-8063, USA
* Corresponding author.
E-mail address: salley.pels@yale.edu

Hematol Oncol Clin N Am 25 (2011) 311–322
doi:10.1016/j.hoc.2011.01.005
0889-8588/11/$ – see front matter © 2011 Elsevier Inc. All rights reserved.

cerebral edema, increased intracranial pressures, seizures, and coma. These severe neurologic symptoms may be seen at lower-than-expected pressures because of the widespread endothelial dysfunction.[2] Women with severe preeclampsia may also go on to develop a hemolytic anemia and thrombocytopenia. HELLP, as the acronym implies, is diagnosed in patients who present with hypertension, elevated levels of transaminases, and thrombocytopenia. Patients may also have hemolytic anemia, disseminated intravascular coagulation, and other organ dysfunctions, even though liver dysfunction is often the predominant feature.

TTP and HUS are rare conditions in the general population, occurring in between 4 and 11 patients per million.[3] TTP has a female to male predominance of 3:2.[4] HUS typically occurs in children, and its incidence is approximately 0.64 of 100,000 in children younger than 15 years.[5] Together, TTP-HUS occurs in 1 in 25,000 pregnancies.[6] The association between TTP-HUS and pregnancy is in part due to the female predominance of the disease; however, pregnancy is thought to precipitate the disease as either a first occurrence or a recurrence in a patient with a history of TTP. In a review of published cases from 1964 to 2002, the frequency of pregnancy among women diagnosed with TTP-HUS was 13%.[7]

Preeclampsia is much more common than TTP-HUS and affects approximately 5% to 8% of pregnancies.[8] Whereas HELLP occurs in 0.5% to 0.9% of pregnancies, it affects 10% to 20% of cases affected by severe preeclampsia.[9]

PATHOPHYSIOLOGY

The hallmark of the microangiopathic disorders is the development of microthrombi in the small vasculature leading to thrombocytopenia, hemolysis, and specific multiorgan damage. Although TTP, HUS, and preeclampsia/HELLP syndrome are all microangiopathic disorders seen in pregnancy, the pathophysiologic mechanisms underlying each condition are different.

TTP

The development of microthrombi in TTP is now attributed to a deficiency in the von Willebrand factor (vWF) cleaving enzyme a disintegrin and metalloprotease thrombospondin type 1 repeats 13 (ADAMTS13).[10–12] A deficiency of this metalloprotease, either inherited or acquired with autoantibody, leads to ultralarge vWF multimers that promote platelet aggregation within the microcirculation.[13] The complex interaction of ADAMTS13 and vWF has been studied extensively, and shear stress is important for unfolding of the vWF protein, revealing the cleavage sites for ADAMTS13.[14] This type of shear stress is found under normal conditions in arterioles and capillaries and promotes vWF-platelet interaction leading to aggregation and thrombus formation.[15] The presence of ADAMTS13 is thus essential for the maintenance of normal hemostasis in the microvasculature. The severe thrombocytopenia that often occurs in TTP is a result of consumption in the microthrombi. Microangiopathic hemolytic anemia subsequently occurs due to mechanical injury within the thrombosed microvasculature.

Deficiency of ADAMTS13 may be either inherited or acquired. Numerous mutation types have been identified, including missense, nonsense, insertions, deletions, and splice-site variations. These mutations present with varying clinical severity, and approximately 90% of patients with either homozygous or compound heterozygous mutations have symptomatic TTP.[13] For patients with no family history or known mutation, autoimmune inhibitors to ADAMTS13 are frequently observed. Of patients with a diagnosis of TTP, approximately 31% to 38% have a detectable inhibitor.[4,16]

The causal relationship of pregnancy to the development or exacerbation of TTP is not fully understood. TTP is more frequent in women of childbearing age, perhaps this association is coincidental; however, some have argued that pregnancy can trigger these conditions. Although normal pregnancy is certainly a prothrombotic state with increases in levels of fibrinogen, vWF, and factor VIII (FVIII), there are also reductions in the level of ADAMTS13 to between 52% and 64% of the normal levels.[17,18] For patients with a history of TTP and baseline lower levels of ADAMTS13, there is theoretically an increased propensity toward recurrence during this time. In a review of a case series in 2003, 14 women from 8 families with known familial TTP-HUS had their initial presentation during pregnancy.[7] Whether pregnancy would prompt a relapse in a known patient with TTP or would induce inhibitor development in a patient with no prior history remains unclear.

HUS

Unlike TTP, HUS is thought to be associated with several abnormalities of the complement cascade, leading to the development of microthrombi, primarily in the renal parenchyma. The following 3 distinct types of HUS have now been described: typical HUS (or D+ HUS) often seen in children as a result of a preceding *Escherichia coli* diarrheal illness, atypical HUS (or D− HUS) often seen in adults and caused by a variety of mutations of proteins in the complement cascade (factor H, factor I), and an autoimmune form of HUS characterized by antibodies to factor H or related proteins.[19]

Factor H is a regulatory protein of the alternative complement pathway, and it functions to protect self-cells from attack by the complement system. Decreased levels of factor H, because of mutations or inhibitors, result in subsequent endothelial cell damage and thrombus formation at the site of exposed subendothelium.[20] Similar to factor H is factor I, another regulator of the complement system. Factor I is a serine protease that cleaves C3b (an essential C3 cleavage product of the alternative complement pathway); its cofactors include factor H, C4-binding protein, and membrane cofactor protein (CD46).[21] These abnormalities in the complement system have been theorized to be problematic for the renal vasculature, specifically because of the inherent presence of fenestrations within the capillary endothelium of the glomerulus, leaving the subendothelium more exposed and therefore vulnerable to complement attack.[22]

The pathophysiologic mechanisms underlying D+ HUS are less well understood. A preceding diarrheal illness is often caused by *E coli* O157:H7, although other strains of *E coli*, *Shigella*, and *Campylobacter* have also been implicated because of the known production of the Shiga toxin. The Shiga toxin binds to Gb3, a glycosphingolipid receptor found on endothelial cells, podocytes, and tubular cells.[23] There is evidence that the Shiga toxin induces the release of ultralarge vWF multimers from endothelial cells and inhibits their cleavage by ADAMTS13, resulting in enhanced platelet adhesion in in vitro experiments.[24]

Diarrheal illnesses are not the only known infectious cause of HUS. Streptococcal pneumonia–related HUS is found in approximately 5% of children diagnosed with HUS and is presumed to be caused by the exposure of the Thomsen-Friedenreich (TF) antigen. This cryptic antigen is found on the surface of red cells, platelets, and glomerular endothelial cells and is normally hidden by neuraminic acid. *Streptococcus* sp produce the enzyme neuraminidase, thus allowing for the exposure of the TF antigen, which is then recognized by the immune system as foreign, triggering immune system response against those cells and leading to the development of HUS.[25]

Histopathologic investigations of both TTP and HUS have been performed, and although these disorders often share a common clinical picture, the pathology of these

2 disorders are distinguishable. Autopsy specimens from patients with TTP contain platelet-rich thrombi within the microvasculature, whereas the tissues from patients with HUS have fibrin and red cell–rich thrombi. In addition, the frequency of which specific organs were found to have microthrombi was noted to be different in each of these diseases. The microthrombi of TTP were found in the heart, pancreas, kidney, adrenal gland, and brain. In HUS, these findings were primarily within the kidney and only infrequently found in the pancreas, adrenal gland, brain, and heart.[26] This distribution of microthrombi speaks both to the clinical picture of these diseases and to the current understanding of the pathophysiology of each of these diseases, with TTP having a deficiency of circulating vWF cleaving protein leading to platelet microthrombi and multiorgan involvement and HUS resulting from a dysfunctional complement cascade, damage to renal vascular endothelium, and the triggering of thrombus formation through the coagulation cascade and subsequent acute renal failure.

Preeclampsia/HELLP

The pathophysiologic mechanisms behind the initial development of severe preeclampsia and HELLP are beginning to be better understood. Abnormal placental/maternal vascularization, inflammatory responses, and maternal hypercoagulability have each been theorized to play critical roles in the pathogenesis of these disorders.

Studies of the placentas from preeclamptic/HELLP pregnancies have shown abnormal vasculature development and areas of placental hypoperfusion and ischemia.[8,27,28] Maternal-placental vascular endothelial dysfunction has also been demonstrated to play a central role. Both these events lead to platelet activation, which results in circulating microthrombi and organ damage/dysfunction.

Several placenta-derived factors have also been implicated in the development of preeclampsia, including the soluble Fms-like tyrosine kinase 1 (sFlt1) and soluble endoglin.[29] Placenta-derived sFlt1 binds to circulating vascular endothelial growth factor (VEGF) and placental growth factor. These factors are essential for the normal development and vascularization of the placenta as well as normal glomerular endothelial function. In patients treated with VEGF antagonists, used in cancer therapy, hypertension and proteinuria have been reported.[30] Soluble endoglin is also an antiangiogenic factor, inhibiting the normal binding of transforming growth factor βto its cellular receptors, leading to impaired capillary angiogenesis. In a study of pregnant rats, rats with elevation of either sFlt1 or endoglin levels had evidence of hypertension and proteinuria; however, in animals with increased levels of both factors there were significant nephritic levels of proteinuria, severe hypertension, elevated L-lactate dehydrogenase, abnormal liver functions, and thrombocytopenia, all clinical evidence of the development of HELLP syndrome.[31] Increased levels of sFlt1 and soluble endoglin in pregnant women have also been shown to be predictive of the development of severe preeclampsia.[32–35]

Beyond the antiangiogenic factors, numerous additional studies of gene expression profiling of placental tissue from preeclamptic and HELLP pregnancies have also implicated alterations in inflammatory responses. Increases in the levels of proinflammatory cytokines tumor necrosis factor α, interleukin (IL)-6, and IL-8 have been documented, as well as significant increases in leukocyte activation.[36]

As a protective mechanism against delivery-associated hemorrhage, pregnancy is also a hypercoagulable state. Many alterations in factors involved in coagulation are observed in normal pregnancy, such as increased levels of fibrinogen; factor VII factor X, and FVIII; and vWF.[37] Levels of fibrinogen, FVIII, and vWF can increase up to 3-fold by the third trimester.[7] ADAMTS13 activity levels also decrease during pregnancy, averaging approximately 94% of the normal in the first trimester and 64% in the second and third trimesters.[18]

The hypercoagulability of a normal pregnancy is enhanced in severe preeclampsia and HELLP not only due to endothelial damage and dysfunction leading to platelet activation but also due to elevated circulating levels of thrombomodulin, vWF, and plasminogen activator inhibitor-1.[1,38] Additional studies comparing patients with severe preeclampsia and HELLP versus normal patients have shown that there is enhanced endothelial cell activation and decreased levels of ADAMTS13.[39,40] ADAMTS13 activity is further reduced to a median of 31% in pregnant women with HELLP compared with 71% in normal pregnant women and 101% in nonpregnant women. While these changes result in an expected increased level of vWF in patients with both severe preeclampsia and HELLP as compared with normal healthy pregnant volunteers, ultralarge multimers are not found in these patients.[40] The findings of decreased ADAMTS13 and increased vWF activity are supportive evidence that coagulopathic changes occur in these disease processes; however, these changes may not be causative and most likely represent consumption of the metalloprotease by ongoing thrombus formation and the vascular damage resulting in excessive release of vWF from endothelial stores.

DIAGNOSTIC EVALUATION

Outside the first trimester, in which preeclampsia and HELLP syndromes do not occur, the difficult task of distinguishing between preeclampsia, HELLP, TTP, and HUS can be both challenging and essential to obtaining a good maternal/fetal outcome. Obtaining rapid results of ADAMTS13 activity and von Willebrand multimeric analysis is unrealistic in most institutions, and the treating physician is left to make treatment decisions without these key pieces of information. Clinical features often widely overlap with each of these entities (**Box 1**); however, treatment and subsequent outcomes are quite dependent on appropriate diagnosis. TTP is considered in patients presenting with severe thrombocytopenia, microangiopathic hemolytic anemia, neurologic abnormalities, and mild renal dysfunction (serum creatinine levels <3 mg/dL). HUS also presents with severe thrombocytopenia and microangiopathic hemolytic anemia; however, renal function is often more severely compromised with serum creatinine levels greater than 3 mg/dL, whereas neurologic abnormalities are less common. TTP-HUS can occur during any stage of pregnancy; however, data suggest that there is a higher incidence in the second and third trimesters, resulting in significant overlap with the preeclamptic disorders.[41] Preeclampsia/HELLP may present with microangiopathic hemolytic anemia and severe thrombocytopenia is accompanied by hypertension and significant elevations in levels of liver enzymes. In preeclampsia/HELLP, these processes often resolve after delivery of the placenta. However, for patients in whom TTP/HUS is suspected, this prompt resolution will not occur.

A better understanding of the pathophysiologic mechanisms underlying each entity has led to the study of ADAMTS13 and vWF multimers in patients with suspected severe preeclampsia and HELLP in an attempt to distinguish it from TTP.[38–40] Whereas these patients do have mild reductions in ADAMTS13 and elevation in vWF, women with HELLP do not have ultralarge vWF multimers. Because none of the patients with HELLP had ultralarge vWF multimers, undetectable ADAMTS13, or presence of antibodies, TTP was ruled out in each of these cases; however, if a patient were to have an ADAMTS13 activity of less than 10%, TTP would have been the correct diagnosis.[40]

Ultralarge multimers, however, may not always be found in patients with TTP. Initially, the vWF may be consumed in microthrombi, and once treatment starts and

---

Box 1
Common presenting signs and symptoms of microangiopathic disorders of pregnancy

TTP

- Thrombocytopenia (often severe <50,000)
- Hemolytic anemia
- Neurologic dysfunction
- Renal dysfunction (creatinine level <3mg/dL)
- Fever

HUS

- Thrombocytopenia
- Hemolytic anemia
- Renal failure (creatinine level >3mg/dL)
- Hypertension

Severe preeclampsia

- Hypertension
- Proteinuria
- Neurologic dysfunction (headache, blurred vision)
- Thrombocytopenia
- Hemolytic anemia

HELLP

- Thrombocytopenia (often mild <100,000, but may be <50,000)
- Hemolytic anemia
- Liver dysfunction

ADAMTS13 levels begin to increase, it may be cleaved as usual thus producing relatively normal-sized multimers.[42]

Distinguishing TTP from HUS is often based on clinical presentation. However, patients with atypical HUS are more challenging. vWF multimeric patterns in patients with HUS often show decreases in large multimers, which is secondary to the enhanced sheer stress that the protein experiences in the microvasculature, whereas the ADAMTS13 levels and activity remain near normal.[42] Adding to the complexity of this situation are studies documenting that the Shiga toxin can induce secretion of ultralarge vWF multimers from endothelial cells and simultaneously impair ADAMTS13 function.[24]

TREATMENT
TTP

Without treatment, the mortality rate of TTP is more than 90%. Since the advent of plasma transfusions and plasmapheresis, this rate is down to approximately 20%.[43] Both plasma exchange and infusion therapy have been shown to be effective treatments for TTP. Protocols typically dictate that the plasma exchange or infusion be performed daily until platelet count and neurologic status is recovered and often for several days after resolution. A randomized controlled trial comparing plasma exchange to infusion was done by the Canadian Apheresis Study Group in 102 patients (male and female). Patients receiving plasma exchange demonstrated both higher initial response to therapy with improved platelet counts (47% vs 25%, $P = .025$) and improved mortality (4% vs 16%, $P = .035$).[44] These results were confirmed in a French study in which mortality rates were higher overall; however, the survival in the plasmapheresis group was 85% compared with only 57% in the plasma infusion group.[45] These responses to plasma-based therapies are logical based on the current understanding of the pathophysiology of TTP. The plasma product contains the missing ADAMTS13 protease, and for patients in whom an inhibitor is the cause, it may be assumed that plasma exchange and subsequent removal of the offending antibody would be more effective than simple transfusion. One concern about the use of fresh frozen plasma is that it also contains vWF multimers that are known to play a significant role in the thrombotic microangiopathy of TTP. Studies evaluating the use of an alternative product from which vWF multimers are removed, cryoprecipitate-poor (or cryosupernatant) plasma, have thus far been unable to show a superiority of this product at improving either laboratory parameters or overall mortality.[46,47]

The treatment of pregnancy-associated TTP is also based on plasma infusion/exchange. Before its institution, the mortality rate among affected women was 58%, whereas maternal mortality is currently less than 10%.[41] For women who respond to plasma exchange, but have declining platelet counts during a pregnancy affected by TTP, plasma infusions or exchange have been performed on an every 1- to 2-week schedule to maintain remission.[48–50] Delivery does not resolve symptoms, thus it is not indicated unless there is associated fetal distress.

For many patients with TTP, steroids are often initiated before plasma exchange or infusion. Adequate randomized controlled trials of the effectiveness of steroids versus plasma exchange or infusion have not been performed because of the dramatically improved patient survival since the introduction of plasma-based therapies. Steroids, however, have been reported to induce remission alone, especially in mild cases of TTP, thus they are often started up front.[51]

An assortment of other chemotherapeutic, anticoagulant, and immunomodulatory agents, including vincristine,[52] aspirin and dipyramidole,[53] cyclosporine,[54,55] rituximab,[56,57] and intravenous immunoglobulin[58] have been used for refractory patients with varying successes. Although the effects of these therapies have not been adequately studied in randomized controlled trials and several of these agents are also not used in pregnant women because of their potential risks to the fetus, they may be considered for severe refractory disease after delivery.

HUS

The treatment of typical HUS has traditionally centered on dialysis for renal failure and supportive care. Plasma therapy for pediatric patients with HUS has not been demonstrated to be superior to supportive care.[59,60] However, patients with atypical presentation may benefit from plasma therapy, which would target either an inhibitor or the inherent deficiencies in the normal complement pathway.[61] Once the diagnosis of atypical HUS has been made, current recommendations are for immediate initiation of plasma exchange.[62] Refractory patients may also benefit from the complement inhibitor eculizumab, a humanized monoclonal antibody to the terminal complement, which has had a reported benefit in patients with atypical HUS.[63] There are currently no reports of the use of eculizumab in pregnancy-associated HUS; however, it has been used safely in several pregnancies in women affected by paroxysmal nocturnal hemoglobinuria.[64]

Patients with atypical HUS are often combined with those diagnosed with TTP in therapeutic studies due in part to the rarity of these conditions and also the significant clinical overlap of the 2 conditions. The evaluation of the use of steroids in these disease processes is one such study in which steroids alone were reported to induce remission in mild cases of TTP-HUS.[51] Investigations into the utility of steroids for typical HUS, however, have shown no significant improvement when compared with placebo.[65]

Severe Preeclampsia/HELLP

The mainstay of therapy for hypertension in pregnancy is delivery, however, this has led to a large number of premature infants with a wide variety of poor pulmonary, cardiovascular, and neurodevelopmental outcomes. For patients who present after 34 weeks' gestation, prompt delivery is indicated. For women who develop severe preeclampsia or HELLP between 20 and 34 weeks' gestation, the management is much more difficult. Conservative management with delay of delivery may lead to worsening of disease processes and devastating outcomes. Patients are routinely given steroids to advance fetal lung development. Women with preeclampsia and HELLP may have severe hypertension and should be treated symptomatically with appropriate antihypertensives.

Steroids have also been studied extensively for patients with HELLP. A recent Cochrane review of 11 trials comparing either steroids to placebo or one steroid to another showed no significant improvements in either maternal or fetal mortality. One parameter that was affected was platelet count, which improved more quickly with steroids and dexamethasone than betamethasone.[66]

Plasma exchange has been reported for patients with persistent disease post partum; however, patients who have continued symptoms beyond delivery may be suspected to have TTP-HUS, which is effectively treated with plasma therapies. In a study of predelivery plasma exchange in an attempt to prolong gestation, there was no beneficial effect in the treatment group.[67]

The coagulopathy associated with preeclampsia and the HELLP syndrome plays an important role in patient morbidity. Studies of preeclamptic women have revealed that there is a decreased plasma level of antithrombin III (ATIII), making it a potential target for the treatment of these processes.[68] A randomized controlled trial of ATIII for use in women with severe preeclampsia before 35 weeks showed that patients who received ATIII had a significantly longer gestation and lower incidence of low-birth-weight infants.[69]

SUMMARY

The microangiopathic disorders in pregnancy are simultaneously clinically similar and pathophysiologically diverse. Prompt evaluation, diagnosis, and initiation of appropriate therapies are essential for obtaining satisfactory outcomes. Preeclampsia and HELLP often present in the latter half of pregnancy and are alleviated after delivery of the fetus and placenta. However, the conditions may persist in the immediate postpartum period. TTP and HUS are rare disorders that may occur any time during pregnancy, are not relieved by delivery, and require intense supportive and medical care, thus the recognition of these disorders as separate from preeclampsia and HELLP are critical. Although testing for specific markers (eg, ADAMTS13, factor H, soluble endoglin, and sFlt1) is intriguing, the availability of these tests and reliability of results needs to be determined and provides a major focus for future clinical and translational research.

REFERENCES

1. Baumwell S, Karumanchi SA. Pre-eclampsia: clinical manifestations and molecular mechanisms. Nephron Clin Pract 2007;106(2):c72–81.
2. Kaplan PW. The neurologic consequences of eclampsia. Neurologist 2001;7(6): 357–63.
3. Terrell DR, Williams LA, Vesely SK, et al. The incidence of thrombotic thrombocytopenic purpura-hemolytic uremic syndrome: all patients, idiopathic patients, and patients with severe ADAMTS-13 deficiency. J Thromb Haemost 2005;3:1432–6.
4. Vesely SK, George JN, Lämmle B, et al. ADAMTS13 activity in thrombotic thrombocytopenic purpura-hemolytic uremic syndrome: relation to presenting features and clinical outcomes in a prospective cohort of 142 patients. Blood 2003;102(1):60–8.
5. Elliott EJ, Robins-Browne RM, O'Loughlin EV, et al. Nationwide study of haemolytic uraemic syndrome: clinical, microbiological, and epidemiological features. Arch Dis Child 2001;85(2):125–31.
6. Dashe JS, Ramin SM, Cunningham FG. The long-term consequences of thrombotic microangiopathy (thrombotic thrombocytopenic purpura and hemolytic uremic syndrome) in pregnancy. Obstet Gynecol 1998;91(5 Pt 1):662–8.
7. George JN. The association of pregnancy with thrombotic thrombocytopenic purpura-hemolytic uremic syndrome. Curr Opin Hematol 2003;10(5):339–44.
8. Kanasaki K, Kalluri R. The biology of preeclampsia. Kidney Int 2009;76(8):831–7.
9. Haram K, Svendsen E, Abildgaard U. The HELLP syndrome: clinical issues and management. A review. BMC Pregnancy Childbirth 2009;9:8.
10. Furlan M, Robles R, Galbusera M, et al. von Willebrand factor-cleaving protease in thrombotic thrombocytopenic purpura and the hemolytic-uremic syndrome. N Engl J Med 1998;339(22):1578–84.
11. Tsai HM, Lian EC. Antibodies to von Willebrand factor-cleaving protease in acute thrombotic thrombocytopenic purpura. N Engl J Med 1998;339(22):1585–94.
12. Levy GG, Nichols WC, Lian EC, et al. Mutations in a member of the ADAMTS gene family cause thrombotic thrombocytopenic purpura. Nature 2001; 413(6855):488–94.
13. Tsai HM. Pathophysiology of thrombotic thrombocytopenic purpura. Int J Hematol 2010;91(1):1–19.
14. Tsai HM, Sussman II, Nagel RL. Shear stress enhances the proteolysis of von Willebrand factor in normal plasma. Blood 1994;83:2171–9.
15. Schneider SW, Nuschele S, Wixforth A, et al. Shear-induced unfolding triggers adhesion of von Willebrand factor fibers. Proc Natl Acad Sci U S A 2007; 104(19):7899–903.
16. Veyradier A, Obert B, Houllier A, et al. Specific von Willebrand factor-cleaving protease in thrombotic microangiopathies: a study of 111 cases. Blood 2001; 98(6):1765–72.
17. Sánchez-Luceros A, Farías CE, Amaral MM, et al. von Willebrand factor-cleaving protease (ADAMTS13) activity in normal non-pregnant women, pregnant and post-delivery women. Thromb Haemost 2004;92(6):1320–6.
18. Mannucci PM, Canciani MT, Forza I, et al. Changes in health and disease of the metalloprotease that cleaves von Willebrand factor. Blood 2001;98(9):2730–5.
19. Zipfel PF, Heinen S, Skerka C. Thrombotic microangiopathies: new insights and new challenges. Curr Opin Nephrol Hypertens 2010;19(4):372–8.
20. Józsi M, Heinen S, Hartmann A, et al. Factor H and atypical hemolytic uremic syndrome: mutations in the C-terminus cause structural changes and defective recognition functions. J Am Soc Nephrol 2006;17(1):170–7.

21. Fremeaux-Bacchi V, Dragon-Durey MA, Blouin J, et al. Complement factor I: a susceptibility gene for atypical haemolytic uraemic syndrome. J Med Genet 2004;41(6):e84.
22. Noris M, Remuzzi G. Atypical hemolytic-uremic syndrome. N Engl J Med 2009; 361(17):1676–87.
23. Psotka MA, Obata F, Kolling GL, et al. Shiga toxin 2 targets the murine renal collecting duct epithelium. Infect Immun 2009;77(3):959–69.
24. Nolasco LH, Turner NA, Bernardo A, et al. Hemolytic uremic syndrome-associated Shiga toxins promote endothelial-cell secretion and impair ADAMTS13 cleavage of unusually large von Willebrand factor multimers. Blood 2005;106(13):4199–209.
25. Keir L, Coward RJ. Advances in our understanding of the pathogenesis of glomerular thrombotic microangiopathy. Pediatr Nephrol 2010. [Epub ahead of print].
26. Thrombotic thrombocytopenic purpura and hemolytic uremic syndrome are distinct pathologic entities. A review of 56 autopsy cases. Arch Pathol Lab Med 2003;127(7):834–9.
27. Smulian J, Shen-Schwarz S, Scorza W, et al. A clinicohistopathologic comparison between HELLP syndrome and severe preeclampsia. J Matern Fetal Neonatal Med 2004;16(5):287–93.
28. Vinnars MT, Wijnaendts LC, Westgren M, et al. Severe preeclampsia with and without HELLP differ with regard to placental pathology. Hypertension 2008; 51(5):1295–9.
29. Banks RE, Forbes MA, Searles J, et al. Evidence for the existence of a novel pregnancy-associated soluble variant of the vascular endothelial growth factor receptor, Flt-1. Mol Hum Reprod 1998;4(4):377–86.
30. Kappers MH, van Esch JH, Sleijfer S, et al. Cardiovascular and renal toxicity during angiogenesis inhibition: clinical and mechanistic aspects. J Hypertens 2009;27(12):2297–309.
31. Venkatesha S, Toporsian M, Lam C, et al. Soluble endoglin contributes to the pathogenesis of preeclampsia. Nat Med 2006;12(6):642–9.
32. Levine RJ, Maynard SE, Qian C, et al. Circulating angiogenic factors and the risk of preeclampsia. N Engl J Med 2004;350(7):672–83.
33. Hertig A, Berkane N, Lefevre G, et al. Maternal serum sFlt1 concentration is an early and reliable predictive marker of preeclampsia. Clin Chem 2004;50(9):1702–3.
34. Moore Simas TA, Crawford SL, Solitro MJ, et al. Angiogenic factors for the prediction of preeclampsia in high-risk women. Am J Obstet Gynecol 2007;197(3):244. e1–8.
35. Maynard SE, Moore Simas TA, Bur L, et al. Soluble endoglin for the prediction of preeclampsia in a high risk cohort. Hypertens Pregnancy 2010;29(3):330–41.
36. Borzychowski AM, Sargent IL, Redman CW. Inflammation and pre-eclampsia. Semin Fetal Neonatal Med 2006;11(5):309–16.
37. Grandone E, Tomaiuolo M, Colaizzo D, et al. Role of thrombophilia in adverse obstetric outcomes and their prevention using antithrombotic therapy. Semin Thromb Hemost 2009;35(7):630–43.
38. Thorp JM Jr, White GC, Moake JL, et al. von Willebrand factor multimeric levels and patterns in patients with severe preeclampsia. Obstet Gynecol 1990;75(2): 163–7.
39. Hulstein JJ, van Runnard Heimel PJ, Franx A, et al. Acute activation of the endothelium results in increased levels of active von Willebrand factor in hemolysis, elevated liver enzymes and low platelets (HELLP) syndrome. J Thromb Haemost 2006;4(12):2569–75.

40. Lattuada A, Rossi E, Calzarossa C, et al. Mild to moderate reduction of a von Willebrand factor cleaving protease (ADAMTS-13) in pregnant women with HELLP microangiopathic syndrome. Haematologica 2003;88(9):1029–34.
41. Martin JN Jr, Bailey AP, Rehberg JF, et al. Thrombotic thrombocytopenic purpura in 166 pregnancies: 1955–2006. Am J Obstet Gynecol 2008;199(2):98–104.
42. Tsai HM. Thrombotic thrombocytopenic purpura: a thrombotic disorder caused by ADAMTS13 deficiency. Hematol Oncol Clin North Am 2007;21(4):609–32.
43. Michael M, Elliott EJ, Ridley GF, et al. Interventions for haemolytic uraemic syndrome and thrombotic thrombocytopenic purpura. Cochrane Database Syst Rev 2009;1:CD003595.
44. Rock GA, Shumak KH, Buskard NA, et al. Comparison of plasma exchange with plasma infusion in the treatment of thrombotic thrombocytopenic purpura. Canadian Apheresis Study Group. N Engl J Med 1991;325(6):393–7.
45. Henon P. Treatment of thrombotic thrombopenic purpura. Results of a multicenter randomized clinical study. Presse Med 1991;20(36):1761–7.
46. Rock G, Anderson D, Clark W, et al. Does cryosupernatant plasma improve outcome in thrombotic thrombocytopenic purpura? No answer yet. Br J Haematol 2005;129(1):79–86.
47. Zeigler ZR, Shadduck RK, Gryn JF, et al. Cryoprecipitate poor plasma does not improve early response in primary adult thrombotic thrombocytopenic purpura (TTP). J Clin Apher 2001;16(1):19–22.
48. Gunther K. Successful pregnancy despite thrombotic thrombocytopenic purpura in the first trimester. Transfusion 2006;46(8):1456–7.
49. Ilter E, Haliloglu B, Temelli F, et al. Thrombotic thrombocytopenic purpura and pregnancy treated with fresh-frozen plasma infusions after plasmapheresis: a case report. Blood Coagul Fibrinolysis 2007;18(7):689–90.
50. Scully M, Starke R, Lee R, et al. Successful management of pregnancy in women with a history of thrombotic thrombocytopaenic purpura. Blood Coagul Fibrinolysis 2006;17(6):459–63.
51. Bell WR, Braine HG, Ness PM, et al. Improved survival in thrombotic thrombocytopenic purpura-hemolytic uremic syndrome. Clinical experience in 108 patients. N Engl J Med 1991;325(6):398–403.
52. Espinoza F, Leal JL, Arenas G. Successful treatment of thrombotic thrombocytopenic purpura with vincristine report of one case. Rev Med Chil 2007;135(12):1572–6.
53. Bobbio-Pallavicini E, Gugliotta L, Centurioni R, et al. Antiplatelet agents in thrombotic thrombocytopenic purpura (TTP). Results of a randomized multicenter trial by the Italian Cooperative Group for TTP. Haematologica 1997;82(4):429–35.
54. Cataland SR, Jin M, Lin S, et al. Cyclosporin and plasma exchange in thrombotic thrombocytopenic purpura: long-term follow-up with serial analysis of ADAMTS13 activity. Br J Haematol 2007;139(3):486–93.
55. Cataland SR, Jin M, Lin S, et al. Effect of prophylactic cyclosporine therapy on ADAMTS13 biomarkers in patients with idiopathic thrombotic thrombocytopenic purpura. Am J Hematol 2008;83(12):911–5.
56. Gutterman LA, Kloster B, Tsai HM. Rituximab therapy for refractory thrombotic thrombocytopenic purpura. Blood Cells Mol Dis 2002;28(3):385–91.
57. Elliott MA, Heit JA, Pruthi RK, et al. Rituximab for refractory and or relapsing thrombotic thrombocytopenic purpura related to immune-mediated severe ADAMTS13-deficiency: a report of four cases and a systematic review of the literature. Eur J Haematol 2009;83(4):365–72.

58. Moore JC, Arnold DM, Leber BF, et al. Intravenous immunoglobulin as an adjunct to plasma exchange for the treatment of chronic thrombotic thrombocytopenic purpura. Vox Sang 2007;93(2):173–5.
59. Rizzoni G, Claris-Appiani A, Edefonti A, et al. Plasma infusion for hemolytic-uremic syndrome in children: results of a multicenter controlled trial. J Pediatr 1988;112(2):284–90.
60. Loirat C, Sonsino E, Hinglais N, et al. Treatment of the childhood haemolytic uraemic syndrome with plasma. A multicentre randomized controlled trial. The French Society of Paediatric Nephrology. Pediatr Nephrol 1988;2(3):279–85.
61. Sánchez-Corral P, Melgosa M. Advances in understanding the aetiology of atypical Haemolytic Uraemic Syndrome. Br J Haematol 2010;150(5):529–42.
62. Ariceta G, Besbas N, Johnson S, et al. Guideline for the investigation and initial therapy of diarrhea-negative hemolytic uremic syndrome. Pediatr Nephrol 2009;24(4):687–96.
63. Köse O, Zimmerhackl LB, Jungraithmayr T, et al. New treatment options for atypical hemolytic uremic syndrome with the complement inhibitor eculizumab. Semin Thromb Hemost 2010;36(6):669–72.
64. Marasca R, Coluccio V, Santachiara R, et al. Pregnancy in PNH: another eculizumab baby. Br J Haematol 2010;150(6):707–8.
65. Perez N, Spizzirri F, Rahman R, et al. Steroids in the hemolytic uremic syndrome. Pediatr Nephrol 1998;12(2):101–4.
66. Woudstra DM, Chandra S, Hofmeyr GJ, et al. Corticosteroids for HELLP (hemolysis, elevated liver enzymes, low platelets) syndrome in pregnancy. Cochrane Database Syst Rev 2010;9:CD008148.
67. Martin JN Jr, Perry KG Jr, Roberts WE, et al. Plasma exchange for preeclampsia: II. Unsuccessful antepartum utilization for severe preeclampsia with or without HELLP syndrome. J Clin Apher 1994;9(3):155–61.
68. Mangione S, Giarratano A. The role of antithrombin III in critical patients in obstetrics. Minerva Anestesiol 2002;68(5):449–53.
69. Maki M, Kobayashi T, Terao T, et al. Antithrombin therapy for severe preeclampsia: result of a double-blind, randomized, placebo-controlled trial. Thromb Haemost 2000;84:583–90.

Thrombophilias in Pregnancy

E.M. Battinelli, MD, PhD[a],*, K.A. Bauer, MD[b,c]

KEYWORDS

- Thrombophilias • Venous thromboembolic events • Pregnancy
- Hypercoagulable • Anticoagulation

Thrombophilic conditions are associated with an increased risk of venous thromboembolic events (VTE) during pregnancy. Thrombophilic disorders are either acquired, as in antiphospholipid syndrome, or inherited, as in factor V Leiden. Both are associated with VTE but acquired disorders can also increase the risk of arterial events. However, there is controversy as to whether they may adversely affect other pregnancy outcomes including pregnancy loss, placental abruption, severe preeclampsia, and stillbirth. This article discusses the effect of thrombophilias on pregnancy.

EPIDEMIOLOGY AND RISKS FOR VTE

The risk of having a thromboembolic event during pregnancy in the general population is approximately 200 per 100,0000 deliveries.[1] The risk is higher during the postpartum period, with an incidence of approximately 500 per 100,000, with a clinical presentation of deep vein thrombosis (DVT) occurring more frequently than pulmonary embolism (PE). The risk seems to increase with age; it is 1.38-fold higher for women who are older than 35 years during their pregnancy.[2] Many factors increase the risk of having a thromboembolic event, including having concomitant diseases such as systemic lupus erythematosus or sickle cell disease, obesity, postpartum complications, or the presence of an underlying thrombophilic disorder. Most thrombotic events are venous, with arterial clots accounting for 20%, which includes stroke and myocardial infarction.[3,4] Most thrombotic events occur at the time of delivery, with one-third of DVTs and 50% of PEs occurring during the postpartum period. PE remains the leading cause of maternal death in developed countries and accounts for 20% of pregnancy-related deaths.[5]

Financial disclosures and/or conflicts: E.M. Battinelli has nothing to disclose.
[a] Division of Hematology, Brigham and Women's Hospital, Harvard Medical School, 1 Blackfan Circle, Karp 5, Boston, MA 02115, USA
[b] Division of Hematology/Oncology, Beth Israel Deaconess Medical Center, Harvard Medical School, Boston, MA, USA
[c] Department of Hematology/Oncology, VA Boston Healthcare System, Harvard Medical School, Boston, MA, USA
* Corresponding author.
E-mail address: ebattinelli@partners.org

Hematol Oncol Clin N Am 25 (2011) 323–333
doi:10.1016/j.hoc.2011.02.003
0889-8588/11/$ – see front matter

The reasons for the increased risk for VTE during pregnancy are multifactorial. The increases in hormone levels can decrease venous outflow from the lower extremities, and more venous thrombotic events occur in the left leg than the right because of mechanical issues; this is related to the course of the right iliac artery, which courses over, and can compress, the left iliac vein.[6–8] There is also increased pressure over the pelvic veins from the gravid uterus. As with patients who are not pregnant, decreased mobility can also put a patient at increased risk of having a clotting event, as can a history of a prior thrombotic event or a history of smoking.[9,10]

Pregnancy itself can also lead to hypercoagulability. Many hemostatic changes occur during pregnancy that can affect the normal clotting mechanisms. The levels of many coagulation factors, including factor VII, factor VIII, factor X, von Willebrand factor, and fibrinogen, are increased, whereas free protein S is decreased.[11] Other alterations include increased resistance to activated protein C in the second and third trimesters, and increased levels of fibrinolytic inhibitors including thrombin activatable fibrinolytic inhibitor (TAFI) and plasminogen activator inhibitor-1 and inhibitor-2 (PAI-1 and PAI-2).[11–13] Although these changes may be essential for maintaining adequate hemostasis and preventing blood loss during delivery, they all potentially contribute to a hypercoagulable state, thereby increasing the risk of having a thromboembolic event during pregnancy that persists into the postpartum period.

There have been many studies of the factors that increase a patient's risk of having a VTE during pregnancy. Patients who have had a previous VTE have a higher incidence of developing a second event compared with those without a past history of a clotting event. The highest risk during pregnancy occurs in women who have had a spontaneous clotting event in the past, with a recurrence rate of 10.9% during pregnancy.[14] Although constant throughout pregnancy, the risk seems to be highest during the postpartum period.[15] Apart from having a history of thrombosis, thrombophilia is the most important risk factor for developing thrombotic complications during pregnancy. Both acquired and inherited thrombophilias seem to increase the risk of having an event during pregnancy.[2]

INHERITED AND ACQUIRED THROMBOPHILIAS
Inherited Disorders

The inherited thrombophilias include deficiencies of the natural anticoagulant proteins, protein C, protein S, and antithrombin. Two gain-of-function mutations occur in genes encoding the procoagulant proteins, factor V and prothrombin. Factor V Leiden results from the replacement of arginine (Arg) by glutamine (Gln) at position 506 in the protein, leading to impaired inactivation of factor Va by activated protein C (ie, the phenomenon of activated protein C resistance). Prothrombin G20210A is a mutation in the 3′-nontranslated region of the prothrombin gene, and heterozygotes have approximately 30% higher plasma levels of prothrombin than noncarriers. Factor V Leiden is the most common genetic risk factor in pregnant women, occurring in up to 44% of those with a history of VTE.[16] The prothrombin G20210A mutation is found in 17% of women with venous thrombosis during pregnancy.[17] Heterozygosity for the factor V Leiden or prothrombin G20210A mutations are common in healthy white populations, with prevalence of about 5% and 2%, respectively.[18–20] Because, in normal pregnancy, there is increased activated protein C resistance, the presence of the factor V Leiden abnormality worsens this phenomenon and likely accounts for the increased thrombotic diathesis.

More controversial than the inherited thrombotic disorders is homozygosity for the thermolabile variant (C677T) of 5,10-methylene tetrahydrofolate reductase (MTHFR). It is associated with higher levels of homocysteine in the general population and often occurs in individuals who have low folate levels. Homocysteine plays an essential role in the metabolism of vitamin B12 and folate. During pregnancy, it has been shown that homocysteine decreases with time.[21] Recent data from many studies have suggested that there is no significant increase in VTE risk in individuals who harbor homozygous mutations in the MTHFR gene.[22,23] For this reason, it is not usually considered when assessing a patient's thrombotic risk, especially in light of the folate supplementation that is routine in pregnancy and offers a means of reducing homocysteine levels.

Acquired Disorders

An acquired disorder in pregnant women leading to thrombosis or pregnancy loss is antiphospholipid antibody. For a patient to be diagnosed with antiphospholipid syndrome, several criteria must be met. The clinical criteria include having had at least 1 arterial or venous thrombotic episode or pregnancy-associated morbidity. The latter include unexplained fetal loss after 10 weeks' gestation; 1 or more premature births of a morphologically normal neonate before gestational age 34 weeks that results from eclampsia, preeclampsia, or placental insufficiency; or having had 3 or more unexplained miscarriages before the tenth week of gestation. There are also laboratory criteria that must be present to assign a diagnosis of antiphospholipid syndrome. These criteria include the presence of a lupus anticoagulant, increased levels of cardiolipin (immunoglobulin G or immunoglobulin M), or β 2 glycoprotein 1 antibodies. In order for the criteria to be met, lupus anticoagulant must be positive, or cardiolipin or β 2 glycoprotein 1 must be of medium or high titer on 2 or more laboratory blood draws at least 12 weeks apart.

THROMBOPHILIA AND THE RISK OF VTE DURING PREGNANCY

Either an acquired or inherited thrombophilia can be identified in 20% to 50% of white women who have a venous thromboembolic event during pregnancy or the postpartum period.[16,24] To better understand the importance of thrombophilia in pregnancy, Robertson and colleagues[25] conducted a systemic review of previously published studies evaluating the importance of thrombophilia in pregnancy-associated VTE. The risk seems to be greatest for those with homozygosity for the factor V Leiden mutation, with an odds ratio (OR) of 34.4. Heterozygosity for factor V Leiden confers an OR of 8.32. Mutations in the prothrombin gene are also highly associated with increased risk with homozygosity and heterozygosity being associated, with ORs of 26.3 and 6.8, respectively. The risk of having a venous thromboembolic event has been estimated to be 1:500 for those who are heterozygous for factor V Leiden, 1:200 for those who are heterozygous for prothrombin G20210A, and 4.6:100 for compound heterozygotes who carry the factor V Leiden and prothrombin gene mutations. The risk with protein C deficiency is 1:113 and 1:42 for antithrombin deficiency type 2 and 1:2.8 for antithrombin deficiency type I.[26] Therefore, the women with the greatest risk are those who are homozygous for factor V Leiden, prothrombin, double heterozygous individuals, and those with antithrombin deficiency.

The acquired disorder of antiphospholipid antibody syndrome also has been associated with increased risk of VTE. Although there is still much controversy, it has been estimated that the OR is 15.8.[2] Antiphospholipid antibodies are present in approximately 5% of pregnant women and in 37% of women who are pregnant and have systemic lupus erythematosus.[27] One study found that the persistence of the increased cardiolipin antibodies was associated with the strongest association for an increased risk of pregnancy-related thrombotic events, although it is generally believed that the presence of a persistent lupus anticoagulant is a stronger risk factor.[28]

Because the risk of having a thromboembolic event during pregnancy is still low in women with the most commonly encountered thrombophilic disorders, most women who harbor thrombophilias in the absence of a history of venous thromboembolism or fetal loss do not generally receive anticoagulation as a preventative measure. The women who gain the most benefit from antithrombotic prophylaxis before and after giving birth are those with a history of a prior thrombotic event.

THROMBOPHILIAS AND PREGNANCY

There is concern that the thrombophilias can lead to adverse outcomes in pregnancy other than venous thromboembolism or fetal loss. Studies that have evaluated the risk of thrombophilias in adverse pregnancy outcome are difficult to interpret because of heterogeneity in study design, including issues with inclusion criteria, sample size, population selection, and diagnostic criteria. The disorders have been linked to poor obstetric outcomes in association with thrombophilia, including preeclampsia, placental abruption, intrauterine growth delay, and fetal loss.

Preeclampsia

In the general population, the incidence of preeclampsia has been estimated at 26 per 1000 births.[29] There seems to be an even higher risk of preeclampsia and the associated conditions of severe preeclampsia and hypertension, increased liver function tests, low platelets (HELLP) syndrome in those with thrombophilia. One study found that 40% of women who develop preeclampsia harbor a thrombophilic defect.[30,31] Meta-analyses have been performed to establish whether there is an association between thrombophilia and preeclampsia. However, it is difficult to interpret these results because there was significant statistical heterogeneity in the results of the different studies. Some studies did suggest an association. One large meta-analysis of the role of factor V Leiden in preeclampsia found that it was associated with an OR of 2.5 for severe hypertension during pregnancy.[32] However, other studies were not able to confirm this observation. Studies of a link between the presence of the factor V Leiden mutation and preeclampsia have only found small differences in risk.[33–35] Other studies have not consistently shown an association between preeclampsia and presence of mutations in prothrombin gene.[36–38] However, there may be a role for hyperhomocysteinemia as an adverse risk factor for preeclampsia.[39] Meta-analyses have also shown a link between preeclampsia and having either protein S or protein C deficiency, with ORs of 12.7 and 21.5, respectively.[40] In general, it is unclear how to interpret these studies because many small studies were included in these analyses, which weakens the statistical significance of the analysis. In conclusion, it is believed that there is not a strong link between preeclampsia and thrombophilia.

Thrombophilia and Placental Abruption

There may be a link between the presence of thrombophilia and the occurrence of placental abruption. A study by Roque and colleagues[41] established that there was a significant dose-dependent increased risk of abruption in those who carry thrombophilic conditions, with the highest risk established for those who carry a deficiency in antithrombin. The association between the prothrombin gene mutation and placental abruption is controversial, with one study suggesting an association based on meta-analyses but no clear-cut association by prospective cohort study.[38]

Hyperhomocysteinemia is believed to be associated with placental abruption based on a large cohort study and support from a meta-analysis study.[39,40] These findings suggest an association between antithrombin deficiency and hyperhomocysteinemia as risk factors for placental abruption.

Pregnancy Outcome in Women with Thrombophilia

There is controversy as to whether there is an association between recurrent pregnancy loss in early as well as late pregnancy and the inherited thrombophilias. Two major studies provide an overview of the evidence linking pregnancy outcome and hypercoagulability. A meta-analysis by Rey and colleagues[42] of 31 case-control, cohort, and cross-sectional studies found that there were some associations. Protein C and antithrombin deficiencies were not associated with fetal loss, whereas protein S was associated with late fetal loss that was not recurrent. Prothrombin gene mutation was linked to both early recurrent and late nonrecurrent loss. Factor V Leiden was also associated with loss throughout pregnancy in women with recurrent and nonrecurrent fetal loss. Meinardi and colleagues[43] confirmed that women with factor V Leiden mutations have an increased incidence of fetal loss, whereas Tormene and colleagues[44] did not find this. Other prospective studies have evaluated the association of the factor V Leiden and prothrombin gene mutations and with pregnancy. In one study that evaluated more than 5000 women, presence of factor V Leiden significantly increased the risk of stillbirth, with an ORs of 10.9.[45] The same association was not found for early fetal loss and no clear role of the prothrombin gene mutation was identified in early or late fetal loss. Another study of more than 100 patients with pregnancy loss found that, of those who had had stillbirth, there was a significant association with either the factor V Leiden or prothrombin gene mutations. However, this result was not found for recurrent early pregnancy loss.[46]

The only prospective and controlled study of thrombophilia and fetal loss was performed by the European Prospective Cohort on Thrombophilia (EPCOT) study, which showed no significant risk of fetal loss in women with thrombophilia in comparison with the general population.[47] This study evaluated 843 women with thrombophilia , 571 of whom had 1524 pregnancies compared with 541 control women, 395 of whom had 1019 pregnancies. The rate of fetal loss was increased in women with thrombophilia (29 vs 23); however the OR was statistically significant only for stillbirth. Having multiple thrombophilic disorders was associated with a higher risk of stillbirths, with an OR of 14.3. There was a trend toward an increased risk of stillbirth or late fetal loss for all of the thrombophilias. However, for miscarriage, the only clear-cut association that emerged was for antithrombin deficiency.

Overall, carrying a thrombophilic condition increases the risk of having a late fetal loss or a stillbirth, but does not increase the risk of early pregnancy loss. These results were recently confirmed by a cohort study of more than 490 patients with thrombophilia who had suffered late pregnancy loss.[41] In this study, the presence of 1 or more thrombophilic conditions was associated with an increased risk of pregnancy loss in the second and third trimester. This study also revealed that having a thrombophilic tendency protected patients from experiencing losses in the early stages of pregnancy.

There is also controversy as to whether the thrombophilias can lead to intrauterine growth delay and low birth weight infants, which is believed to be caused by altered oxygen distribution with low blood flow through the placental circulation. However, there does not seem to be a strong association between the presence of a thrombophilic disorder and fetal growth restriction. One meta-analysis specifically of the role of the factor V Leiden and prothrombin gene mutations and MTHFR homozygosity in intrauterine growth restriction, which included analyses of both case-control and cohort studies, found no evidence of any association between these disorders and growth restriction.[46] Another study with a small sample size suggested that there may be an association between protein S deficiency and fetal growth delay, with an OR of 10.2, but wide confidence intervals reduced the study's validity.[40]

INDICATIONS FOR TREATMENT WITH ANTICOAGULATION
Prevention of Venous Thromboembolism

The studies discussed earlier can be used to influence current thinking about anticoagulation to prevent venous thromboembolism in pregnancy. As anticoagulation itself carries a risk of increased bleeding, its use should be limited to those who would clearly benefit. The most consistent benefit of anticoagulation is in those who have previously had a thrombotic event. Patients with a history of thrombophilia may also benefit depending on the type of disorder. It is clear from studies regarding VTE that patients who are at highest risk for clotting issues during pregnancy include those with antithrombin deficiency, those who are homozygous for factor V Leiden or prothrombin, and those who carry compound heterozygous mutations for factor V Leiden and prothrombin gene mutations.[25] Women with heterozygous factor V Leiden or prothrombin gene mutations or protein C or S deficiency are considered to be at lower risk. However, when considering anticoagulation, the personal clotting history of the patient must also become part of the discussion. Women who have had personal or strong family histories of thrombotic events or who carry other thrombotic risk factors, such as obesity or periods of immobilization, must also be assessed. Asymptomatic women who harbor thrombophilic conditions, but have never manifested clinical manifestations, do not require anticoagulation during the pregnancy unless they are at increased risk for clotting such as after delivery by cesarean section. If the patient does have a prior history of clotting and carries a thrombophilic condition, anticoagulation is warranted. This opinion is supported by 2 studies that showed that the incidence of thrombosis during pregnancy in women who have a hypercoagulable state and a previous history of VTE is higher than in the general population.[48,49]

The most conclusive recommendations regarding who would benefit from anticoagulation to prevent VTE in pregnancy and how it should be administered is provided by the American College of Chest Physicians.[50] In summary, pregnant women with thrombophilia with no prior history of VTE do not require anticoagulation; those with thrombophilia and prior history of VTE should be anticoagulated.

Prevention of Poor Pregnancy Outcome

Management of patients with a history of prior adverse pregnancy outcomes is still controversial. It is not clear that harboring a hereditary thrombophilic defect leads to increased risk of recurrent pregnancy loss in the early first trimester, and therefore the use of anticoagulation is not recommended.[41,51]

However, those who do have a prior history of adverse pregnancy outcomes, especially those with late second and third trimester fetal loss, may warrant the use of anticoagulation. This view is supported by several studies that have evaluated the use of anticoagulation in pregnancy in patients with thrombophilia. Gris and colleagues[52] conducted a randomized trial involving 160 women who carried a hypercoagulable disorder, including heterozygosity for factor V Leiden or prothrombin gene mutation or protein S deficiency, and who had had 1 unexplained pregnancy loss that occurred after the tenth week of pregnancy. In this study, half of the patients were given low-dose aspirin and the other half were given prophylactic doses of enoxaparin for the duration of the pregnancy until the 37th week of gestation. Women who were in the enoxaparin group had a higher rate of live births, at 86%, in comparison with those treated with aspirin, who had a rate of 28%. The use of enoxaparin in this study was associated with other improvements for pregnancy outcome, including less intra-uterine growth delay and higher birth weight babies. However, there were some concerns in this study that make it difficult to base treatment decisions on its data. First, it was not a blinded trial and, second, the low birth rate in the aspirin-only group was lower than expected.

Another study also suggested a benefit, especially in selected disorders including antithrombin, protein C, and protein S deficiency.[53] Heparin was given to both groups starting soon after pregnancy was confirmed. Women who received anticoagulation overall had a significantly lower rate of fetal loss than women who did not receive anti-coagulation, with fetal loss rates of 0% in deficient women who had received throm-bophylaxis compared with 45% in those who were not anticoagulated. Again, this study is difficult to interpret because it was small, not blinded, and was not a random-ized study. Adding more controversy to the data, 1 study even found that women with either factor V Leiden or the prothrombin gene mutation who had suffered a first preg-nancy loss were able to have good outcomes in subsequent pregnancies, with live birth rates in the 70% range, without receiving any anticoagulation.[54]

The most striking association between pregnancy loss and thrombophilia is for women with antiphospholipid antibody syndrome; it is in this population that the use of anticoagulation can greatly affect outcome. A randomized control trial, including women with increased levels of antiphospholipid antibodies and previous recurrent fetal loss, showed that the outcomes were greatly improved by combining 75 mg of aspirin and unfractionated heparin. The rate of live births was 71% compared with 42% in the women who just took aspirin.[55] Similar findings were shown in other studies that showed that women who received both aspirin and heparin had an almost 50% increased rate of delivering a live birth in the presence of antiphospholipid syndrome.[56] However, more recent studies have suggested that the benefit is not clear-cut. Another trial by Farquharson and colleagues[57] did not show an additional benefit to treating women with antiphospholipid syndrome with heparin in addition to aspirin; similar rates of live births were seen in those who received aspirin alone, with no additional benefit from the use of heparin. It therefore remains unclear whether it is useful to add low-molecular-weight heparin (LMWH) to improve pregnancy outcomes in women with antiphospholipid syndrome.

Based on these studies of pregnant women with thrombophilia, the American College of Chest Physicians has established guidelines that can be summarized based on the type of thrombophilia present.[50] For women who have antiphospholipid syndrome and recurrent pregnancy loss, prophylactic dose of anticoagulation combined with low-dose aspirin is recommended. The use of anticoagulation prophy-laxis in women with inherited thrombophilias and previous pregnancy loss is less convincing and further studies are needed before recommendations can be made. For women with thrombophilia and previous late fetal loss, placental abruption, or fetal growth delay, it is controversial whether antithrombotic therapy should be adminis-tered, and decisions need to be made on a case-by-case basis.

Because studies suggest that anticoagulation can be useful to achieve live births, others have tried to extend its use to women without thrombophilias who experience recurrent pregnancy loss. The benefit does not seem to apply to these cases.[58–61] Recently, a study by Mantha and colleagues[62] tried to address this further. In this study, a systematic review of randomized controlled trials was performed to determine whether there was a benefit to LMWH in achieving live births for women with recurrent or late nonrecurrent pregnancy loss in the absence of antiphospholipid syndrome. This study concluded that there is insufficient evidence to support the routine use of LMWH in this group to improve outcomes from women with a history of pregnancy loss and recommended that additional studies be performed.

Based on all the controversies and lack of statistical robustness, it is difficult to make definitive clinical recommendations at this time. More studies are needed to address the role of anticoagulation in patients with thrombophilia. Until that time, decisions must be made based on the individual circumstances of the patient.

SUMMARY

This article addresses the risk of thromboembolism during pregnancy in women with thrombophilia. Women are especially at risk for VTE in the postpartum period. The importance of thrombophilia in adverse pregnancy outcomes and its complications is controversial, and more studies are needed before definitive recommendations can be made. Until more information is available, anticoagulation should be reserved for those who have a history of venous thromboembolism, a recent clot, or thrombophilia and a history of a previous poor pregnancy outcome.

REFERENCES

1. Heit JA, Kobbervig CE, James AH, et al. Trends in the incidence of venous thromboembolism during pregnancy or postpartum: a 30-year population-based study. Ann Intern Med 2005;143(10):697–706.
2. James AH, Jamison MG, Brancazio LR, et al. Venous thromboembolism during pregnancy and the postpartum period: incidence, risk factors, and mortality. Am J Obstet Gynecol 2006;194(5):1311–5.
3. James AH, Bushnell CD, Jamison MG, et al. Incidence and risk factors for stroke in pregnancy and the puerperium. Obstet Gynecol 2005;106(3):509–16.
4. James AH, Jamison MG, Biswas MS, et al. Acute myocardial infarction in pregnancy: a United States population-based study. Circulation 2006;113(12): 1564–71.
5. Ronsmans C, Graham WJ. Maternal mortality: who, when, where, and why. Lancet 2006;368(9542):1189–200.
6. Macklon NS, Greer IA, Bowman AW. An ultrasound study of gestational and postural changes in the deep venous system of the leg in pregnancy. Br J Obstet Gynaecol 1997;104(2):191–7.
7. Goldhaber SZ, Tapson VF. A prospective registry of 5,451 patients with ultrasound-confirmed deep vein thrombosis. Am J Cardiol 2004;93(2):259–62.
8. Ginsberg JS, Brill-Edwards P, Burrows RF, et al. Venous thrombosis during pregnancy: leg and trimester of presentation. Thromb Haemost 1992;67(5):519–20.
9. Kovacevich GJ, Gaich SA, Lavin JP, et al. The prevalence of thromboembolic events among women with extended bed rest prescribed as part of the treatment for premature labor or preterm premature rupture of membranes. Am J Obstet Gynecol 2000;182(5):1089–92.
10. Danilenko-Dixon DR, Heit JA, Silverstein MD, et al. Risk factors for deep vein thrombosis and pulmonary embolism during pregnancy or post partum: a population-based, case-control study. Am J Obstet Gynecol 2001;184(2):104–10.
11. Bremme KA. Haemostatic changes in pregnancy. Best Pract Res Clin Haematol 2003;16(2):153–68.
12. Antovic JP, Rafik Hamad R, Antovic A, et al. Does thrombin activatable fibrinolysis inhibitor (TAFI) contribute to impairment of fibrinolysis in patients with

preeclampsia and/or intrauterine fetal growth retardation? Thromb Haemost 2002;88(4):644–7.

13. Cerneca F, Ricci G, Simeone R, et al. Coagulation and fibrinolysis changes in normal pregnancy. Increased levels of procoagulants and reduced levels of inhibitors during pregnancy induce a hypercoagulable state, combined with a reactive fibrinolysis. Eur J Obstet Gynecol Reprod Biol 1997;73(1):31–6.

14. Pabinger I, Grafenhofer H, Kyrle PA, et al. Temporary increase in the risk for recurrence during pregnancy in women with a history of venous thromboembolism. Blood 2002;100(3):1060–2.

15. Pabinger I, Grafenhofer H, Kaider A, et al. Risk of pregnancy-associated recurrent venous thromboembolism in women with a history of venous thrombosis. J Thromb Haemost 2005;3(5):949–54.

16. Gerhardt A, Scharf RE, Beckmann MW, et al. Prothrombin and factor V mutations in women with a history of thrombosis during pregnancy and the puerperium. N Engl J Med 2000;342(6):374–80.

17. Middeldorp S, Libourel EJ, Hamulyak K, et al. The risk of pregnancy-related venous thromboembolism in women who are homozygous for factor V Leiden. Br J Haematol 2001;113(2):553–5.

18. Bertina RM, Koeleman BP, Koster T, et al. Mutation in blood coagulation factor V associated with resistance to activated protein C. Nature 1994;369(6475):64–7.

19. Ridker PM, Miletich JP, Stampfer MJ, et al. Leiden and risks of recurrent idiopathic venous thromboembolism. Circulation 1995;92(10):2800–2.

20. Poort SR, Rosendaal FR, Reitsma PH, et al. A common genetic variation in the 3'-untranslated region of the prothrombin gene is associated with elevated plasma prothrombin levels and an increase in venous thrombosis. Blood 1996;88(10):3698–703.

21. Cotter AM, Molloy AM, Scott JM, et al. Elevated plasma homocysteine in early pregnancy: a risk factor for the development of severe preeclampsia. Am J Obstet Gynecol 2001;185(4):781–5.

22. van der Meer FJ, Koster T, Vandenbroucke JP, et al. The Leiden Thrombophilia Study (LETS). Thromb Haemost 1997;78(1):631–5.

23. Ray JG, Shmorgun D, Chan WS. Common C677T polymorphism of the methylenetetrahydrofolate reductase gene and the risk of venous thromboembolism: meta-analysis of 31 studies. Pathophysiol Haemost Thromb 2002;32(2):51–8.

24. Dilley A, Austin H, El-Jamil M, et al. Genetic factors associated with thrombosis in pregnancy in a United States population. Am J Obstet Gynecol 2000;183(5):1271–7.

25. Robertson L, Wu O, Langhorne P, et al. Thrombophilia in pregnancy: a systematic review. Br J Haematol 2006;132(2):171–96.

26. Benedetto C, Marozio L, Tavella AM, et al. Coagulation disorders in pregnancy: acquired and inherited thrombophilias. Ann N Y Acad Sci 2010;1205:106–17.

27. Kutteh WH. Antiphospholipid antibodies and reproduction. J Reprod Immunol 1997;35(2):151–71.

28. Long AA, Ginsberg JS, Brill-Edwards P, et al. The relationship of antiphospholipid antibodies to thromboembolic disease in systemic lupus erythematosus: a cross-sectional study. Thromb Haemost 1991;66(5):520–4.

29. Saftlas AF, Olson DR, Franks AL, et al. Epidemiology of preeclampsia and eclampsia in the United States, 1979–1986. Am J Obstet Gynecol 1990;163(2):460–5.

30. Brenner B, Lanir N, Thaler I. HELLP syndrome associated with factor V R506Q mutation. Br J Haematol 1996;92(4):999–1001.

31. van Pampus MG, Dekker GA, Wolf H, et al. High prevalence of hemostatic abnormalities in women with a history of severe preeclampsia. Am J Obstet Gynecol 1999;180(5):1146–50.

32. Kosmas IP, Tatsioni A, Ioannidis JP. Association of Leiden mutation in factor V gene with hypertension in pregnancy and pre-eclampsia: a meta-analysis. J Hypertens 2003;21(7):1221–8.

33. Dudding TE, Attia J. The association between adverse pregnancy outcomes and maternal factor V Leiden genotype: a meta-analysis. Thromb Haemost 2004; 91(4):700–11.

34. Lin J, August P. Genetic thrombophilias and preeclampsia: a meta-analysis. Obstet Gynecol 2005;105(1):182–92.

35. Dudding T, Heron J, Thakkinstian A, et al. Factor V Leiden is associated with pre-eclampsia but not with fetal growth restriction: a genetic association study and meta-analysis. J Thromb Haemost 2008;6(11):1869–75.

36. D'Elia AV, Driul L, Giacomello R, et al. Frequency of factor V, prothrombin and methylenetetrahydrofolate reductase gene variants in preeclampsia. Gynecol Obstet Invest 2002;53(2):84–7.

37. Morrison ER, Miedzybrodzka ZH, Campbell DM, et al. Prothrombotic genotypes are not associated with pre-eclampsia and gestational hypertension: results from a large population-based study and systematic review. Thromb Haemost 2002; 87(5):779–85.

38. Silver RM, Zhao Y, Spong CY, et al. Prothrombin gene G20210A mutation and obstetric complications. Obstet Gynecol 2010;115(1):14–20.

39. Ray JG, Laskin CA. Folic acid and homocyst(e)ine metabolic defects and the risk of placental abruption, pre-eclampsia and spontaneous pregnancy loss: a systematic review. Placenta 1999;20(7):519–29.

40. Alfirevic Z, Roberts D, Martlew V. How strong is the association between maternal thrombophilia and adverse pregnancy outcome? A systematic review. Eur J Obstet Gynecol Reprod Biol 2002;101(1):6–14.

41. Roque H, Paidas MJ, Funai EF, et al. Maternal thrombophilias are not associated with early pregnancy loss. Thromb Haemost 2004;91(2):290–5.

42. Rey E, Kahn SR, David M, et al. Thrombophilic disorders and fetal loss: a meta-analysis. Lancet 2003;361(9361):901–8.

43. Meinardi JR, Middeldorp S, de Kam PJ, et al. Increased risk for fetal loss in carriers of the factor V Leiden mutation. Ann Intern Med 1999;130(9):736–9.

44. Tormene D, Simioni P, Prandoni P, et al. The risk of fetal loss in family members of probands with factor V Leiden mutation. Thromb Haemost 1999;82(4):1237–9.

45. Kocher O, Cirovic C, Malynn E, et al. Obstetric complications in patients with hereditary thrombophilia identified using the LCx microparticle enzyme immunoassay: a controlled study of 5,000 patients. Am J Clin Pathol 2007;127(1):68–75.

46. Sottilotta G, Oriana V, Latella C, et al. Genetic prothrombotic risk factors in women with unexplained pregnancy loss. Thromb Res 2006;117(6):681–4.

47. Preston FE, Rosendaal FR, Walker ID, et al. Increased fetal loss in women with heritable thrombophilia. Lancet 1996;348(9032):913–6.

48. Simioni P, Tormene D, Prandoni P, et al. Pregnancy-related recurrent events in thrombophilic women with previous venous thromboembolism. Thromb Haemost 2001;86(3):929.

49. Brill-Edwards P, Ginsberg JS, Gent M, et al. Safety of withholding heparin in pregnant women with a history of venous thromboembolism. Recurrence of Clot in This Pregnancy Study Group. N Engl J Med 2000;343(20):1439–44.

50. Bates SM, Greer IA, Pabinger I, et al. Venous thromboembolism, thrombophilia, antithrombotic therapy, and pregnancy: American College of Chest Physicians Evidence-Based Clinical Practice Guidelines (8th Edition). Chest 2008;133(Suppl 6):844S–86S.

51. Hohlagschwandtner M, Unfried G, Heinze G, et al. Combined thrombophilic polymorphisms in women with idiopathic recurrent miscarriage. Fertil Steril 2003; 79(5):1141–8.

52. Gris JC, Mercier E, Quere I, et al. Low-molecular-weight heparin versus low-dose aspirin in women with one fetal loss and a constitutional thrombophilic disorder. Blood 2004;103(10):3695–9.

53. Folkeringa N, Brouwer JL, Korteweg FJ, et al. Reduction of high fetal loss rate by anticoagulant treatment during pregnancy in antithrombin, protein C or protein S deficient women. Br J Haematol 2007;136(4):656–61.

54. Coppens M, Folkeringa N, Teune MJ, et al. Outcome of the subsequent pregnancy after a first loss in women with the factor V Leiden or prothrombin 20210A mutations. J Thromb Haemost 2007;5(7):1444–8.

55. Rai R, Cohen H, Dave M, et al. Randomised controlled trial of aspirin and aspirin plus heparin in pregnant women with recurrent miscarriage associated with phospholipid antibodies (or antiphospholipid antibodies). BMJ 1997;314(7076):253–7.

56. Kutteh WH. Antiphospholipid antibody-associated recurrent pregnancy loss: treatment with heparin and low-dose aspirin is superior to low-dose aspirin alone. Am J Obstet Gynecol 1996;174(5):1584–9.

57. Farquharson RG, Quenby S, Greaves M. Antiphospholipid syndrome in pregnancy: a randomized, controlled trial of treatment. Obstet Gynecol 2002;100(3): 408–13.

58. Badawy AM, Khiary M, Sherif LS, et al. Low-molecular weight heparin in patients with recurrent early miscarriages of unknown aetiology. J Obstet Gynaecol 2008; 28(3):280–4.

59. Warren JE, Simonsen SE, Branch DW, et al. Thromboprophylaxis and pregnancy outcomes in asymptomatic women with inherited thrombophilias. Am J Obstet Gynecol 2009;200(3):281.e1–5.

60. Dolitzky M, Inbal A, Segal Y, et al. A randomized study of thromboprophylaxis in women with unexplained consecutive recurrent miscarriages. Fertil Steril 2006; 86(2):362–6.

61. Laskin CA, Spitzer KA, Clark CA, et al. Low molecular weight heparin and aspirin for recurrent pregnancy loss: results from the randomized, controlled HepASA Trial. J Rheumatol 2009;36(2):279–87.

62. Mantha S, Bauer KA, Zwicker JI. Low molecular weight heparin to achieve live birth following unexplained pregnancy loss: a systematic review. J Thromb Haemost 2010;8(2):263–8.

Von Willebrand Disease in Pregnancy

Brea C. Lipe, MD[a], Maura A. Dumas, RN, MSN[b],
Deborah L. Ornstein, MD[b,c],*

KEYWORDS

- von Willebrand disease • Bleeding disorder • Women
- Pregnancy • Delivery

CASE PRESENTATION

A 24-year-old woman pregnant with her first child presents for her first prenatal obstetric visit at 16 weeks' gestation. She reports a history of von Willebrand disease (VWD) that she believes was diagnosed after she experienced excessive bleeding after a tonsillectomy as a child, but is unable to provide further details. She is otherwise healthy and has had no other significant hemostatic challenges in life. Her pregnancy has been unremarkable thus far, and she has a normal obstetric examination. She is subsequently referred to a hematologist for clarification of the nature of her bleeding disorder and for recommendations for hemostasis support during labor and delivery. Laboratory testing for VWD, however, identifies no abnormalities. Cases like these, commonly seen in hematology practice, pose several challenges for the hematologist, including ruling in or ruling out a diagnosis of VWD during pregnancy, management of the labor and delivery, and extending optimum postpartum care when uncertainty about what, if any, bleeding disorder exists. In this article the authors review VWD in pregnancy with special attention to current evidence-based guidelines as they pertain to the pregnant patient with suspected or confirmed VWD, as well as areas of uncertainty and controversy in the diagnosis and management in this frequently encountered condition are highlighted.

VWD results from a deficiency of or qualitative abnormality in the large plasma glycoprotein, von Willebrand factor (VWF). VWF serves two critical functions in hemostasis: (1) it mediates initial adhesion of platelets to sites of vascular endothelial

The authors have no relevant disclosures.
[a] Section of Hematology/Oncology, Dartmouth-Hitchcock Medical Center, One Medical Center Drive, Lebanon, NH 03756, USA
[b] Section of Hematology/Oncology, Hemophilia and Thrombosis Center, Dartmouth-Hitchcock Medical Center, One Medical Center Drive, Lebanon, NH 03756, USA
[c] Department of Medicine, Dartmouth Medical School, Hanover, Rope Ferry Road, NH 03755, USA
* Corresponding author. Hemophilia and Thrombosis Center, Dartmouth-Hitchcock Medical Center, One Medical Center Drive, Lebanon, NH 03756.
E-mail address: dlornstein@dartmouth.edu

Hematol Oncol Clin N Am 25 (2011) 335–358
doi:10.1016/j.hoc.2011.01.006
0889-8588/11/$ – see front matter © 2011 Published by Elsevier Inc.

hemonc.theclinics.com

damage, and (2) it binds and chaperones coagulation factor VIII, thus stabilizing and prolonging its circulating half-life as well as localizing factor VIII activity to the site of vascular injury.[1] Estimates of the prevalence of VWD vary widely and depend on case definitions used in the various studies that have investigated this subject. Surveys of symptomatic patients followed at hemostasis centers arrive at a prevalence of symptomatic VWD of around 0.01%, while a recent study of the pediatric primary care population estimated a 10-fold higher prevalence of 0.1%.[2] Older population-based studies, on the other hand, have yielded even higher prevalence estimates of up to 1.3%.[3] While prevalence estimates differ, there is general agreement that VWD is likely the most common hereditary bleeding disorder, affecting both sexes and all ethnic groups. Women are at increased risk for bleeding complications with the hemostatic challenges of menstruation and childbirth, thus VWD can be expected to affect women disproportionately.[4] Over 4 million births were recorded in the United States in 2009,[5] of which as many as 50,000 may be expected to have occurred in women with VWD according to disease prevalence estimates. Given the scope of the disease, therefore, the public health implications are obvious, and the consequences of missing or ignoring the diagnosis may be catastrophic.

DIAGNOSIS AND CLASSIFICATION OF VON WILLEBRAND DISEASE

VWD is a hereditary disorder, and the spectrum of VWF gene mutations leading to the condition is broad. Genetic testing is costly, not widely available, and impractical for the initial diagnosis of VWD. Routine screening coagulation laboratory tests such as the prothrombin time, activated partial thromboplastin time, bleeding time, and PFA-100 lack sensitivity for VWD. The diagnostic evaluation for VWD in a person with a personal and/or a family history of abnormal bleeding, therefore, is best accomplished with laboratory testing aimed at measuring the quantity and functionality of the VWF protein.[6,7] Moreover, such testing characterizes the nature of the defect in VWF and allows rational classification of VWD. A typical initial VWD screening test panel includes assays for VWF antigen (VWF:Ag), VWF activity (ristocetin cofactor activity; VWF:RCo), and factor VIII coagulant activity (FVIII:C). The VWF:Ag test is a quantitative immunoassay that measures the concentration of VWF protein in plasma, whereas the VWF:RCo is a functional test that assays the ability of VWF to interact with platelets and mediate platelet agglutination via the antibiotic, ristocetin. Abnormalities in these tests should prompt a multimer analysis, a gel electrophoresis study that assesses the quantity and composition of the various VWF multimers. The ristocetin-induced platelet aggregation (RIPA) test provides additional diagnostic information, as the ability of ristocetin to mediate platelet aggregation in vitro is proportional to the level of VWF in plasma. At a high dose of ristocetin, platelet aggregation will be decreased in types 1 and 3 VWD and in most type 2 variants (see later discussion). Low-dose ristocetin is ineffective at causing platelet aggregation in vitro in normal subjects and in most VWD variants, but will mediate platelet aggregation in type 2B VWD. The VWF collagen-binding (VWF:CB) measures the ability of VWF to bind to collagen, and is abnormal in individuals with defects in the VWF collagen binding sites. This test is not routinely performed for the evaluation of VWD but may identify the occasional patient with VWD when the other tests are normal. In-depth discussion of diagnostic testing is beyond the scope of this article, but a summary of useful initial diagnostic tests for evaluating patients with suspected VWD is provided in **Box 1**, and readers are directed to excellent reviews on the topic for more information.[6,7]

At present, 3 major categories of VWD are recognized and are summarized in **Table 1**.[6,7] Each type of VWD exhibits autosomal inheritance, thus affecting both

---

Box 1
Initial diagnostic evaluation of patients with suspected VWD

Initial Tests

    General hemostasis screening

        Complete blood count with platelet count

        Prothrombin time

        Partial thromboplastin time

        Thrombin time or fibrinogen

    VWD screening

        von Willebrand factor antigen (VWF:Ag)

        von Willebrand factor activity (VWF:RCo)

        Factor VIII coagulant activity (FVIIIC)

Second-Tier Tests if Abnormalities are Found in Initial Tests

    Abnormal prothrombin time and/or isolated abnormal activated partial thromboplastin

        Mixing study and evaluation for coagulation factor deficiency(ies) as appropriate

    Low platelet count

        Evaluation for causes of thrombocytopenia (including VWD, type 2B)

    Abnormal VWD screening tests

        Repeat VWD screening tests to confirm

        VWF multimer analysis

        Ristocetin-induced platelet aggregation (RIPA)

Third-Tier Tests

    If VWD suspected based on initial testing, but subtype in question

        VWF:collagen-binding (VWF:CB)

        Factor VIII binding (VWF:FVIIIB; if type 2N suspected)

    If history suggests a defect in primary hemostasis but testing does not suggest VWD

        Platelet function testing (aggregation, secretion assays)

Adapted from Nichols WL, Hultin MB, James AH, et al. von Willebrand disease (VWD): evidence-based diagnosis and management guidelines, the National Heart, Lung, and Blood Institute (NHLBI) Expert Panel report (USA). Haemophilia 2008;14(2):171–232; and Pruthi RK. A practical approach to genetic testing for von Willebrand disease. Mayo Clin Proc 2006;81(5):679–91.

---

men and women. Types 1 and 3 result from quantitative deficiencies in the VWF protein, whereas type 2 VWD results from qualitative and functional abnormalities in VWF protein. Type 1 VWD accounts for 70% to 80% of symptomatic cases, and is a consequence of a partial deficiency of structurally and functionally normal VWF. The abnormality in type 1 VWD confers a generally mild to moderate bleeding risk. Type 2 VWD accounts for the majority of the remainder of symptomatic cases and imparts a moderate to moderately severe bleeding phenotype. Type 2 VWD is further divided into 4 subtypes depending on the nature of the qualitative defect in VWF. Type 2A is the most common of the qualitative VWF disorders and arises as a result of a reduction in the larger, more active VWF multimers. Types 2B and 2M are due to

Table 1
Summary of laboratory test results in von Willebrand disease subtypes

VWD Subtype	VWF:Ag (IU/dL)	VWF:RCo (IU/dL)	FVIIIC	RIPA	LD-RIPA	Platelet Count	VWF Multimer Pattern	VWF:FVIIIB
Type 1	<30	<30	D or N	N or slightly D	A	N	N	N
Type 2A	<30–200	<30	D or N	D	A	N	HMW forms D	N
Type 2B	<30–200	<30	D or N	Usually N	Markedly I	N or D	HMW forms D	N
Type 2M	<30–200	<30	D or N	D	A	N	N	N
Type 2N	<30–200	30–200	D	N	A	N	N	D
Type 3	A	A	Markedly D	A	A	N	A	A
"Low VWF"	30–50	30–50	N or Slightly D	Usually N	A	N	N	N
Normal	50–200	50–200	N	N	N	N	N	N

Abbreviations: A, absent; D, decreased; FVIIIC, factor VIII coagulant activity; HMW, high molecular weight; I, increased; LD, low dose; N, normal; RIPA, ristocetin-induced platelet aggregation; VWD, von Willebrand disease; VWF:Ag, von Willebrand factor antigen; VWF:FVIIIB, von Willebrand factor:factor VIII binding activity; VWF:RCo, von Willebrand factor ristocetin cofactor activity.

Data from Nichols WL, Hultin MB, James AH, et al. von Willebrand disease (VWD): evidence-based diagnosis and management guidelines, the National Heart, Lung, and Blood Institute (NHLBI) Expert Panel report (USA). Haemophilia 2008;14(2):171–232.

missense mutations in VWF that lead either to increased (2B) or decreased (2M) platelet binding via the GPIb binding site. Type 2B VWD is caused by a gain-of-function mutation in VWF such that there is enhanced binding between VWF and platelet receptor GPIb, leading to thrombocytopenia as platelet-VWF aggregates are sequestered by the microcirculation. Type 2N is caused by a mutation that leads to impaired binding of factor VIII to VWF, resulting in increased proteolysis of factor VIII and decreased circulating factor VIII levels on the order of those seen with mild hemophilia A. Type 2N VWD should be suspected in a woman presenting with a low factor VIII level with normal levels of VWF, and can be distinguished from hemophilia A carriership by the VWF-factor VIII binding assay. Type 3 disease is rare, is caused by a complete absence of VWF, and results in a severe bleeding disorder.

Genetic transmission of VWD types 1 and 2A, 2B, and 2M is characterized by an autosomal dominant inheritance pattern with variable penetration. VWD type 2N has an autosomal recessive inheritance pattern, as do rare cases of types 2A and 2M. VWD type 3 is also an autosomal recessive disease, resulting from either compound heterozygosity of 2 VWF gene mutations or homozygosity for a single gene defect.[8]

In the recently updated VWD classification scheme, a distinction is made between genetic type 1 VWD and low levels of VWF that may occur as a result of population variation.[6] For example, ABO blood group influences VWF levels, with type O individuals having mean levels that are roughly 25% lower than individuals with other ABO types.[9,10] Racial differences have also been reported, with African Americans having higher levels than other groups.[11,12] The accepted normal range for VWF:Ag is 50 to 200 IU/dL. In general, very low levels of VWF (ie, <20–30 IU/dL) correlate well with VWF gene mutations, bleeding symptoms, and a family history of bleeding (reviewed in Ref.[6]); however, levels of 30 to 50 IU/dL, while below the "normal range," do not reliably correlate with genetic VWD and often occur in healthy individuals with type O blood. Levels of VWF between 30 and 50 IU/dL, while not diagnostic of the disease per se, nevertheless constitute a mild risk factor for bleeding. Many clinicians, therefore, elect to refer to these otherwise healthy patients as having "low VWF" rather than labeling them with a disease, which potentially carries adverse psychological, social, and insurance ramifications.[6,13] The laboratory characteristics of the subtypes of VWD are summarized in **Table 1**.

CLINICAL MANIFESTATIONS

VWD is suspected in individuals with a personal history of unexplained spontaneous bleeding or with excessive bleeding after seemingly minor insults. Of note, although VWD is a hereditary disorder, often there may be no relevant family history of bleeding, due to variability in expression of symptoms, especially in milder forms of the disorder. Many patients with types 1 and 2 VWD are asymptomatic in everyday life but may experience mild to moderate bleeding after hemostatic challenges such as trauma or surgery. The character of bleeding in patients with VWD is generally mucocutaneous, with epistaxis and easy bruisability as frequent manifestations. Affected individuals will describe bleeding that persists after injury or surgery, thus indicating a defect in primary hemostasis rather than that which stops initially and starts up again later as is typical with defects in secondary hemostasis or the fibrinolytic pathway. In women, menstruation is a monthly hemostatic challenge, and menorrhagia is common in those with VWD. Patients with type 2N or type 3 VWD experience more severe bleeding that can resemble that of patients with factor VIII deficiency. These patients are more often at risk for deep tissue and joint bleeds, intracranial hemorrhage, or gastrointestinal bleeding.[6,14]

VON WILLEBRAND FACTOR LEVELS DURING PREGNANCY

Complex physiologic adaptations occur in the maternal hemostatic system during pregnancy (reviewed in Ref.[15]). Establishment of the uteroplacental circulation occurs early, and its maintenance is critical to fetal survival. The integrity of the uteroplacental circulation is dependent on local conditions, and mandates that the maternal hemostatic system be readily responsive to bleeding or thrombotic events that pose a threat to normal blood flow. By the third trimester the hemostatic adaptations result in a net prothrombotic state that is designed to mitigate life-threatening bleeding at parturition. At the time of delivery uterine myometrial contractions initially limit bleeding associated with parturition, while at the cessation of contractions a hypertophied hemostatic system takes over to form clots in injured blood vessels. As a consequence of the physiologic changes in the coagulation system in response to the hemostatic demands of pregnancy and parturition, normal pregnancy and the puerperium are associated with an increased risk for both bleeding and thrombosis.

Levels of many of the coagulation factors increase during a normal pregnancy under the influence of an increasing level of estradiol. Both VWF and factor VIII levels start to increase during the second trimester (and possibly as early as 6 weeks' gestation for VWF:Ag), peak at term, and return to baseline levels shortly after delivery in normal women as well in the majority of those with VWD.[16–20] Although the magnitude of the increase in coagulation factors is variable, some investigators have documented an average twofold increase for factor VIII and a threefold increase for VWF,[21,22] while others have noted lesser increases throughout the pregnancy.[19] Most women with type 1 VWD will experience a progressive climb in VWF:Ag, VWF:RCo, and factor VIII levels throughout pregnancy, such that they notice an improvement in their baseline bleeding symptoms as the pregnancy progresses. This phenomenon is responsible for the difficulty in making a diagnosis of type 1 VWD in pregnancy, as VWF levels increase into the normal range in all but the most severe cases. Although women with type 2 VWD may show increased levels of VWF:Ag and factor VIII, this reflects an increase in the level of abnormal VWF protein and does not necessarily produce a concurrent increase in VWF:RCo activity. In fact, type 2B VWD is reported to worsen during pregnancy as increased levels of abnormal VWF result in progressive thrombocytopenia. Accordingly, type 2B VWD should be ruled out in any pregnant woman presenting with thrombocytopenia, especially if there is a family history of abnormal bleeding.[16,23,24] Although factor VIII levels have been reported to increase and normalize in pregnant women with type 2N disease,[25] often they do not despite increased levels of both VWF:Ag and VWF:RCo (reviewed in Ref.[16]). Most women with type 3 VWD will have no improvement in VWF or factor VIII levels in pregnancy.[16]

VWF and factor VIII levels decline after delivery and there is substantial interindividual variability in the rate at which the factors return to their baseline levels.[16] Although levels of VWF and factor VIII generally begin to decline 1 week postpartum and return to baseline by 4 to 6 weeks,[15,19,21] the decrease can be precipitous and has been reported as early as 24 hours after delivery.[16]

PRECONCEPTION CONSIDERATIONS

To prevent pregnancy complications in patients with VWD, correct identification of individuals at risk is crucial. Practicing gynecologists surveyed in Georgia in one study reported that 8% of their patients complain of menorrhagia.[26] Although VWD is estimated to be present in 5% to 20% of women with menorrhagia,[27] almost half of the respondents to the Georgia survey reported never having seen a patient with a bleeding disorder, and only 3% had ever referred patients with menorrhagia for specialty evaluation. A recent survey of British gynecologists reported increased familiarity with bleeding disorders, with 91% of practitioners reporting having managed patients with bleeding disorders. Nevertheless, survey respondents underestimated prevalence of VWD at less than 1% among women with menorrhagia.[28] To help identify women at risk, an international expert panel convened to formulate recommendations for diagnosis and management.[29] The panel recommended that assessment for a bleeding disorder be performed by a hematologist in patients with a history of menorrhagia since menarche, a family history of a bleeding disorder, or personal history of one or more of the following: prolonged epistaxis (usually bilateral), bruising without injury, unexpected bleeding after surgery or dental extractions, unexplained bleeding from the gastrointestinal tract, bleeding from a minor wound lasting more than 5 minutes, postpartum hemorrhage, hemorrhage that requires transfusions, or hemorrhage from corpus luteum cysts. The recommended initial evaluation of patients with a suspected bleeding disorder includes a complete blood count, prothrombin time, activated partial thromboplastin time, fibrinogen level, VWF:Ag, VWF:RCo, and FVIII:C, with further testing performed as indicated and outlined in **Box 1**.[29]

It is preferable that women with documented VWD who wish to have children begin to plan for a pregnancy prior to conception.[30,31] Such planning should include discussions with an obstetrician and a hematologist to review the bleeding risks associated with pregnancy, labor, and delivery, and the various management options. Women with bleeding disorders are also advised to receive vaccinations against both hepatitis A and B viruses because of the increased risk of exposure to blood products. Because these vaccinations are considered category C medications (ie, animal reproduction studies have not been conducted and it is not known whether the product is harmful to an unborn fetus), it is recommended that they be administered prior to pregnancy if possible. Meeting with a pediatric hematologist may be helpful to review the evaluation and care of an infant at risk for VWD in the perinatal period. In addition, prenatal genetic counseling should be offered to discuss the inheritance pattern of VWD. As most patients have only mild to moderate disease, prenatal diagnosis is generally best reserved only for pregnancies at risk for the type 3 variant. Moreover, there are many molecular defects responsible for type 1 disease and determination of the exact genetic defect within a family may be difficult, whereas gene defects associated with type 3 disease generally consist of large deletions that are not subtle.[32] Genetic diagnosis is generally accomplished via tandem repeat or restriction fragment length polymorphism analysis of the fetal VWF gene, provided there is an informative gene mutation documented within the family. Several methods for obtaining fetal DNA are currently available. Preimplantation analysis is possible with in vitro fertilization procedures, while chorionic villous sampling can be performed at 10 to 12 weeks' gestation and amniocentesis at 16 to 18 weeks. Percutaneous umbilical cord vein sampling (cordocentesis) may be performed at 17 to 20 weeks, and provides a direct measurement of VWF antigen levels.[33]

Fertility issues are important to patients with VWD wishing to conceive. Women with VWD have an increased incidence of endometriosis, endometrial hyperplasia and polyps, uterine fibroids, and ovarian cysts as compared with healthy female counterparts.[34] In addition, hemorrhagic ovarian cysts are more frequently encountered in women with VWD than in the general population.[35] Both endometriosis and hemorrhage into ovarian cysts may lead to primary infertility, therefore one might speculate that women with VWD are at higher than average risk for infertility on this basis. The limited data available on this subject, however, suggest that these women do not in fact have substantially increased rates of infertility or miscarriage than women without bleeding disorders.[16,36–39]

There are few data on the implications of fertility therapy and assisted reproduction in women with VWD; however, it is reasonable to assume that the acknowledged complications associated with these technologies might be amplified in women with bleeding disorders. For example, ovarian hyperstimulation syndrome may complicate the use of medications used to induce ovulation.[40] Ovarian hyperstimulation is characterized by cystic enlargement of the ovaries and fluid shifts that result in third space fluid accumulation. Although ovarian hyperstimulation syndrome is often associated with hypercoagulability, ovarian rupture with subsequent hemorrhage is seen, and this may cause catastrophic hemorrhage in women with bleeding disorders such as VWD. Invasive fertility treatments such as oocyte retrieval similarly pose a risk to women with VWD,[41] and should be performed only with appropriate hemostatic support. Nevertheless, successful in vitro fertilization in a woman with VWD and a history of recurrent massive hemoperitoneum associated with induced ovulation has been reported.[42]

ANTEPARTUM MANAGEMENT

Management of a pregnant woman with VWD is best performed by a multidisciplinary medical team.[43] In general, the patient should be followed throughout the pregnancy by an obstetrician and a hematologist with expertise in coagulation disorders, and consultation with an anesthesiologist in the second or third trimester is helpful for planning for analgesia during labor and delivery. The role of the hematologist before delivery is to monitor VWF and factor VIII levels to assess the risk for bleeding at the time of parturition and to formulate a plan for optimizing hemostasis. There is, however, no consensus on the appropriate schedule for monitoring coagulation factor levels during pregnancy. The authors' practice is to follow VWF:RCo and FVIII:C levels routinely at least once per trimester and within 2 weeks of the expected delivery date in an uncomplicated pregnancy to ensure appropriate increases in these parameters. If complications arise or invasive procedures are required, coagulation factor levels are checked more frequently. Most women have type 1 VWD, and will experience an increase in VWF and factor VIII levels such that they frequently increase into the normal range by the time of delivery. Women with type 3 VWD will experience no increase, and women with type 2 disease will exhibit variable increases in VWF and factor VIII, as outlined previously.

Antepartum pregnancy complications apart from bleeding do not appear to be more common in women with VWD than in those without the disorder. In fact, studies of antepartum bleeding rates in women with VWD have shown conflicting results even on that point. A recent epidemiologic study evaluated pregnancy complications in 4067 women with a diagnosis of VWD among 16,824,897 deliveries between 2000 and 2003 reported in a United States database.[38] Although women with VWD were 10 times more likely to experience antepartum bleeding than women who did not carry a VWD diagnosis in this study, they were no more likely to develop preeclampsia, eclampsia, placental abruption, intrauterine growth restriction, intrauterine fetal demise, or preterm labor. In another, albeit much smaller, study women with VWD had a rate of antepartum bleeding (6%) similar to that of women without bleeding disorders.[44]

Although the incidence of spontaneous miscarriage does not appear to be increased in women with VWD, they are nevertheless at increased risk for bleeding complications should placental abruption, miscarriages, or elective terminations occur, especially early on in the pregnancy before VWF levels have begun to increase.[16] Moreover, invasive diagnostic and fetal monitoring procedures may be associated with bleeding in women with VWD. In the absence of such hemostatic challenges, however, antenatal bleeding is infrequent, and routine treatment of women with VWD with hemostatic agents is usually not required prior to labor and delivery.

LABOR AND DELIVERY

The periods of highest risk for bleeding in women with VWD are during parturition and in the postpartum period. The risk of bleeding during either surgical or vaginal delivery is small, and neuraxial anesthesia is safe when the levels of VWF:RCo and FVIII:C are 50 IU/dL or greater,[29,45] as will be the case at term without the use of hemostatic augmentation for many women with VWD, especially those with mild type 1 disease. FVIII:C is the parameter best correlated with postoperative hemostasis, and some experts advocate expectant management of women with VWD whose FVIII:C has exceeded the 50 IU/dL threshold at term even if the VWF:RCo has not, as data suggest that FVIII:C of greater than 50 IU/dL provides adequate protection from postpartum hemorrhage irrespective of the VWF:RCo (reviewed in Refs.[46,47]). Although the authors individualize the management of each woman, they often supplement those whose VWF:RCo remains below 50 IU/dL at term with an appropriate hemostatic agent at the time of delivery or shortly thereafter, notwithstanding a normalized FVIII:C, particularly if a surgical delivery is forthcoming (see the section on hemostatic agents).

Women with mild type 1 VWD who have hemostatic levels of VWF:RCo and FVIII:C at term are generally safely delivered in community hospital settings with guidance from a hematologist. For patients with severe type 1 and most women with types 2 and 3 disease, however, the authors recommend delivery at a center with a high-risk obstetric service, availability of on-site hematology consultation (both pediatric and adult), coagulation laboratory facilities with the capability to perform VWF:RCo and/or FVIII:C determinations, adequate pharmacy and transfusion support, and ready availability of appropriate hemostatic agents. Most women with type 1 VWD do not require prophylactic treatment with hemostatic agents for delivery, whereas all women with type 3 disease require prophylactic treatment.[45] Type 2 VWD is variable, and many women do not require prophylaxis unless there is a surgical delivery or perineal trauma. There are several options for augmenting VWF:RCo and FVIII:C for delivery should they fail to rise to the 50 IU/dL threshold at term. The specific agents and their use are reviewed in the section entitled "Hemostatic agents" and are summarized in **Table 2**. Examples of formal guidelines that the authors provide to the obstetric team for delivery of patients with mild and moderate to severe VWD, respectively, are shown in **Figs. 1** and **2**. These guidelines can be developed as templates and can be readily customized to the individual patient.

The mode of delivery is normally dictated by obstetric considerations, as vaginal delivery and cesarean section appear to be equally safe for mother and baby provided that maternal coagulation factors are in the hemostatic range.[45] For example, in a recently published series of 19 neonates born with either type 1 or type 2 VWD, all were born vaginally without bleeding complications.[48] Intracranial hemorrhage in neonates with VWD is rare, even in cases of type 3 disease; nevertheless, certain precautions should be undertaken.[49] Delivery should occur by the least traumatic method, with active management to avoid a prolonged second stage of labor and early progression to cesarean section if necessary.[45,50] In addition, invasive scalp monitoring and forceps and vacuum extraction should be avoided in a potentially affected fetus to minimize the risk for scalp hematoma and intracranial hemorrhage.[16,30,31,43,45]

Table 2
Hemostatic agents for treatment of von Willebrand disease in pregnancy

Drug Class	Appropriate for Use in Which VWD Subtypes	Dose Range/Schedule
Desmopressin	Type 1 Some type 2 Avoid in type 2B	IV: 0.3 µg/kg (limit: 25–30 µg) Intranasal: 300 µg (2 nasal inhalations) May administer every 24 h up to 2 to 3 doses

Fibrinolytic agents	All	Aminocaproic acid
		  IV: Loading dose, 5 g followed by
		    continuous infusion of 1 g/h
		  PO: 50 mg/kg up to every 6 h
		Tranexamic acid
		  IV: 10 mg/kg every 6–8 h
		  PO: 1300 mg every 8 h

Plasma-derived factor VIII-VWF concentrates	All	Alphanate SD/HT, Humate P, Wilate
		  IV Loading dose: 40–60 IU/kg
		  IV Maintenance dose: 20–40 IU/kg
		    every 8–24 h

Abbreviations: g, grams; IV, intravenous; PO, by mouth.

VWD need not be a contraindication to administering neuraxial/regional anesthesia for labor and delivery.[51,52] A regional block, that is, epidural or combined spinal/epidural, is more effective than systemically administered analgesics for managing the pain associated with labor (reviewed in Ref.[53]) and is the preferred method of analgesia for operative deliveries, given its association with lower maternal mortality and blood loss than general anesthesia.[54,55] The authors' anesthesiologist colleagues are occasionally reluctant to perform a regional block in patients with VWD for fear of bleeding complications, despite spontaneous normalization or augmentation of VWF levels at term. Although there are few studies on this subject, available data suggest that regional anesthesia is safe in women with VWD whose coagulation factor levels have either normalized spontaneously or have been supplemented with hemostatic agents before performing the procedure. For example, in one retrospective study of labor and delivery, a regional block was accomplished in 41 pregnancies involving 37 women with bleeding disorders (including 14 pregnancies in 13 women with VWD) without major bleeding complications.[51] All of the women with VWD had spontaneous normalization of VWF at term, and although there was one "bloody tap" among the VWD patients, no further bleeding in that patient was observed. A recent systematic review of neuraxial techniques in patients with bleeding disorders identified 74 procedures performed on 72 patients with VWD, including 71 with type 1, 2 with type 2, and 1 with type 3 disease.[52] The majority (n = 64) had normalization of VWF levels before needle insertion, and no hemostatic treatment was provided. The remaining patients received hemostatic augmentation before needle insertion, and there were no complications reported in any of the 72 patients under review.

The use of ultrasound guidance for administering regional anesthesia is becoming increasingly popular, and guidelines for its use have been published.[56,57] Ultrasound guidance for administering regional blocks has the advantage of more precise placement of the local anesthetic agent while avoiding needle contact with vital structures such as nerves and blood vessels.[58] A study in pregnancy using this technique demonstrated that the initial success rate for administering epidural analgesia was improved among anesthesiology trainees using ultrasound guidance compared with those trainees randomized to perform catheter insertion by relying only on anatomic landmarks for proper placement.[59] The use of ultrasound to guide placement of epidural catheters therefore holds promise for improving efficacy and reducing complications for women with and without bleeding disorders alike.

In the authors' view, there is no legitimate reason to deny a laboring woman with VWD access to effective regional analgesia when VWF levels have normalized spontaneously or when effective hemostatic agents are used. Whenever possible, however, the authors recommend an antenatal consultation with an obstetric anesthesiologist for analgesia planning. The authors have found that providing a detailed hemostatic plan for labor and delivery to both the anesthesiologist and obstetrician in advance goes a long way toward assuaging an exaggerated fear of bleeding complications.

POSTPARTUM MANAGEMENT

Older case-control studies have reported postpartum hemorrhage rates ranging from 23% to 59% in women with VWD compared with 10% to 26% in controls.[34,39,44,60,61] A recent report,[38] however, documented lower rates of postpartum hemorrhage (6% vs 4% in women with and without VWD, respectively), likely as a result of improved prophylactic care in women with VWD during delivery. Nevertheless, women with VWD are at a 2- to 3-fold higher risk for postpartum hemorrhage than women without bleeding disorders, and have up to a fivefold increased risk of receiving a blood transfusion.[38,62] Furthermore, women with VWD who have experienced a postpartum hemorrhage are at risk for recurrence with a subsequent delivery.[63]

The risk for postpartum hemorrhage correlates inversely with VWF levels in women with VWD, with most postpartum bleeding episodes occurring in women in whom VWF and factor VIIIC levels are less than 50 IU/dL.[64] Although most women with VWD will have coagulation factor levels in the normal range at the time of delivery that gradually decrease to prepregnancy baseline levels over the course of a week, VWF levels may decline rapidly after delivery and should be monitored for up to the first 3 to 5 days postpartum. Bleeding complications may be minimized by ensuring that levels are maintained above 50 IU/dL in the postpartum period with the use of hemostatic agents if necessary (see next section).

It is important to account for nonhematologic factors associated with postpartum hemorrhage. Although the presence of a bleeding disorder increases the risk of postpartum hemorrhage, the vast majority of severe hemorrhages associated with delivery are due to anatomic factors including uterine atony, retained placental fragments, and trauma.[62] Accordingly, obstetricians must sometimes be reminded not to overlook these causes of immediate postpartum hemorrhage in patients with VWD in whom the hematologist has ensured hemostatic levels of VWF. In fact, women with VWD are at highest risk for postpartum hemorrhage later on in the puerperium when VWF levels decline to their baseline levels. In one study the average time of presentation with postpartum hemorrhage in women with VWD was 15.7 ± 5.2 days,[65] thus mandating close postpartum follow-up.

TREATMENT WITH HEMOSTATIC AGENTS

Most women with VWD will not require hemostatic agents for labor and delivery. For those women who do require hemostatic support during delivery and the postpartum period there are several options available, which are summarized in **Table 2** and are reviewed here. Both plasma-derived and pharmaceutical agents are available. Each product has advantages and disadvantages, thus the choice of product(s) should be individualized. A combination of agents may be required in some cases, and careful

Hemostasis Treatment Protocol

Patient Name:_____ Date: _____ Date of birth:_____ Medical Record

#:_____

Ms. X is a 25-year old woman who is 38 weeks pregnant with an estimated delivery date of July 15, 2010. She

has mild type 1 von Willebrand disease, but normal von Willebrand factor (VWF) and coagulation factor VIII

(F8) levels have been documented throughout her pregnancy as follows: Her current weight is 80 kg.

Lab parameter	Test results		Normal range
	24 weeks gestation	38 weeks gestation	
VWF:RCo Activity	76	138	50 – 200 IU/dL
VWF Antigen	80	144	50 – 200 IU/dL
Factor VIII (F8)	82	176	50 – 150 IU/dL

It is common for both VWF and factor VIII levels to normalize and rise beyond the normal hemostatic range by

the third trimester and to remain elevated for several weeks following delivery. A small percentage of patients

experience a rapid decrease in VWF and F8 soon after delivery, however, and may have significant post-partum

hemorrhage. A plan to support hemostasis for labor and delivery is outlined below:

Upon Admission for Delivery:

No hemostatic treatment is required before or during labor as the VWF and F8 levels are within the range

required for normal hemostasis. Insertion of an epidural catheter for regional anesthesia is safe based on these

coagulation factor levels. Please notify hematologist on call of the admission (XXX-XXX-XXXX).

Delivery and Post-partum

For bleeding that, in the opinion of the attending obstetrician, is within the expected range after a normal

delivery, no hemostatic agents are required. We do not recommend empiric administration of hemostatic agents

in the absence of bleeding, as this may increase the risk for thrombosis.

For moderate to severe bleeding (not life threatening) that is, in the opinion of the attending obstetrician,

unexpected, not due to uterine atony and not amenable to treatment with uterotonic agents or local measures:

- Notify hematologist on call (XXX-XXX-XXXX)
- Send blood in blue top specimen tube STAT to coagulation lab for VWF antigen and F8

  determinations.

Fig. 1. Sample labor and delivery plan for a patient with mild type 1 or suspected VWD hemostasis treatment protocol.

attention must be paid to surgical and local measures to ensure hemostasis. In addition, care should be taken to avoid administering medications that may impair hemostasis. For example, the authors discourage the use of most nonsteroidal anti-inflammatory agents for postpartum analgesia, as the antiplatelet effects of these

- Options for enhancing hemostasis include:
  - Desmopressin (DDAVP) infusion, 0.3 mcg/kg in 50 mL of normal saline over 30 minutes (do not exceed 25 mcg in single dose and do not administer more often than once every 24 hours). Monitor blood pressure during infusion. Desmopressin may cause hyponatremia, thus it is recommended to restrict fluid intake to 2/3 the usual maintenance amount for 24 hours after the infusion. Due to possible effects on the neonate (e.g., hyponatremia) desmopressin should be used with caution, OR
  - Aminocaproic acid, 5 gram loading dose IV followed by continuous infusion at a rate of 1 gram/hour until bleeding is controlled, OR
  - Tranexamic acid, 10 mg/kg IV every 6 to 8 hours until bleeding controlled

For severe/life threatening bleeding:

- Notify hematologist on call (XXX-XXX-XXXX)
- Send blood in blue top specimen tube STAT to coagulation lab for VWF antigen and F8 determinations.
- Infuse F8-VWF concentrate (BRAND), 40 – 50 IU/kg IV. Aminocaproic acid or tranexamic acid may be used as above as adjunctive treatment if necessary.
- Employ standard treatments, including confirmation of surgical hemostasis & infusion of blood products as indicated and dictated by CBC and laboratory coagulation parameters.

CC: OB, Labor & Delivery, Hematology, Anesthesiology, Pharmacy, Coagulation Laboratory, Blood Bank, Patient

Fig. 1. (continued)

drugs exacerbate bleeding risk. Selective cyclooxygenase-2 inhibitors lack antiplatelet activity and, from a bleeding standpoint, are safe to use in women with VWD.

Desmopressin

For women with type 1 VWD who do not achieve the minimum level of VWF:RCo and FVIII:C of 50 IU/dL at term, desmopressin is recommended as the first-line treatment to raise coagulation factor levels before insertion of an epidural catheter or delivery. Desmopressin (1-deamino-8-D-arginine vasopressin; DDAVP) is a synthetic analogue of antidiuretic hormone that acts via type 2 vasopressin receptors to release VWF and factor VIII into the systemic circulation from storage sites within vascular endothelial cells. Desmopressin generally results in a 2- to 5-fold increase in VWF and factor VIII in the plasma, and although the effect varies among individuals, the response is generally consistent over time in a given individual.[47,66] Desmopressin is a pregnancy category B drug; that is, animal reproduction studies have failed to demonstrate a risk to the fetus, but there are no adequate and well-controlled studies in pregnant women. Small, retrospective studies suggest, however, that the drug is safe for pregnant women and fetuses.[67,68] A theoretical concern is that desmopressin may cause placental insufficiency via arterial vasoconstriction or uterine contraction via an oxytocin effect, but this is unlikely inasmuch as desmopressin lacks significant activity at type 1 vasopressin receptors through which these effects are mediated. Reassuringly, these problems have not been observed in animal or human studies.[67,68] Desmopressin, however, has potent antidiuretic effects via V2 receptors and can lead to fluid retention and hyponatremia if fluid restriction is not employed, and some controversy remains over the use of desmopressin in pregnancy because of a risk of fetal hyponatremia.[45] To avoid maternal hyponatremia, the authors limit fluid intake to two-thirds the usual maintenance volume for the 24 hours after a dose of desmopressin is administered. Other common side effects of desmopressin include tachycardia, flushing, headache, and nausea, which are generally mild.

Hemostasis Treatment Protocol

Patient Name:_____ Date: _____ Date of birth:_____ Medical Record
#:_____

Ms. X is a 25-year old woman who is 38 weeks pregnant with an estimated delivery date of July 15, 2010. She has type 2A von Willebrand disease (VWD) with coagulation factor levels documented throughout her pregnancy as follows: Her current weight is 80 kg.

Lab parameter	Test results			
	24 weeks gestation	38 weeks gestation	Onset of labor	Normal range
VWF:RCo Activity	10	10	10	50 – 200 IU/dL
VWF Antigen	38	63	92	50 – 200 IU/dL
Factor VIII (F8)	35	72	115	50 – 150 IU/dL

It is common for both VWF antigen and coagulation factor VIII (F8) levels to normalize and rise beyond the normal hemostatic range by the third trimester and to remain elevated for several weeks following delivery; whereas, the VWF:RCo activity may not increase in type 2 VWD. VWF:RCo and F8 levels >50 IU/dL are generally safe for administration of neuraxial anesthesia and for delivery. A small percentage of patients experience a rapid decrease in VWF and F8 soon after delivery, however, and may experience significant post-partum hemorrhage. A plan to support hemostasis during labor and delivery is outlined below:

Upon Admission for Delivery:

Please notify hematologist on call of the admission (XXX-XXX-XXXX). If regional anesthesia is to be used, infuse F8-VWF concentrate (BRAND) at a dose of 40 IU/kg just prior to insertion of the epidural catheter.

Delivery and Post-partum

For bleeding that, in the opinion of the attending obstetrician, is within the expected range after a normal delivery, no additional hemostatic agents are required. We do not recommend empiric administration of additional hemostatic agents in the absence of bleeding, as this may increase the risk for thrombosis. In the absence of abnormal bleeding, further hemostatic agents will be administered according to VWF:RCo and F8 levels which should be obtained immediately and 12 hours after delivery (send blood in blue top specimen tube to coagulation laboratory).

For moderate to severe bleeding (not life-threatening) that is, in the opinion of the attending obstetrician, unexpected, not due to uterine atony and not amenable to treatment with uterotonic agents or local measures:

- Notify hematologist on call immediately (XXX-XXX-XXXX)
- Send blood in blue top specimen tube STAT to coagulation lab for VWF:RCo and F8 determinations.
- Options for enhancing hemostasis include:
  - Infuse F8-VWF concentrate (BRAND), 20 – 40 IU/kg IV, OR
  - Aminocaproic acid, 5 gram loading dose IV followed by continuous infusion at a rate of 1 gram/hour until bleeding is controlled, OR
  - Tranexamic acid, 10 mg/kg IV every 6 to 8 hours until bleeding controlled

Fig. 2. Sample labor and delivery plan for a patient with severe VWD hemostasis treatment protocol.

For severe/life threatening bleeding:

- Notify hematologist on call immediately (XXX-XXX-XXXX)
- Send blood in blue top specimen tube STAT to coagulation lab for VWF:RCo and F8 determinations.
- Infuse F8-VWF concentrate (BRAND), 40 – 50 IU/kg IV. Aminocaproic acid or tranexamic acid may be used as above as adjunctive treatment if necessary.
- Employ standard treatments including confirmation of surgical hemostasis & infusion of blood products as indicated and dictated by CBC and laboratory coagulation parameters.

CC: OB, Labor & Delivery, Hematology, Anesthesiology, Pharmacy, Coagulation Laboratory, Blood Bank, Patient

Fig. 2. (*continued*)

Desmopressin may be administered intravenously at a dose of 0.3 μg per kilogram of body weight, and the authors generally cap the dose at 25 to 30 μg. Alternatively, a high-concentration nasal spray is available (Stimate); the intranasal dose for adults weighing more than 50 kg is 300 μg, consisting of 2 metered-dose inhalations of 150 μg each. It is critical that the appropriate desmopressin product be administered to patients with VWD. The various oral formulations and nasal sprays that are used to treat diabetes insipidus and nocturnal eneuresis are insufficiently potent to produce a hemostatic effect, and cannot be used for that purpose. This fact must be specified clearly in the delivery plan to avoid confusion. The peak effect on coagulation factor levels occurs 30 to 60 minutes after an intravenous dose and 90 to 120 minutes after an intranasal dose. All VWD patients should be evaluated for response to desmopressin before using the medication for hemostatic effect to ensure an appropriate increase in VWF and factor VIIIC. The authors administer a test dose of either intravenous or intranasal desmopressin in the outpatient clinic, and measure VWF:Ag, VWF:RCo and FVIII:C at baseline and 1 and/or 2 hours after a dose to evaluate the peak effect and at 4 hours to gather information about the rate of clearance. Plasma levels of VWF and factor VIIIC are sustained for 8 to 10 hours in most people, but tachyphylaxis often develops. Although desmopressin may be effective when administered every 12 hours, the authors try to limit the frequency to not more than once every 24 hours to reduce the risk for hyponatremia, and use no more than 2 or 3 doses per course. VWF-containing plasma products are recommended thereafter should prolonged hemostatic levels of VWF be required. Desmopressin does not appear to pass into breast milk and is therefore safe for nursing mothers.

Desmopressin is effective for most women with type 1 VWD. Occasional women with type 2A, 2M, or 2N disease may have a hemostatic response to desmopressin, but this should always be confirmed with a test dose prior to use. Women with type 2B VWD should not generally be treated with this drug, and it is ineffective in type 3 disease.

Plasma-Derived Products

The preferred agent for all women with type 3 VWD, most women with type 2 VWD, and occasional women with type 1 VWD who do not achieve an adequate response to desmopressin is a plasma-derived, factor VIII-VWF concentrate, also referred to as an intermediate-purity factor VIII concentrate by virtue of the presence of VWF "contaminating" the factor VIII product. Examples of plasma-derived factor VIII-VWF concentrates available in the United States include Alphanate SD/HT, Humate-P, and Wilate. These agents differ in the method used to inactivate viruses and in the ratio of VWF:RCo to FVIII:C in the preparation, but all have been shown to be safe in humans and none has been proven to be superior to the others for clinical use. All of currently available factor VIII-VWF concentrates are designated as pregnancy category C agents. Nevertheless, adverse fetal events have not been reported, and the benefit to both the mother and baby of using one of these products to prevent serious bleeding complications in women with severe VWD likely outweighs the risk to the fetus.

Humate-P and Wilate are labeled with both the VWR:RCo and FVIII:C content, whereas Alphanate is labeled with only the FVIII:C content. On average, the response to factor VIIIC-VWF concentrates is an approximately 2 IU/dL increase in factor VIII and VWF:RCo for every 1 IU per kilogram of body weight infused. Accordingly, in women with baseline FVIII:C and/or VWF:RCo of 10 IU/dL or less, a dose of 40 to 60 IU/kg administered before delivery followed by doses of 20 to 40 IU/kg every 8 to 24 hours for 3 to 5 days postpartum will be expected to maintain trough levels above 50 IU/dL and reduce the risk for postpartum hemorrhage. Proportionally lower doses can be administered to women with VWF:RCo levels higher than 10 IU/dL. Adverse reactions to the plasma-derived products are infrequent, and most commonly consist of mild allergic reactions. Severe allergic reactions and anaphylaxis, while rare, have been reported.

The ready availability of factor VIII-VWF concentrates obviates the need for the use of fresh frozen plasma or cryoprecipitate in routine situations. In emergencies in which an appropriate factor VIII-VWF product is not available, however, plasma or cryoprecipitate can be infused, with cryoprecipitate being the preferred product because of the higher concentration of both factor VIII and VWF. A reasonable dose is one bag of cryoprecipitate per 10 kg of body weight, but it should be emphasized that an intermediate-purity, plasma-derived product is the treatment of choice with a lower risk for viral transmission than either fresh frozen plasma or cryoprecipitate. Platelet concentrates may be administered if bleeding persists despite restoration of hemostatic levels of VWF and factor VIII. Platelet concentrates contain a small amount of VWF but, more importantly, appear to transport and direct VWF to the site of vascular injury.[69]

Antifibrinolytic Agents

The antifibrinolytic amino acids, aminocaproic acid and tranexamic acid, inhibit fibrinolytic enzymes, thus preventing fibrin degradation by plasmin and stabilizing formed fibrin clot. Although these drugs exert no appreciable effect on VWF and factor VIII levels, their mechanism of action makes them useful adjuncts for treating bleeding in areas of high fibrinolytic activity such as the oropharynx and uterus. These agents are both available in oral and intravenous formulations, and aminocaproic acid is a pregnancy category C drug while tranexamic acid is included in category B. Antifibrinolytic medications reduce perioperative blood loss and decrease allogeneic blood transfusion requirements in randomized surgical trials,[70] and have shown similar favorable effects on reducing postpartum blood loss.[71] Aminocaproic acid can be administered intravenously as a 5 g loading dose followed by a continuous infusion at a rate of 1 g per hour until bleeding stops. A total dose of 24 g per 24 hours should not be exceeded. Alternatively, an oral dose of 50 to 60 mg/kg every 6 hours can be given. Side effects including nausea, vomiting, abdominal pain, diarrhea, headache, dizziness, hallucinations, and tinnitus limit the oral dose of aminocaproic acid in the authors' experience. One gram of tranexamic acid administered intravenously has been used successfully in several small studies before cesarean section as well as after vaginal delivery to reduce postpartum blood loss,[71] and is currently being evaluated in a large, international, prospective randomized trial (the WOMAN trial; http//www.thewomantrial.Lshtm.ac.uk). Tranexamic acid is also available as a 650-mg oral formulation that is approved for the treatment of menorrhagia at a dose of 1300 mg every 8 hours. The use of tranexamic acid to manage antenatal bleeding has been reported, and appears to be effective without posing an increased risk for maternal thrombosis.[72,73] Antifibrinolytic medications should not be used in patients with hematuria, as clot stabilization may result in ureteral obstruction.

LABORATORY MONITORING

The frequency with which laboratory parameters should be monitored during pregnancy and after delivery will depend on each woman's individual circumstances. The authors perform laboratory monitoring at least once per trimester and close to term in uncomplicated cases. After delivery, laboratory monitoring should be performed at least once or twice daily while hemostatic agents are being administered. Laboratory monitoring may be done by measuring either VWF:RCo or FVIII:C; however, many laboratories are not equipped to measure VWF:RCo, and FVIII:C correlates well with surgical hemostasis and is thus appropriate for monitoring the hemostatic effect of therapeutic agents used to treat VWD (reviewed in Ref.[47]). Although hemostatic agents should be administered when FVIII:C is less than 50 IU/dL after delivery, laboratory monitoring should be used to avoid a supranormal FVIII:C, which increases the risk for venous thromboembolism. Treatment with hemostatic agents and laboratory monitoring may be required for up to 2 weeks or more postpartum.

THROMBOSIS

Pregnancy is associated with an increased risk of venous thromboembolism, and thrombotic pulmonary embolism remains a major cause of maternal mortality in the United States.[74] Women with VWD, especially those with mild forms of the disorder, are not exempt from this increased risk given that numerous individual factors influence thrombosis risk during pregnancy. For example, obesity, advance maternal age, smoking, surgical delivery, immobilization, and the concurrent presence of hereditary or acquired thrombophilia increase the risk for thrombotic complications during pregnancy and the puerperium.[75] The presence of these risk factors may overshadow any protection that may be afforded by low VWF levels, especially in women with mild VWD whose VWF levels normalize as the pregnancy proceeds. It is important, therefore, not to add to the problem by overreacting to a perceived bleeding risk in patients who carry a diagnosis of VWD. In the authors' experience, overzealous obstetricians or anesthesiologists occasionally insist on treating a pregnant woman with hemostatic agents empirically despite normalization of VWF levels at term. This practice is potentially dangerous, as the markedly high levels of factor VIIIC and VWF that often result after a dose of desmopressin is administered to a woman with normal coagulation factor levels may predispose to thrombotic complications.[47] This practice underscores the need for scrupulous communication between the hematologist and the other members of the medical team as well as for a clear labor and delivery plan outlined well in advance. Moreover, standard thromboprophylaxis must be provided for women with VWD who undergo operative deliveries or receive other surgical interventions.

EVALUATION OF THE BABY

The diagnosis of VWD in a newborn may not be straightforward, especially in mild cases. While severe cases are easily diagnosed by measuring VWF levels after birth from an umbilical cord blood specimen, VWF:Ag levels increase during birth, and a normal umbilical cord blood sample result does not rule out a mild case of VWD. Testing should be repeated when the child is older if normal results are obtained at birth. A pediatric hematology specialist should be available for consultation following the birth of a child with suspected VWD. Elective procedures (eg, circumcision) should be deferred until the coagulation status of the infant is confirmed and appropriate arrangements for hemostatic support are in place. An example of a formal hemostasis protocol for an infant with suspected VWD is provided in **Box 2**.

MATERNAL POSTPARTUM FOLLOW-UP

Women with VWD are at risk for delayed postpartum hemorrhage, therefore an outpatient hemostasis plan must be in place before hospital discharge and close follow-up by telephone and/or office visits for at least the first 2 weeks after delivery must be arranged. Options for prevention and treatment of delayed postpartum hemorrhage are similar to those for hemorrhage in the immediate postpartum period. Formulations of desmopressin (Stimate) and antifibrinolytic agents for outpatient use are readily available, and the authors recommend that women with mild VWD have current prescriptions for either or both at home during the postpartum period for use if needed. Women with types 2 and 3 VWD will require treatment with factor VIII-VWF concentrates for delayed postpartum hemorrhage, but will also likely benefit from treatment with an antifibrinolytic agent adjunctively. Prophylactic treatment with hemostatic agents is indicated for women whose VWF:RCo and/or FVIII:C drop below the hemostatic range. If it is not feasible to follow VWF:RCo and FVIII:C in the postpartum period after hospital discharge, then empiric use of prophylactic hemostatic agents should be considered.

Women in whom the diagnosis of VWD is in doubt during pregnancy, such as the patient in the case presentation at the beginning of this article, should be followed up postpartum for definitive testing. Levels of VWF and factor VIII generally return to prepregnancy, baseline levels by 4 to 6 weeks postpartum, and repeat testing can be performed at the 6-week postpartum visit. Occasionally, however, coagulation factor levels will remain mildly elevated at the 6-week point and if the diagnosis is in doubt, laboratory testing should be repeated several weeks or months hence. Patients who appear to have a bleeding diathesis but whose testing in the nonpregnant state fails to document VWD should undergo more comprehensive testing, which should

---

Box 2
Sample protocol for managing a newborn with suspected VWD

1. Notify the pediatric hematologist of the birth of an infant with suspected VWD.

2. At the time of delivery, draw umbilical cord blood specimen into a blue top tube for determination of VWF antigen and factor VIII levels by coagulation laboratory test.

3. Elective surgical procedures (eg, circumcision) should be deferred until VWF and factor VIII levels are obtained and are determined by the pediatric hematologist to be within the hemostatic range.

4. Intramuscular injections may be administered unless the infant's pediatrician specifically advises otherwise. Intramuscular injections carry a risk of hematoma formation for patients with bleeding disorders; therefore, as a precautionary measure, a fine-gauge needle ($\leq$23 gauge) should be used and steady pressure should be held at the site for at least 3 to 5 minutes afterward.

include an evaluation of platelet function. Mild qualitative platelet disorders are common,[76] and the authors frequently encounter patients who carry a diagnosis of VWD who, on further evaluation, have a qualitative platelet disorder in addition to or instead of VWD.

CASE REVIEW

Although, in the ideal situation, women at risk for VWD would have their bleeding disorder status determined before becoming pregnant, the authors' experience is that women present frequently much as the woman profiled in the introduction to this article. Obstetrician colleagues commonly will refer a pregnant woman when, during the first prenatal visit, she discloses a history of VWD or other bleeding disorder, or if such a disorder is suspected based on personal or family history. Because most VWD is type 1, by the time the patient is evaluated by a hematologist during the pregnancy, the VWF level has normalized and confirming the diagnosis is

---

Box 3
Key points in the management of VWD in pregnancy

Antepartum

- Follow VWF and factor VIII levels once per trimester and near term
- No routine hemostatic agents for uncomplicated antenatal course
- Consider hemostatic agents for early miscarriage, termination or bleeding
- Hematology, anesthesiology consultations
- Formulate and distribute written hemostasis plan

Labor and Delivery

- No routine hemostatic agents if VWF:RCo and FVIII:C have normalized at term
- Administer desmopressin (type 1 VWD) or factor VIII-VWF concentrates (types 2 and 3) if VWF:RCo and/or FVIII:C <50 IU/dL at term

  Institute fluid restriction if desmopressin administered

  Limit desmopressin to no more than 3 doses at intervals no closer than 24 hours
- No contraindication to regional/neuraxial anesthesia if VWF:RCo and/or FVIII:C >50 IU/dL either due to spontaneous normalization or supplementation with factor VIII-VWF concentrates
- Avoid fetal scalp monitoring, operative vaginal delivery, prolonged second stage of labor

Postpartum

- Follow VWF:RCo and/or FVIII:C through day 5 and maintain levels >50 IU/dL
- Close outpatient follow-up for up to 2 or more weeks
- Options for prevention/treatment of delayed postpartum hemorrhage:

  Intranasal desmopressin (Stimate) for type 1 VWD

  Factor VIII-VWF concentrates for types 2 and 3 VWD and type 1 VWD not responsive to desmopressin

  Antifibrinolytic agents can be used as adjunct for prevention and treatment of bleeding in all types of VWD
- Return >6 weeks postpartum for definitive VWD testing in equivocal cases

not possible. Although many patients who profess to have been diagnosed with VWD will not actually have the disorder, the authors nevertheless consider the worst-case scenario and assume they have either VWD or another bleeding disorder, and manage them accordingly. The authors follow VWF levels and FVIII:C in these women antepartum and at term to ensure appropriate augmentation, and often perform platelet function testing antepartum because qualitative platelet disorders may not normalize during pregnancy. The authors put a labor and delivery plan in place with a recommendation for the use of desmopressin or antifibrinolytic agents empirically as general hemostatic agents for excessive and unexpected bleeding not attributable to anatomic causes. Close postpartum follow-up is provided, and each patient with a suspected bleeding disorder is given a prescription for an oral fibrinolytic agent for use at home in the event of excessive postpartum bleeding. Finally, the laboratory testing is repeated at the 2- or 3-month point postpartum after coagulation factor levels have returned to baseline.

SUMMARY

Although with modern obstetric care and hematologic support most women with VWD can expect to have normal pregnancies that result in the birth of healthy babies, the potential for catastrophic bleeding complications still exists. Ensuring optimal outcomes for pregnant women with VWD, therefore, requires a multidisciplinary approach with meticulous advanced planning and effective communication among all parties who may be located in different hospitals at the time of delivery. This article outlines a general approach to managing VWD in pregnancy, which is summarized in **Box 3**. It cannot be overemphasized, however, that care must be individualized and hemostatic plans devised that have sufficient flexibility to be adapted to often rapidly changing circumstances.

REFERENCES

1. De Meyer SF, Deckmyn H, Vanhoorelbeke K. von Willebrand factor to the rescue. Blood 2009;113(21):5049–57.
2. Bowman M, Hopman WM, Rapson D, et al. A prospective evaluation of the prevalence of symptomatic von Willebrand disease (VWD) in a pediatric primary care population. Pediatr Blood Cancer 2010;55(1):171–3.
3. Werner EJ, Broxson EH, Tucker E, et al. Prevalence of von Willebrand disease in children: a multiethnic study. J Pediatr 1993;123(6):893–8.
4. James AH. Von Willebrand disease in women: awareness and diagnosis. Thromb Res 2009;124(Suppl 1):S7–10.
5. Arias E, Rostron BL, Tejada-Vera B. United States life tables, 2005. Natl Vital Stat Rep 2010;58(10):1–132.
6. Nichols WL, Hultin MB, James AH, et al. von Willebrand disease (VWD): evidence-based diagnosis and management guidelines, the National Heart, Lung, and Blood Institute (NHLBI) Expert Panel report (USA). Haemophilia 2008;14(2):171–232.
7. Pruthi RK. A practical approach to genetic testing for von Willebrand disease. Mayo Clin Proc 2006;81(5):679–91.
8. Goodeve AC. The genetic basis of von Willebrand disease. Blood Rev 2010; 24(3):123–34.
9. Favaloro EJ, Soltani S, McDonald J, et al. Reassessment of ABO blood group, sex, and age on laboratory parameters used to diagnose von Willebrand

disorder: potential influence on the diagnosis vs the potential association with risk of thrombosis. Am J Clin Pathol 2005;124(6):910–7.

10. Gill JC, Endres-Brooks J, Bauer PJ, et al. The effect of ABO blood group on the diagnosis of von Willebrand disease. Blood 1987;69(6):1691–5.

11. Lutsey PL, Cushman M, Steffen LM, et al. Plasma hemostatic factors and endothelial markers in four racial/ethnic groups: the MESA study. J Thromb Haemost 2006;4(12):2629–35.

12. Miller CH, Dilley A, Richardson L, et al. Population differences in von Willebrand factor levels affect the diagnosis of von Willebrand disease in African-American women. Am J Hematol 2001;67(2):125–9.

13. Sadler JE. Von Willebrand disease type 1: a diagnosis in search of a disease. Blood 2003;101(6):2089–93.

14. Mannucci PM, Federici AB, James AH, et al. von Willebrand disease in the 21st century: current approaches and new challenges. Haemophilia 2009;15(5): 1154–8.

15. Hellgren M. Hemostasis during normal pregnancy and puerperium. Semin Thromb Hemost 2003;29(2):125–30.

16. Kujovich JL. von Willebrand disease and pregnancy. J Thromb Haemost 2005; 3(2):246–53.

17. Sie P, Caron C, Azam J, et al. Reassessment of von Willebrand factor (VWF), VWF propeptide, factor VIII: C and plasminogen activator inhibitors 1 and 2 during normal pregnancy. Br J Haematol 2003;121(6):897–903.

18. Wickstrom K, Edelstam G, Lowbeer CH, et al. Reference intervals for plasma levels of fibronectin, von Willebrand factor, free protein S and antithrombin during third-trimester pregnancy. Scand J Clin Lab Invest 2004;64(1):31–40.

19. Sanchez-Luceros A, Meschengieser SS, Marchese C, et al. Factor VIII and von Willebrand factor changes during normal pregnancy and puerperium. Blood Coagul Fibrinolysis 2003;14(7):647–51.

20. Kadir RA, Lee CA, Sabin CA, et al. Pregnancy in women with von Willebrand's disease or factor XI deficiency. Br J Obstet Gynaecol 1998;105(3):314–21.

21. Kjellberg U, Andersson NE, Rosen S, et al. APC resistance and other haemostatic variables during pregnancy and puerperium. Thromb Haemost 1999;81(4): 527–31.

22. Ramsahoye BH, Davies SV, Dasani H, et al. Obstetric management in von Willebrand's disease: a report of 24 pregnancies and a review of the literature. Haemophilia 1995;1(2):140–4.

23. Casonato A, Sartori MT, Bertomoro A, et al. Pregnancy-induced worsening of thrombocytopenia in a patient with type IIB von Willebrand's disease. Blood Coagul Fibrinolysis 1991;2(1):33–40.

24. Rick ME, Williams SB, Sacher RA, et al. Thrombocytopenia associated with pregnancy in a patient with type IIB von Willebrand's disease. Blood 1987;69(3): 786–9.

25. Castaman G, Bertoncello K, Bernardi M, et al. Pregnancy and delivery in patients with homozygous or heterozygous R854Q type 2N von Willebrand disease. J Thromb Haemost 2005;3(2):391–2.

26. Dilley A, Drews C, Lally C, et al. A survey of gynecologists concerning menorrhagia: perceptions of bleeding disorders as a possible cause. J Womens Health Gend Based Med 2002;11(1):39–44.

27. James AH, Ragni MV, Picozzi VJ. Bleeding disorders in premenopausal women: (another) public health crisis for hematology? Hematology Am Soc Hematol Educ Program 2006;474–85.

28. Chi C, Shiltagh N, Kingman CE, et al. Identification and management of women with inherited bleeding disorders: a survey of obstetricians and gynaecologists in the United Kingdom. Haemophilia 2006;12(4):405–12.

29. James AH, Kouides PA, Abdul-Kadir R, et al. Von Willebrand disease and other bleeding disorders in women: consensus on diagnosis and management from an international expert panel. Am J Obstet Gynecol 2009;201(1):12.e1–8.

30. American College of Obstetricians and Gynecologists Committee on Adolescent Health Care, American College of Obstetricians and Gynecologists Committee Gynecologic Practice. ACOG Committee Opinion no. 451: Von Willebrand disease in women. Obstet Gynecol 2009;114(6):1439–43.

31. James AH, Manco-Johnson MJ, Yawn BP, et al. Von Willebrand disease: key points from the 2008 National Heart, Lung, and Blood Institute guidelines. Obstet Gynecol 2009;114(3):674–8.

32. Federici AB. Diagnosis of inherited von Willebrand disease: a clinical perspective. Semin Thromb Hemost 2006;32(6):555–65.

33. Shetty S, Ghosh K. Robustness of factor assays following cordocentesis in the prenatal diagnosis of haemophilia and other bleeding disorders. Haemophilia 2007;13(2):172–7.

34. Kirtava A, Drews C, Lally C, et al. Medical, reproductive and psychosocial experiences of women diagnosed with von Willebrand's disease receiving care in haemophilia treatment centres: a case-control study. Haemophilia 2003;9(3):292–7.

35. Radakovic B, Grgic O. Von Willebrand disease and recurrent hematoperitoneum due to the rupture of haemorrhagic ovarian cysts. Haemophilia 2009;15(2):607–9.

36. Smith S, Pfeifer SM, Collins JA. Diagnosis and management of female infertility. JAMA 2003;290(13):1767–70.

37. Bick RL, Hoppensteadt D. Recurrent miscarriage syndrome and infertility due to blood coagulation protein/platelet defects: a review and update. Clin Appl Thromb Hemost 2005;11(1):1–13.

38. James AH, Jamison MG. Bleeding events and other complications during pregnancy and childbirth in women with von Willebrand disease. J Thromb Haemost 2007;5(6):1165–9.

39. Lak M, Peyvandi F, Mannucci PM. Clinical manifestations and complications of childbirth and replacement therapy in 385 Iranian patients with type 3 von Willebrand disease. Br J Haematol 2000;111(4):1236–9.

40. Vloeberghs V, Peeraer K, Pexsters A, et al. Ovarian hyperstimulation syndrome and complications of ART. Best Pract Res Clin Obstet Gynaecol 2009;23(5): 691–709.

41. Moayeri SE, Coutre SE, Ramirez EJ, et al. Von Willebrand disease presenting as recurrent hemorrhage after transvaginal oocyte retrieval. Am J Obstet Gynecol 2007;196(4):e10–1.

42. Brabec C, Vogt M, Wilson JM, et al. Successful in vitro fertilization with anonymous donor oocytes in a patient with recurrent massive hemoperitoneum following spontaneous and induced ovulation. Fertil Steril 2002;77(4):836–7.

43. MASAC guidelines for perinatal management or women with bleeding disorders and carriers of hemophilia A and B. In: National Hemophilia Foundation, editors. MASAC document #192. New York; 2009. Available at: http://www.hemophilia. org/NHFWeb/MainPgs/MainNHF.aspx?menuid=57&contentid=1436. Accessed March 3, 2011.

44. Siboni SM, Spreafico M, Calo L, et al. Gynaecological and obstetrical problems in women with different bleeding disorders. Haemophilia 2009;15(6):1291–9.

45. Lee CA, Chi C, Pavord SR, et al. The obstetric and gynaecological management of women with inherited bleeding disorders–review with guidelines produced by a taskforce of UK Haemophilia Centre Doctors' Organization. Haemophilia 2006; 12(4):301–36.

46. Kouides PA. Current understanding of von Willebrand's disease in women—some answers, more questions. Haemophilia 2006;12(Suppl 3):143–51.

47. Mannucci PM. Treatment of von Willebrand's disease. N Engl J Med 2004;351(7): 683–94.

48. Castaman G, Tosetto A, Rodeghiero F. Pregnancy and delivery in women with von Willebrand's disease and different von Willebrand factor mutations. Haematologica 2010;95(6):963–9.

49. Wetzstein V, Budde U, Oyen F, et al. Intracranial hemorrhage in a term newborn with severe von Willebrand disease type 3 associated with sinus venous thrombosis. Haematologica 2006;91(Suppl 12):ECR60.

50. Pacheco LD, Costantine MM, Saade GR, et al. von Willebrand disease and pregnancy: a practical approach for the diagnosis and treatment. Am J Obstet Gynecol 2010;203(3):194–200.

51. Chi C, Lee CA, England A, et al. Obstetric analgesia and anaesthesia in women with inherited bleeding disorders. Thromb Haemost 2009;101(6):1104–11.

52. Choi S, Brull R. Neuraxial techniques in obstetric and non-obstetric patients with common bleeding diatheses. Anesth Analg 2009;109(2):648–60.

53. Hawkins JL. Epidural analgesia for labor and delivery. N Engl J Med 2010; 362(16):1503–10.

54. Guay J. The effect of neuraxial blocks on surgical blood loss and blood transfusion requirements: a meta-analysis. J Clin Anesth 2006;18(2):124–8.

55. Hawkins JL. Anesthesia-related maternal mortality. Clin Obstet Gynecol 2003; 46(3):679–87.

56. Ecimovic P, Loughrey JP. Ultrasound in obstetric anaesthesia: a review of current applications. Int J Obstet Anesth 2010;19(3):320–6.

57. Sites BD, Chan VW, Neal JM, et al. The American Society of Regional Anesthesia and Pain Medicine and the European Society of Regional Anaesthesia and Pain Therapy joint committee recommendations for education and training in ultrasound-guided regional anesthesia. Reg Anesth Pain Med 2010;35(2 Suppl): S74–80.

58. Griffin J, Nicholls B. Ultrasound in regional anaesthesia. Anaesthesia 2010; 65(Suppl 1):1–12.

59. Grau T, Bartusseck E, Conradi R, et al. Ultrasound imaging improves learning curves in obstetric epidural anesthesia: a preliminary study. Can J Anaesth 2003;50(10):1047–50.

60. Kouides PA, Phatak PD, Burkart P, et al. Gynaecological and obstetrical morbidity in women with type I von Willebrand disease: results of a patient survey. Haemophilia 2000;6(6):643–8.

61. Silwer J. von Willebrand's disease in Sweden. Acta Paediatr Scand Suppl 1973; 238:1–159.

62. Al-Zirqi I, Vangen S, Forsen L, et al. Prevalence and risk factors of severe obstetric haemorrhage. BJOG 2008;115(10):1265–72.

63. Kominiarek MA, Kilpatrick SJ. Postpartum hemorrhage: a recurring pregnancy complication. Semin Perinatol 2007;31(3):159–66.

64. Kadir RA. Women and inherited bleeding disorders: pregnancy and delivery. Semin Hematol 1999;36(3 Suppl 4):28–35.

65. Roque H, Funai E, Lockwood CJ. von Willebrand disease and pregnancy. J Matern Fetal Med 2000;9(5):257–66.
66. Mannucci PM. Desmopressin (DDAVP) in the treatment of bleeding disorders: the first twenty years. Haemophilia 2000;6(Suppl 1):60–7.
67. Mannucci PM. Use of desmopressin (DDAVP) during early pregnancy in factor VIII-deficient women. Blood 2005;105(8):3382.
68. Sanchez-Luceros A, Meschengieser SS, Turdo K, et al. Evaluation of the clinical safety of desmopressin during pregnancy in women with a low plasmatic von Willebrand factor level and bleeding history. Thromb Res 2007;120(3):387–90.
69. Castillo R, Escolar G, Monteagudo J, et al. Hemostasis in patients with severe von Willebrand disease improves after normal platelet transfusion and normalizes with further correction of the plasma defect. Transfusion 1997;37(8):785–90.
70. Henry DA, Carless PA, Moxey AJ, et al. Anti-fibrinolytic use for minimising perioperative allogeneic blood transfusion. Cochrane Database Syst Rev 2007; 4:CD001886.
71. Ferrer P, Roberts I, Sydenham E, et al. Anti-fibrinolytic agents in post partum haemorrhage: a systematic review. BMC Pregnancy Childbirth 2009;9:29.
72. Lindoff C, Rybo G, Astedt B. Treatment with tranexamic acid during pregnancy, and the risk of thrombo-embolic complications. Thromb Haemost 1993;70(2): 238–40.
73. Tetruashvili NK. Hemostatic therapy for hemorrhages during first and second trimesters. Anesteziol Reanimatol 2007;6:46–8.
74. Berg CJ, Callaghan WM, Syverson C, et al. Pregnancy-related mortality in the United States, 1998 to 2005. Obstet Gynecol 2010;116(6):1302–9.
75. Jacobsen AF, Skjeldestad FE, Sandset PM. Ante- and postnatal risk factors of venous thrombosis: a hospital-based case-control study. J Thromb Haemost 2008;6(6):905–12.
76. Hayward CP, Rao AK, Cattaneo M. Congenital platelet disorders: overview of their mechanisms, diagnostic evaluation and treatment. Haemophilia 2006;12(Suppl 3): 128–36.

Factor Deficiencies in Pregnancy

Gillian N. Pike, MBChB, MRCP,
Paula H.B. Bolton-Maggs, DM, FRCP, FRCPath*

KEYWORDS

• Factor deficiencies • Pregnancy • Obstetric • Hemorrhage

Women with inherited coagulation factor deficiencies face particular hemostatic challenges during pregnancy, childbirth, and the puerperium. Most of these disorders are rare and are inherited in an autosomal recessive fashion. The incidence is increased in countries and ethnic groups where consanguineous marriages are more prevalent. In several of the disorders the bleeding risk does not correlate well with measured factor levels and, in some, abnormal bleeding can also occur in heterozygotes, adding to the complexity of management of these patients. Guidelines have been written about the obstetric management of women with factor deficiencies[1,2]; however, information is limited in some of the disorders because of their rarity, and it has mainly been derived from case reports and case series. This article provides general recommendations about the management of pregnancy, delivery, and the puerperium in women with inherited factor deficiencies, and gives more detailed information about each factor deficiency in turn.

GENERAL RECOMMENDATIONS

All patients with factor deficiencies should be registered with a hemophilia center. Women should be offered genetic counseling before conception in order to discuss the inheritance of their bleeding disorder, prenatal diagnosis, and, for some disorders, the option of preimplantation diagnosis may be available. Prenatal diagnosis is possible but is only recommended in couples who have had previous severely affected children or who are known to both be heterozygous carriers and at risk of having a severely affected child. In order to carry out prenatal diagnosis, the causative gene mutations or informative markers must first be identified in the parents, which can take time and should ideally be done before conception. Prenatal diagnosis can

The authors have nothing to disclose.
Department of Clinical Haematology, Manchester Royal Infirmary, Oxford Road, Manchester M13 9WL, UK
* Corresponding author.
E-mail address: paula.bolton-maggs@manchester.ac.uk

Hematol Oncol Clin N Am 25 (2011) 359–378
doi:10.1016/j.hoc.2011.01.007   hemonc.theclinics.com

be carried out via chorionic villus sampling (CVS), amniocentesis, or fetal cord blood sampling (cordocentesis).[1–4]

Pregnancy in women with these disorders should be managed in an obstetric unit within a hospital that has a hemophilia center. The patient should ideally be seen in a joint obstetric hematology clinic and be managed by a multidisciplinary team that includes an obstetrician who is a specialist in high-risk obstetrics and a hematologist with expertise in hemostasis and, where appropriate, a pediatric hematologist. Factor levels should be checked at booking, at 28 and 34 weeks' gestation, and before any invasive procedures.[2,3] More frequent checks may be required if prophylactic factor treatment is being given during pregnancy. When assessing the risk of bleeding in pregnant women with factor deficiencies, a detailed bleeding history, family history, and obstetric history should be obtained in association with factor levels. The management plan should be individualized for each patient and all women should have a written delivery plan made during the third trimester that is made available to all of those involved in the patient's care (including the woman herself). Good communication between hematologists, obstetricians, anesthetists, midwives, and pediatricians is essential for the safe management of labor and delivery.[1–3]

All women with factor deficiencies should deliver in a unit that has easy access to factor treatments and laboratory tests. Factor treatments are described separately for each bleeding disorder in this article. Having a severe bleeding disorder is not in itself an indication for a cesarean section delivery and, in most cases, normal vaginal delivery can be planned. In some cases, cesarean delivery may be deemed safer for obstetric indications. If the fetus is at risk of having a bleeding disorder, invasive monitoring, such as fetal blood sampling, fetal scalp electrodes, and the use of vacuum extraction and midcavity forceps, should be avoided. Prolonged second stage of labor also increases the risk of neonatal hemorrhage and therefore, in cases in which this is likely, an early recourse to cesarean section is recommended. Trauma to the maternal genital and perineal areas should be minimized during delivery.[2–4]

The use of regional anesthesia/analgesia has often been denied to women with bleeding disorders because of the potential risk of spinal/epidural hematoma formation with subsequent spinal cord compression. Regional blocks can be used in women who have normalized their factor levels during pregnancy or who have normal factor levels as a result of treatment, but women should be adequately counseled about the risks and benefits of regional blocks and informed consent obtained. An experienced anesthetist should perform the procedure and the patient should be monitored for any signs of spinal/epidural hematoma, with prompt imaging of the spinal cord if any complications are suspected. Factor levels also need to be maintained in the normal range at the time of catheter removal. Regional blocks should not be used in situations in which hemostasis is not guaranteed, such as in patients with uncorrected severe deficiencies or in whom there is poor correlation between the bleeding risk and factor levels.[3]

Pediatric hematologists and neonatologists need to be informed of the birth of any neonates with possible bleeding disorders. Cord blood samples should be collected if the neonate is at risk of being severely affected by a bleeding disorder, and intramuscular injections and surgery (eg, circumcision) should be delayed until the results are known. Several of the severe factor deficiencies are associated with neonatal cranial hemorrhage, which requires prompt diagnosis and treatment.[1–3]

Women with factor deficiencies are at increased risk of primary and secondary postpartum hemorrhage (PPH). The third stage of labor should be managed actively in order to reduce the risk of PPH. Prophylactic factor replacement should be given to women who have suboptimal factor levels or a significant bleeding history. Treatment is recommended during delivery and for at least 3 days after vaginal delivery and 5 days after cesarean section.[1–3]

INHERITED ABNORMALITIES OF FIBRINOGEN

Inherited abnormalities of fibrinogen can be subdivided into quantitative defects in which there is a complete absence of fibrinogen (afibrinogenemia) or a reduced amount of fibrinogen (hypofibrinogenemia), and qualitative defects in which the fibrinogen produced does not function normally (dysfibrinogenemia). Patients can also have low levels of dysfunctional fibrinogen (hypodysfibrinogenemia). Afibrinogenemia is an autosomal recessive disorder with an estimated prevalence of 1 in 1 million. Hypofibrinogenemia can be inherited in an autosomal recessive or dominant fashion.[5] Dysfibrinogenemia is an autosomal dominant disorder with an unknown incidence.[1,6,7]

Women who have quantitative defects of fibrinogen are at increased risk of miscarriage, placental abruption, and postpartum hemorrhage.[8–12] The ability of fibrinogen to form a stable fibrin network is important in maintaining placental integrity. As pregnancy progresses, fibrinogen turnover increases, with most fibrinogen consumption occurring in the uteroplacental bed.[13–15]

A literature review reveals 22 pregnancies in 10 women with afibrinogenemia, resulting in 12 miscarriages, 2 perinatal deaths, and 8 live births. Fibrinogen replacement was given throughout all of the successful pregnancies.[8,9,12,16–22] A review of the literature on hypofibrinogenemia reported 44 pregnancies in 15 women, resulting in 13 miscarriages, 8 placental abruptions, and 14 postpartum transfusions.[10] All women with afibrinogenemia should commence treatment with either fibrinogen concentrate or cryoprecipitate infusions as soon as pregnancy is confirmed. Fibrinogen concentrate is preferred because cryoprecipitate is not pathogen inactivated.[3] In the first and second trimester, trough fibrinogen levels of greater than 0.5 g L^{-1} and, if possible, greater than 1.0 g L^{-1} should be attempted by giving 2 to 3 g week^{-1}.[23] Fibrinogen levels should be checked weekly along with regular ultrasound assessment to monitor fetal growth and look for placental bleeding.[3] The amount of fibrinogen required will increase throughout pregnancy as the fibrinogen clearance increases.[9] In the later part of the third trimester, a trough level of greater than 1.0 g L^{-1} should be maintained. At the start of labor, a bolus of 4 g of fibrinogen concentrate should be administered followed by a continuous infusion of fibrinogen concentrate, intended to keep levels at more than 1.5 g L^{-1} during delivery and for 24 hours postpartum.[12] Replacement treatment during pregnancy and delivery may also be required in women with hypofibrinogenemia, depending on their bleeding history, previous obstetric history, and fibrinogen levels. All women who have a fibrinogen level of less than 1.5 g L^{-1} or a significant bleeding history should receive replacement treatment intrapartum.[3]

Less commonly, thrombotic events have been reported in association with pregnancy in women with hypofibrinogenemia and afibrinogenemia.[24,25] Early mobilization, maintenance of adequate hydration, and compression stockings are recommended in the postpartum period. If there is a family or personal history of previous thrombotic events, thromboprophylaxis with low molecular weight heparin (LMWH) should be considered.[3]

Dysfibrinogenemia is characterized by a wide variation in clinical phenotype, with both bleeding and thrombotic tendencies reported. A study of 64 pregnancies in 15 women with dysfibrinogenemia reported an increased rate of miscarriage (38%) and stillbirth (9%).[25] Placental abruption, PPH, and thrombosis have also been reported.[1,26] The management of pregnant women with dysfibrinogenemia should be individually tailored, taking into account any family or personal history of bleeding or thrombosis and any previous obstetric history along with fibrinogen levels. Approximately half of patients with this disorder are asymptomatic and do not need any treatment during pregnancy or delivery unless bleeding or thrombosis occurs. Standard postpartum thromboprophylaxis measures should be followed in asymptomatic patients.

In women with a personal or family history of thrombosis, antenatal and postpartum thromboprophylaxis should be given with LMWH and fibrinogen replacement should not be given unless the patient is bleeding. In women who have a history of bleeding or who require a cesarean section, fibrinogen replacement should be given to increase the fibrinogen levels to more than 1 g L^{-1} to cover delivery and should be continued, keeping levels at more than 0.5 g L^{-1} until wound healing has occurred. LMWH prophylaxis is also recommended after cesarean section along with compression stockings, good hydration, and early mobilization. Invasive monitoring during labor and instrumental deliveries should be avoided in case the neonate is affected. In patients who experience recurrent miscarriages, either prophylactic LMWH or fibrinogen concentrate treatment can be tried.[1]

FACTOR II: PROTHROMBIN DEFICIENCY

Prothrombin deficiency is a rare autosomal recessive disorder with a prevalence of 1 per 2 million in the general population.[27] It can be classified into 2 main phenotypes: hypoprothrombinemia (type 1 deficiency, characterized by a concomitant reduction of prothrombin antigen and activity levels), and dysprothrombinemia (type 2 deficiency, characterized by the production of a dysfunctional protein with reduced activity levels and normal antigen levels). Compound heterozygotes with combined defects have also been described.[28] Complete deficiency of prothrombin has not been reported and is believed to be incompatible with life.[29]

Patients with homozygous hypoprothrombinemia usually have prothrombin activity levels of less than 10 IU dL^{-1} and severe bleeding manifestations. In comparison, heterozygotes have levels between 40 and 60 IU dL^{-1} and are usually asymptomatic, but may have excessive bleeding after surgery. Individuals with dysprothrombinemia have both variable bleeding tendencies and prothrombin activity levels (between 1 and 50 IU dL^{-1}).[28]

There are insufficient published data to determine whether patients with prothrombin deficiency are at increased risk of miscarriage or to give definitive guidance on the management of pregnancy in patients with this disorder. Catanzarite and colleagues[30] reported a woman with hypoprothrombinemia (factor [F]II activity <1 IU dL^{-1}) who had had 8 pregnancies. All of the pregnancies were complicated by first trimester bleeding. Four of the pregnancies ended in miscarriage, with 2 having had ultrasound evidence of subchorionic hemorrhage before loss of pregnancy. The patient received prothrombin complex concentrate (PCC) before uterine curettage for all of the miscarriages and had no excessive bleeding. Four of the pregnancies reached term without any replacement treatment. The patient was given fresh frozen plasma (FFP) before delivery of her first child but had a delayed PPH requiring additional FFP, PCC, and blood transfusions. She was given PCC before the next 3 deliveries and had no PPH. An extra infusion of PCC was given after delivery of her fourth child because the placenta was found to have a large marginal clot. PPH has also been reported in a small Iranian series of 14 patients.[27]

It is unknown whether prophylaxis during pregnancy can prevent miscarriages and improve overall outcomes. A prothrombin level of 20 to 30 IU dL^{-1} is believed to be required for normal hemostasis, and it is recommended that a prothrombin level of more than 25 IU dL^{-1} should be achieved during labor and delivery.[1] There are no specific prothrombin concentrates, and therefore PCCs are the treatment of choice; these also contain FIX and FX and some also contain FVII in addition to FII, and therefore there is a potential risk that this treatment could be thrombogenic.[3] There is approximately 1 unit of prothrombin per unit of FIX in vials of PCC, and doses of 20 to 30 IU kg^{-1} should be used. Major surgery or life threatening bleeds may require higher doses. Prothrombin has a long half-life (about 72 hours), allowing dosing every 2 to 3 days, and treatment should be guided by levels.[1] If no PCC is available, virally inactivated FFP should be administered at a dose of 15 to 20 mL kg^{-1}, which will raise the FII level by approximately 25%.[31] Treatment should also be given if there is serious bleeding during pregnancy, before invasive procedures, and if a cesarean section is required.[3] It is uncertain whether treatment is beneficial in threatened miscarriages, but it would be reasonable to consider replacement in this situation.

FV DEFICIENCY

FV deficiency is an autosomal recessive disorder with a prevalence of approximately 1 per 1 million in the general population.[32] Patients with type I deficiency have a quantitative defect (ie, low levels of antigen), and individuals with type II deficiency have a qualitative defect (ie, normal or mildly reduced antigen levels with reduced activity). Patients who are homozygotes or compound heterozygotes for mutations in the FV gene have severe deficiency that is characterized by FV levels of less than 10 to 15 IU dL^{-1}. Individuals with mild to moderate FV deficiency have FV levels of greater than 20% to 30% and are usually heterozygotes.[33] There is limited correlation between the FV activity level and the clinical phenotype in this disorder. A wide variation in bleeding symptoms has been reported in patients with identical FV gene mutations or activity levels, including between related patients with identical genotypes.[34,35] Taking an accurate bleeding history is therefore an important part of assessing the bleeding risk in patients with FV deficiency.

FV levels do not increase significantly during pregnancy. There is no reported increase in rates of miscarriage, premature births, or fetal deaths in patients with FV deficiency,[36] and prophylaxis during pregnancy is not required unless the patient is undergoing an invasive procedure. Patients with severe deficiency are at risk of excessive bleeding at delivery and postpartum. A report of 2 pregnancies in patients with severe FV deficiency and literature review of a further 18 pregnancies showed that, of the 20 pregnancies, 11 (55%) were complicated by excessive bleeding that required transfusion of either FFP or whole blood.[36] Another group reported PPH in 13 of 17 deliveries (76%) in 9 women with FV deficiency.[37] A series of 15 pregnancies in 11 heterozygotic patients resulted in uneventful deliveries with no excessive bleeding without prophylaxis.[36]

Pregnant women with FV deficiency should have a bleeding history review and an FV level checked during the third trimester so that a delivery plan can be made. Labor and delivery can be managed expectantly in women with partial FV deficiency and no significant bleeding history. In women with severe deficiency, FV levels should be increased to more than 15 to 25 IU dL^{-1} during delivery and, if a cesarean section is performed, this should be maintained until wound healing has occurred (ie, 5–7 days).[1,3,36] No FV concentrate is currently available, therefore women should be treated with pathogen-inactivated FFP either in the form of solvent-detergent FFP (SD-FFP) or methylene blue–treated plasma. Because of the plasma processing, FV activity is reduced by 30% in SD-FFP compared with standard FFP and therefore a dose of 15 to 20 mL kg^{-1} of SD-FFP will have a lower posttransfusion increment of FV than standard FFP.[38] It is therefore important to monitor FV levels.[3,38] Plasma should be administered as soon as the patient is in established labor, and further doses given as dictated by the FV levels and clinical need. If a cesarean section is performed, FV levels should be maintained at more than 15 IU dL^{-1} until wound healing has occurred (ie, 5–7 days).[1]

Prenatal diagnosis of FV deficiency is possible in families in which the parents have had a previous severely affected child and the gene mutation has been characterized.[33] Cord blood can be taken at birth to measure FV levels in the baby. Severe and moderate deficiencies can be diagnosed at birth, but blood tests suggestive of a mild deficiency should be repeated when the child is older in order to confirm the diagnosis, because FV levels may not be reliable at birth. Bleeding is uncommon in the neonatal period but intracranial hemorrhage can occur and it is recommended that babies with an FV level of less than 15 IU dL^{-1} may have central nervous system imaging carried out in the first few days of life to exclude this. If bleeding does occur, neonates should be treated with 15 to 20 mL kg^{-1} of pathogen-inactivated plasma in order to increase FV levels to more than 15 IU dL^{-1}. Prophylactic plasma treatment is not required in asymptomatic FV-deficient neonates.[1]

FVII DEFICIENCY

FVII deficiency is the most common of the rare bleeding disorders, with an estimated incidence of 1 in 300,000 to 500,000 in its severe form and 1 in 350 for heterozygotes.[1,39] Clinical heterogeneity is described with little correlation between absolute FVII levels and bleeding risk. Some patients with very low FVII levels are asymptomatic, whereas others experience severe bleeding and some individuals with higher FVII levels may also bleed.[1] Phenotypic heterogeneity has also been described in patients with identical FVII mutations, supporting the theory that other genetic or environmental factors may play an important role in modulating the bleeding risk in FVII deficiency.[40,41] It is therefore important to take a thorough bleeding history when assessing patients with this disorder because a positive bleeding history predicts for bleeding.[42]

Heterozygotes usually have FVII levels of 20 to 60 IU dL^{-1} and homozygotes with severe deficiency have levels of les than 10 IU dL^{-1}.[43,44] Pregnancy induces a hypercoagulable state with increases of several coagulation factors in normal women and, in nondeficient women, FVII levels can increase up to fourfold during pregnancy, delivery, and the puerperium.[45,46] A significant increase in levels has also been reported in pregnant heterozygotes with mild to moderate FVII deficiencies. A study of 10 pregnancies in 4 women who had undiagnosed mild/moderate FVII deficiency at the time of delivery reported that 2 of the pregnancies resulted in early loss requiring surgical evacuation with excessive intraoperative bleeding, suggesting that women with mild/moderate deficiencies may be at increased risk of bleeding early in pregnancy before their FVII levels increase. FVII replacement should therefore be considered for any invasive procedures or bleeding during early pregnancy. From the other 8 pregnancies, 5 resulted in vaginal deliveries and 3 babies were delivered via cesarean section with epidural anesthesia. The baseline FVII levels in these women ranged from 7 to 49 IU dL^{-1}. No anesthetic or major hemorrhagic complications were seen in these women who received no prophylactic treatment.[47] Four pregnancies were reported in 3 women after the diagnosis of mild/moderate FVII deficiency. The FVII levels increased from a mean baseline of 33 IU dL^{-1} to a mean of 73 IU dL^{-1} in these women during pregnancy. Three of the women delivered by cesarean section and 1 by vaginal delivery, with all women receiving treatment with recombinant activated FVII (rFVIIa) before delivery. Three of the deliveries had no major bleeding, but 1 woman had excessive bleeding during a cesarean section.[47]

FVII replacement may not be required before delivery in women with mild/moderate deficiency. A decision regarding treatment should be based on FVII levels in the third trimester, the expected mode of delivery, and, most importantly, the past bleeding history because of the poor correlation between FVII levels and bleeding risk.

No increase in FVII levels occurs in pregnant women with severe FVII deficiency, who usually have levels of less than 10 IU dL^{-1}. Antepartum hemorrhage has been described in 2 women with severe deficiency but there are not enough data to determine whether FVII deficiency increases the risk of miscarriage and antepartum hemorrhage.[44,46] These women should also have FVII levels measured in the third trimester so that a delivery plan can be made. All women with an FVII level of less than 10 to 20 IU dL^{-1} at term, or with a significant bleeding history, should receive prophylaxis before delivery and in the postpartum period. Possible treatments include rFVIIa, or a plasma-derived FVII concentrate, or SD-FFP if concentrates are not available. The treatment of choice is rFVIIa, although the optimal dosing in pregnancy is not known.[1] Several case reports have described the successful use of rFVIIa in pregnant women with severe FVII deficiency using a variety of regimens. Pehlivanov and colleagues[48] reported a pregnant woman with an FVII level of 2% who received 60 μg kg^{-1} of rVIIa at complete dilatation of the cervix and then 30 μg kg^{-1} every 2 hours for 5 doses following vaginal delivery with no complications. Eskandari and colleagues[46] described a pregnant woman with an FVII level of 1% who was given 50 μg kg^{-1} of rFVIIa at complete dilatation of the cervix and a second dose of 35 μg kg^{-1} 4 hours later with no excessive bleeding following vaginal delivery. Muleo and colleagues[49] reported a pregnant woman with an FVII level of 6% who was given 20 μg kg^{-1} of rVIIa before cesarean section and then 10 μg kg^{-1} doses at 6 hourly intervals for 2 days with no excessive bleeding. Jiménez-Yuste and colleagues[50] reported a woman with an FVII level of 3.7 IU dL^{-1} who, after pharmacokinetic studies, was given a bolus of 13.3 μg kg^{-1} of rVIIa before cesarean section, followed by a 3.33 μg kg^{-1} h^{-1} infusion for 48 hours, and then 1.66 μg kg^{-1} h^{-1} infusion for a further 48 hours without any hemorrhagic complications. An FVII level of 10 to 20 IU dL^{-1} is believed to be required to achieve hemostasis after invasive procedures or surgery.[1] A dose of 15 to 30 μg kg^{-1} has been recommended to cover delivery.[3]

Pregnancies in which there is a risk of a severely affected baby delivery should be planned to minimize the risk of bleeding. Diagnosis of FVII deficiency may be difficult in the neonatal period because FVII levels are physiologically low in the newborn, but cord blood should be taken at delivery for FVII levels if severe deficiency is suspected. There is a 15% risk of cerebral hemorrhage in severely affected neonates, and prophylaxis should be considered.[1,46]

CARRIERS OF HEMOPHILIA A AND B

Hemophilia A and B are X-linked disorders that result in deficiencies in FVIII and FIX respectively. The incidence of hemophilia A is 1 in 5000 live male births and 1 in 30,000 live male births in hemophilia B.[51] Female carriers of hemophilia are expected to have clotting factor levels around 50% of normal but, in 10% to 20% of carriers, extreme lyonization of the *FVIII* gene and *FIX* gene results in much lower factor levels (<40%).[52] Carriers of hemophilia may therefore experience bleeding symptoms and may be at risk of bleeding, especially in those with levels of less than 10%.[53]

Hemophilia carriers have a 25% chance of having an affected child, a risk of 1 in 2 for every male child. Prepregnancy counseling and mutation detection should be offered to all women who are possible carriers of hemophilia. This service enables carriership to be confidently diagnosed before pregnancy and allows the patient to be provided with information about reproductive choices and prenatal diagnosis.[2] In a study of pregnant possible hemophilia carriers, those who were unaware of their carrier status at the time of delivery were more likely to have instrumental deliveries that are significant risk factors for intracranial and extracranial hemorrhage in newborn hemophiliacs.[54]

It is not known whether hemophilia carriers have an increased risk of miscarriage or early pregnancy bleeding. Chi and colleagues[4] performed a retrospective review of 41 hemophilia A carriers and 12 hemophilia B carriers who had received obstetric care in a 10-year period. They reported 13 miscarriages in 90 pregnancies (14%) and 2 cases of early pregnancy bleeding that had both occurred in low-factor-level carriers of hemophilia B. Hemorrhage occurred after a termination of pregnancy in a patient with an FVIII level of 42 IU dL^{-1} and after an evacuation of retained products in a carrier with a normal FVIII level. A retrospective survey on pregnancies in 46 hemophilia carriers reported 25 miscarriages in 120 pregnancies (21%). Three of the women (7%) experienced 2 or more miscarriages.[55] Coagulation factor replacement should be considered in patients with low factor levels who have bleeding, miscarriages, terminations of pregnancy, or invasive procedures during pregnancy.[2] There is no evidence of an increased risk of antepartum hemorrhage after 24 weeks' gestation.[54,56]

FVIII levels increase significantly during pregnancy in most hemophilia A carriers; however, a small percentage still have low levels at term. FIX levels do not increase in carriers of hemophilia B during pregnancy.[4,54,56] Factor levels should be checked in pregnant hemophilia carriers at booking and at 28 and 34 weeks' gestation in order to plan the optimal management of labor and delivery.[2] A delivery plan should be formulated in the third trimester. In patients who have opted not to have prenatal diagnosis, it is helpful if the gender of the fetus is determined before delivery either by ultrasound or by assessing free fetal DNA in a maternal blood sample for the presence of Y chromosome–specific DNA.[57] If the fetus is known to be male or the gender is unknown, vacuum extraction, high-cavity and midcavity forceps deliveries, prolonged labor, and invasive monitoring techniques such as the use of fetal scalp electrodes or fetal blood sampling should be avoided. There is a 50% chance that a male fetus will be affected by hemophilia and be at risk of hemorrhagic complications.[2]

FVIII or FIX concentrate (preferably recombinant) should be given during labor if factor levels in the third trimester are less than 50 IU dL^{-1}. Desmopressin (1-desamino-8-D-arginine vasopressin [DDAVP]) can be used to raise FVIII levels in some carriers of hemophilia A but has no effect in hemophilia B. Fluid intake should be restricted for 24 hours following each dose in patients who are given desmopressin because fluid retention can occur. It is safe for women to breast feed following desmopressin administration.

Babies with hemophilia are at risk of severe intracranial bleeding from the birth process and there is debate about the safest mode of delivery. In a review of 117 children born with severe or moderate hemophilia, 23 neonatal bleeds were reported. The risk of cranial bleeding was 64% with vacuum extraction, 15% with cesarean section, and 3% with normal vaginal deliveries. Normal vaginal deliveries were recommended, but there is an increased risk of bleeding in babies if there has been a prolonged second stage of labor.[56,58] An early decision to carry out a cesarean section is recommended in patients who are likely to have prolonged labor or difficult vaginal deliveries.[2] If factor levels are greater than 50 IU dL^{-1}, regional blocks can be used but should be performed by an experienced anesthetist. Intramuscular injections and nonsteroidal anti-inflammatory drugs should not be administered in low-level carriers of hemophilia.[2]

After delivery the pregnancy-induced increase of FVIII rapidly decreases. Hemophilia carriers have increased rates of primary and secondary PPH. In normal women, the rates of primary PPH are 5% to 8%, and 0.8% for secondary PPH.[59,60] In comparison, the incidence of primary PPH and secondary PPH in hemophilia carriers are 22% and 11% respectively.[56] Patients are also at risk of perineal hematomas.[54] Active management of the third stage of labor should be practiced and factor levels should be maintained at more than 50 IU dL^{-1} for 3 days in vaginal deliveries and 5 days after cesarean section. Antifibrinolytic agents should also be considered.[2]

Cord blood samples for factor assays should be taken from all male babies born to hemophilia carriers to allow early identification of hemophiliac neonates.[2] Intracranial hemorrhage occurs in 1% to 4% of neonates affected by hemophilia.[61] Cranial imaging should be arranged for hemophiliac neonates if the labor has been prolonged, the delivery has been traumatic, or if a cerebral bleed is suspected. Factor concentrate should be given to neonates suspected of having a cranial bleed in order to raise the factor level to 100 IU dL^{-1}.[2]

FX DEFICIENCY

FX deficiency is an autosomal recessive disorder with an incidence of 1 per 1 million in the general population. The prevalence of carriers (heterozygotes) for FX deficiency is approximately 1 in 500 people.[62,63] FX deficiency can be subdivided into type I deficiency, which is a quantitative defect with proportionally reduced FX activity and antigen levels, and type II deficiency, which is a qualitative defect characterized by a near normal antigen level but reduced FX activity.[64] Patients have been classified into 3 different groups according to their FX activity levels, but this classification has not been widely validated.[65] Individuals with severe deficiency (FX level <1 IU dL^{-1}) have spontaneous bleeding and are among the most seriously affected individuals with rare bleeding disorders.[65] Patients with moderate deficiency (FX level 1–5 IU dL^{-1}) have fewer spontaneous bleeds but usually bleed after hemostatic challenges (ie, after surgery or trauma). Patients with mild deficiency (FX level 6–10 IU dL^{-1}) and heterozygotes rarely have significant bleeds and can be asymptomatic.[65,66] An FX level of 10 to 20 IU dL^{-1} is required to achieve hemostasis.[67]

In normal individuals, FX levels increase during pregnancy,[68] and this may also occur in some women with FX deficiency.[69] FX levels should therefore be checked in the third trimester to inform the delivery plan. A literature review describes 18 pregnancies in 12 women with FX deficiency.[70–81] Miscarriage,[71] retroplacental hemorrhage,[71,76] and preterm labor[78,80] have been reported; however, because of small numbers, a definitive association between FX deficiency and obstetric complications cannot be made. No clear correlation between FX levels and complication risk has been reported.[69] A woman with an FX level of 1% had a spontaneous miscarriage with her first pregnancy. Her second was a twin pregnancy and she was treated with alternate-day prophylaxis with PCC at a dose of 1000 IU from early pregnancy. Despite this, she experienced vaginal bleeding at 15 and 19 weeks' gestation and a retroplacental hematoma was detected. This condition remained stable for the rest of the pregnancy. She developed preterm labor at 34 weeks' gestation and was delivered by cesarean section with PCC cover. There was no excessive bleeding during delivery or in the postpartum period.[71] Kumar and Mehta[78] reported 4 pregnancies in a woman with severe FX deficiency. The first 2 pregnancies were complicated by preterm labor at 21 and 15 weeks' gestation and both neonates died of problems related to prematurity. In the following 2 pregnancies, the patient received PCC treatment from early pregnancy and she delivered healthy babies at 32 and 34 weeks' gestation. Konje and colleagues[76] described a woman with FX activity of 4% who developed a fundal retroplacental hematoma at 22 weeks with a second hematoma at 37 weeks' gestation. The patient was given PCC to control the bleeding on both occasions with good effect. Successful pregnancies have also been reported in women with severe FX deficiency who have not received prophylaxis.[79,81] Treatment during pregnancy should be considered in women with severe FX deficiency and a history of adverse outcomes.[1] Treatment should also be given in women before invasive procedures and for antepartum bleeding. Women with severe FX deficiency should have close monitoring during pregnancy, with regular clinical and ultrasound assessment if retroplacental bleeding is suspected.[3]

Replacement therapy should be administered to pregnant women with FX deficiency during labor and delivery to prevent excessive bleeding. FX concentrate is available in some countries (CSL Behring, King of Prussia, PA, USA) and a second is in clinical trials (BPL, Elstree, UK) and successful deliveries have been reported using either FFP or PCC treatment.[69,71–73] An FX level of greater than 20 IU dL^{-1} is desirable to cover delivery and can be achieved by an initial dose of 15 to 20 mL kg^{-1} of virally inactivated FFP followed by 3 to 6 mL kg^{-1} twice daily. If PCC is used, a loading dose of 15 to 30 IU kg^{-1} is given with subsequent doses of 10 to 20 IU kg^{-1}. The dose of PCC is calculated from the finding that 1 IU FX kg^{-1} raises the FX level by 1.5% of normal. In all cases, the patient's factor level before treatment and the mode of delivery should be taken into account when calculating the dose required, and FX levels should be monitored. Patients with FX levels of greater than 10 to 20 IU dL^{-1} and no significant bleeding history can be managed expectantly.[1,3]

Although elective cesarean section in women with FX deficiency has previously been recommended to avoid intracranial or abdominal hemorrhage in the newborn,[81] several case reports have described good outcomes from normal vaginal deliveries.[78,79] Elective cesarean section is therefore not recommended for all women with FX deficiency, and each delivery plan should be individualized with input from a multidisciplinary team.

The newborn has low physiologic levels, making the diagnosis of moderate or mild FX deficiency more difficult at birth, but neonates with severe deficiency can be diagnosed from a cord blood sample. Imaging should be performed on neonates with severe deficiency to rule out intracranial hemorrhage, and prophylaxis should be considered.[1]

FXI DEFICIENCY

FXI deficiency is an autosomally inherited disorder. It is particularly common among Ashkenazi Jews and it is estimated that, within this population, 1 in 190 individuals are severely deficient with 2 *FX1* gene mutations, and 1 in 8 are heterozygotes.[82,83] The incidence of severe deficiency within the general population is approximately 1 in 1 million.[84] Severe deficiency is characterized by FXI levels of less than 15 to 20 IU dL^{-1}. Spontaneous hemorrhage is rare, but patients are generally at high risk of postoperative bleeding, particularly in areas of high fibrinolytic activity (ie, the mouth, nose, and genitourinary system).[1] Heterozygotes have a mild or partial deficiency, with levels of 20 to 70 IU dL^{-1}, and a lower risk of bleeding after surgery.[85–88] The bleeding tendency in FXI deficiency does not correlate well with the FXI level and can also vary within an individual and within family members who have the same genotype.[86,87,89,90] Some patients with severe deficiency do not have excessive bleeding, even after surgery, whereas some patients with a mild deficiency report significant hemorrhagic symptoms.[88]

The miscarriage and antepartum hemorrhage rates are not increased in women with FXI deficiency, but bleeding may be severe in women after miscarriages or terminations of pregnancies.[91–93] FXI levels do not increase during pregnancy, and women with severe or partial deficiency can be at risk of excessive bleeding during delivery and in the postpartum period.[91–93] Myers and colleagues[92] performed a retrospective analysis of 105 pregnancies in 33 women with FXI deficiency and divided the women into bleeders and nonbleeders according to criteria used by Bolton-Maggs and colleagues.[89] The PPH rate was increased at 13% (compared with a rate of 5% within the normal population), with most occurring in patients who had been identified as having a bleeding tendency.[92] Kadir and colleagues[91] studied a total of 28 pregnancies in 11 women with FXI deficiency and reported a primary PPH rate of 16% and a secondary PPH rate of 24%. No bleeding was seen in patients who received prophylaxis.

Chi and colleagues[93] carried out a retrospective review of 61 pregnancies in 30 women with FXI deficiency and reported an 11% rate of primary PPH and 11% rate of secondary PPH. Most women who had PPH, and all of the women who had excessive bleeding after miscarriages, had a positive bleeding history. Salomon and colleagues[94] carried out a retrospective study of 164 pregnancies in 62 women with severe FXI deficiency (FXI<17 IU dL^{-1}). Forty-three of the 62 women (69%) had no PPH after a total of 93 deliveries without prophylaxis. When no prophylaxis was given, excessive bleeding was reported in 24% of vaginal deliveries (32/132) and 17% of cesarean sections (2/12). No excessive bleeding was seen in patients treated with FFP before having cesarean sections. This study suggests that not all women with severe deficiency require prophylaxis at delivery. Salomon and colleagues[94] also found that women who had bled with previous hemostatic challenges were more likely to have PPH. There was no correlation between PPH and the FXI level or genotype.

All patients with FXI deficiency should have their FXI levels monitored in the third trimester. The bleeding history is helpful in assessing the bleeding risk and making delivery plans. The decision as to whether or not to use prophylaxis during labor and delivery should be based on the bleeding history and previous response to hemostatic challenges, FXI level, and the proposed mode of delivery. Current guidelines recommend that vaginal deliveries can be managed expectantly in women with no significant bleeding history and FXI levels of 15 to 70 IU dL^{-1}. An antifibrinolytic agent such as tranexamic acid is recommended to cover vaginal deliveries in women with significant bleeding histories or no previous hemostatic challenges and FXI levels of 15 to 70 IU dL^{-1}. The first dose should be given during labor and continued for 3 days. FXI concentrate, or SD-FFP if concentrate is not available, should be given to women with severe FXI deficiency (FXI level of <10–20 IU dL^{-1}) before vaginal deliveries and cesarean sections. Decisions about the use of FXI concentrate treatment in women with partial deficiency (FXI 20–70 IU dL^{-1}) who require cesarean sections should be based on the patient's bleeding history and FXI level.[1]

FXI concentrate should be administered at the start of labor or before cesarean section or planned induction.[2] FXI concentrate has been associated with an increased risk of thrombosis and therefore doses should not exceed 30 IU kg^{-1} and should be designed to achieve a peak FXI level no greater than 70 IU dL^{-1}.[1,95,96] A dose of 10 IU kg^{-1} may be adequate to treat patients with severe FXI deficiency.[3] Prophylaxis can be continued for 3 days after vaginal delivery or 5 days after cesarean section.[2] The half-life of FXI is 52 (±22) hours, therefore daily doses may not be required.[1,97] An antifibrinolytic agent should be given in the postpartum period to prevent PPH and can be administered for up to 2 weeks after delivery. However, it should not be given concomitantly with FXI concentrate in view of possible thrombogenicity.[95,96]

In patients who have developed inhibitors to FXI (generally individuals with termination mutations), rVIIa has been successfully used to prevent bleeding during surgical procedures,[98,99] although it is not currently licensed for this use. It could be used to cover delivery in this rare subset of patients.[3]

The use of epidural or spinal anesthesia in patients with FXI deficiency has generally been discouraged because of the risk of spinal hematoma formation. However, epidurals have been performed in FXI-deficient women without complications and therefore could be used in women who have received therapy and a demonstrable adequate increase in FXI level.[1,2] Prenatal diagnosis is unnecessary for this disorder because the morbidity associated with FXI deficiency is low.[88] There are no reports of spontaneous bleeding or intracranial hemorrhage in neonates with FXI deficiency; however, severe bleeding can occur after circumcision, and severely affected boys having this procedure may need cover with FXI concentrate or antifibrinolytic agents.[1]

FXIII DEFICIENCY

FXIII deficiency Is a rare autosomal recessive disorder with an incidence of 1 in 1 million to 1 in 5 million people.[100] FXIII has the ability to cross-link proteins and plays an important role in clot stabilization, wound healing, and placental attachment.[101,102] Circulating FXIII is a protransglutaminase that is composed of 2 active A subunits and 2 carrier B subunits.[103] FXIII deficiency has been subdivided into XIIIA deficiency (former type 2 deficiency) and XIIIB deficiency (former type 1 deficiency).[104]

FXIII is not essential for ovulation, fertilization, or egg implantation, but it is vital for early placental adhesion.[101,105,106] Through the cross-linkage of fibrin and fibronectin, FXIII enables extravillous cytotrophoblasts to become anchored. At 6 to 8 weeks' gestation, these cells form the cytotrophoblastic shell and Nitabuch layer, which make up the inner and outer surface of the maternal-fetal interface within the placenta.[106] In FXIIIA deficiency, the cytotrophoblastic layer and Nitabuch layer are poorly formed. This deficiency may increase the likelihood of placental detachment and subsequent miscarriage, usually in the first trimester.[101]

Burrows and colleagues[107] collated data from 117 patients with FXIII deficiency, of which 16 were women of reproductive age. Ten of the 16 women with FXIIIA deficiency had recurrent miscarriages. Five out of 7 of women who had successful pregnancies received FXIII replacement during their pregnancy. Asahina and colleagues[103] described a further 8 case reports of successful pregnancies in women with FXIIIA deficiency who had been given FXIII prophylaxis. In comparison, women with FXIIIB deficiency had normal pregnancies without prophylaxis.[107]

All women with FXIIIA deficiency should be started on regular FXIII concentrate replacement treatment as early as possible in pregnancy (ideally before 5–6 weeks' gestation). Women with this disorder should receive prenatal counseling about the importance of early detection of pregnancy. FXIII concentrate is the treatment of choice (rather than FFP or cryoprecipitate), with a target FXIII level of greater than 10 IU dL^{-1}. This level can be achieved by administering 250 IU of FXIII concentrate weekly from pregnancy confirmation up until 22 weeks' gestation, and 500 IU weekly from 23 weeks onwards. At the onset of labor, an additional dose of 1000 IU should be given to increase the FXIII level to greater than 30 IU dL^{-1}.[103] Safe deliveries have been reported in 2 women with FXIII levels of 19 IU dL^{-1} and 36 IU dL^{-1} at the time of delivery.[105,107]

PPH is not commonly seen in women with FXIIIA deficiency. The most likely reason for this is that FXIII treatment given at the time of delivery also reduces the bleeding risk in the postpartum period because the FXIII concentrate has a long half-life of 7 to 13 days.[108] In comparison, women with FXIIIB deficiency do not require FXIII concentrate during pregnancy and delivery, but are at risk of PPH. The postpartum administration of FXIII concentrate should therefore be considered in these patients.[107]

COMBINED DEFICIENCY OF FV AND FVIII

Combined FV and FVIII deficiency is a truly autosomal recessive disorder (heterozygotes have completely normal FV and FVIIIC levels) with an incidence of 1 per 1 million.[32,109] The deficiency results from mutations in either the *LMAN1* or *MCFD2* genes, which encode for proteins involved in the intracellular transport of FV and FVIII.[110,111] The synthesis of FV and FVIII within hepatocytes is normal, but intracellular trafficking and release into the circulation is impaired.[1,110] Patients with this disorder usually have mild to moderate bleeding symptoms and concomitantly low levels of FV and FVIII (between 5% and 20%).[109]

Unless a couple have already had a severely affected child, prenatal diagnosis is not routinely carried out.[112] No published data are available on the optimal management of women with this disorder during pregnancy. The FV level is likely to be the main determinant of bleeding risk at delivery because FVIII levels increase during pregnancy but FV levels remain the same. FV and FVIII levels should be checked during the third trimester so that a delivery plan can be made. During labor, virally inactivated FFP at an initial dose of 15 to 20 mL kg^{-1} should be used to maintain FV levels at more than 15 IU dL^{-1} and recombinant fFVIII concentrate should be used to maintain FVIII levels at more than 50 IU dL^{-1}. If a cesarean section is required, FV levels should be increased to more than 25 IU dL^{-1} and factor replacement should continue until wound healing has occurred.[1,3,112]

INHERITED DEFICIENCY OF THE VITAMIN K–DEPENDENT CLOTTING FACTORS

Vitamin K–dependent clotting factors deficiency (VKCFD) is a rare autosomal recessive disorder described in the literature as case reports in only 21 kindreds worldwide.[23] Two clinically similar variants of this disorder exist: VKCFD1, resulting from point mutations in the γ-glutamyl carboxylase gene (*GGCX*), and VKCFD2, resulting from point mutations in the vitamin K epoxide reductase gene (*VKORC1*).[113,114] The clinical phenotype is variable and can be exacerbated by acquired vitamin K deficiency. The bleeding risk correlates with factor levels, with severe bleeding symptoms occurring when factor levels are less than 5 IU dL^{-1}. FII, FVII, FIX, and FX are affected in this disorder.[23,115]

Pregnant women who are at risk of having a child with VKCFD should receive oral vitamin K supplementation during the third trimester. Prenatal diagnosis is possible but is not normally carried out, because most patients with VKCFD achieve adequate control of hemostasis with vitamin K treatment alone.[115] A single case of a pregnancy in a woman with severe VKCFD has been described. At diagnosis, her FII, FVII, FIX, and FX activities were all less than 3 IU dL^{-1}. She received oral supplementation of vitamin K during her pregnancy (15 mg day^{-1}) and at the time of labor induction her FII, FVII, FIX, and FX activities had risen to 7%, 27%, 29%, and 6% respectively. She had an uneventful pregnancy but had excessive postpartum bleeding from an episiotomy site, which required treatment with FFP.[116]

There is limited guidance in the literature on how best to manage pregnant women with this disorder. All patients with VKCFD are commenced on lifelong vitamin K treatment from diagnosis, and this should be continued throughout pregnancy.[1,3] Most patients have a partial or complete response to vitamin K treatment but, in some kindreds, vitamin K is ineffective.[114–119] Factor levels should be measured in the third trimester in order to plan for delivery. Replacement therapy with either virally inactivated FFP or 4-factor PCCs should be given to treat acute bleeding and should be considered to cover delivery or invasive procedures, especially in severe cases and in patients who do not respond to vitamin K.[1,3] FVII has the shortest half-life of the vitamin K–dependent clotting factors and therefore treatment should be monitored using either the prothrombin time or FVII activity assays.[1,120]

SUMMARY

Pregnancy and childbirth present a major challenge to women with inherited bleeding disorders. All women should be managed by a multidisciplinary team in a center where the expertise, laboratory support, and factor treatment required to care for these patients is available at all times. Women with FXIII or fibrinogen deficiencies are at high risk of recurrent miscarriages and placental abruption, and prophylactic factor replacement should be started early in pregnancy. The risk of antepartum complications in women with other rare bleeding disorders is not fully determined because of the rarity of these disorders and the limited published data. During the third trimester of pregnancy, factor levels should be checked and an individualized management plan for delivery and the postpartum period should be written. Several bleeding disorders are associated with high rates of PPH, and women need to be monitored closely during the puerperium and treated with factor replacement when appropriate. It is hoped that, in the future, more will be learned about the effect of bleeding disorders on pregnancy and the puerperium through data collection about women in international databases of bleeding disorders. These data will provide us with better guidance for the optimal management of these women in pregnancy.

ACKNOWLEDGMENTS

We thank Dr Rezan Kadir for helpful review of the manuscript.

REFERENCES

1. Bolton-Maggs PH, Perry DJ, Chalmers EA, et al. The rare coagulation disorders–review with guidelines for management from the United Kingdom Haemophilia Centre Doctors' Organisation. Haemophilia 2004;10(5):593–628.
2. Lee CA, Chi C, Pavord SR, et al. The obstetric and gynaecological management of women with inherited bleeding disorders–review with guidelines produced by a taskforce of UK Haemophilia Centre Doctors' Organization. Haemophilia 2006; 12(4):301–36.
3. Kadir R, Chi C, Bolton-Maggs P. Pregnancy and rare bleeding disorders. Haemophilia 2009;15(5):990–1005.
4. Chi C, Lee CA, Shiltagh N, et al. Pregnancy in carriers of haemophilia. Haemophilia 2008;14(1):56–64.
5. Menache D. Congenital fibrinogen abnormalities. Ann N Y Acad Sci 1983;408: 121–30.
6. Acharya SS, Dimichele DM. Rare inherited disorders of fibrinogen. Haemophilia 2008;14(6):1151–8.
7. Peyvandi F, Asselta R, Mannucci PM. Autosomal recessive deficiencies of coagulation factors. Rev Clin Exp Hematol 2001;5(4):369–88.

8. Evron S, Anteby SO, Brzezinsky A, et al. Congenital afibrinogenemia and recurrent early abortion: a case report. Eur J Obstet Gynecol Reprod Biol 1985;19(5): 307–11.
9. Kobayashi T, Kanayama N, Tokunaga N, et al. Prenatal and peripartum management of congenital afibrinogenaemia. Br J Haematol 2000;109(2):364–6.
10. Goodwin TM. Congenital hypofibrinogenemia in pregnancy. Obstet Gynecol Surv 1989;44(3):157–61.
11. Ness PM, Budzynski AZ, Olexa SA, et al. Congenital hypofibrinogenemia and recurrent placental abruption. Obstet Gynecol 1983;61(4):519–23.
12. Mensah PK, Oppenheimer C, Watson C, et al. Congenital afibrinogenaemia in pregnancy. Haemophilia 2011;17(1):167–8.
13. Liedholm P, Astedt B. Fibrinolytic activity of the rat ovum, appearance during tubal passage and disappearance at implantation. Int J Fertil 1975;20(1):24–6.
14. Beller FK, Ebert C. The coagulation and fibrinolytic enzyme system in pregnancy and in the puerperium. Eur J Obstet Gynecol Reprod Biol 1982;13(3): 177–97.
15. Fletcher AP, Alkjaersig NK, Burstein R. The influence of pregnancy upon blood coagulation and plasma fibrinolytic enzyme function. Am J Obstet Gynecol 1979;134(7):743–51.
16. Trehan AK, Fergusson IL. Congenital afibrinogenaemia and successful pregnancy outcome. Case report. Br J Obstet Gynaecol 1991;98(7):722–4.
17. Kobayashi T, Asahina T, Maehara K, et al. Congenital afibrinogenemia with successful delivery. Gynecol Obstet Invest 1996;42(1):66–9.
18. Inamoto Y, Terao T. First report of case of congenital afibrinogenemia with successful delivery. Am J Obstet Gynecol 1985;153(7):803–4.
19. Grech H, Majumdar G, Lawrie AS, et al. Pregnancy in congenital afibrinogenaemia: report of a successful case and review of the literature. Br J Haematol 1991; 78(4):571–2.
20. Matsuno K, Mori K, Amikawa H. A case of congenital afibrinogenemia with abortion, intracranial hemorrhage and peritonitis. Jpn J Clin Hematol 1977;18:1438.
21. Dube B, Agarwal SP, Gupta MM, et al. Congenital deficiency of fibrinogen in two sisters. A clinical and haematological study. Acta Haematol 1970;43(2):120–7.
22. Aygoren-Pursun E, Martinez Saguer I, Rusicke E, et al. Retrochorionic hematoma in congenital afibrinogenemia: resolution with fibrinogen concentrate infusions. Am J Hematol 2007;82(4):317–20.
23. Brenner B, Kuperman AA, Watzka M, et al. Vitamin K-dependent coagulation factors deficiency. Semin Thromb Hemost 2009;35:439–46.
24. Roque H, Stephenson C, Lee MJ, et al. Pregnancy-related thrombosis in a woman with congenital afibrinogenemia: a report of two successful pregnancies. Am J Hematol 2004;76(3):267–70.
25. Haverkate F, Samama M. Familial dysfibrinogenemia and thrombophilia. Report on a study of the SSC Subcommittee on Fibrinogen. Thromb Haemost 1995; 73(1):151–61.
26. Edwards RZ, Rijhsinghani A. Dysfibrinogenemia and placental abruption. Obstet Gynecol 2000;95(6 Pt 2):1043.
27. Peyvandi F, Mannucci PM. Rare coagulation disorders. Thromb Haemost 1999; 82:1207–14.
28. Girolami A, Scarano L, Saggiorato G, et al. Congenital deficiencies and abnormalities of prothrombin. Blood Coagul Fibrinolysis 1998;9(7):557–69.
29. Sun WY, Witte DP, Degen JL, et al. Prothrombin deficiency results in embryonic and neonatal lethality in mice. Proc Natl Acad Sci U S A 1998;95(13):7597–602.

30. Catanzarite VA, Novotny WF, Cousins LM, et al. Pregnancies in a patient with congenital absence of prothrombin activity: case report. Am J Perinatol 1997; 14(3):135–8.
31. United Kingdom Haemophilia Centre Doctors' Organisation. Guidelines on the selection and use of therapeutic products to treat haemophilia and other hereditary bleeding disorders. Haemophilia 2003;9(1):1–23.
32. Mannucci PM, Duga S, Peyvandi F. Recessively inherited coagulation disorders. Blood 2004;104(5):1243–52.
33. Asselta R, Peyvandi F. Factor V deficiency. Semin Thromb Hemost 2009;35(4): 382–9.
34. Kalafatis M. Coagulation factor V: a plethora of anticoagulant molecules. Curr Opin Hematol 2005;12(2):141–8.
35. Castoldi E, Lunghi B, Mingozzi F, et al. A missense mutation (Y1702C) in the coagulation factor V gene is a frequent cause of factor V deficiency in the Italian population. Haematologica 2001;86(6):629–33.
36. Girolami A, Scandellari R, Lombardi AM, et al. Pregnancy and oral contraceptives in factor V deficiency: a study of 22 patients (five homozygotes and 17 heterozygotes) and review of the literature. Haemophilia 2005;11(1):26–30.
37. Noia G, De Carolis S, De Stefano V, et al. Factor V deficiency in pregnancy complicated by Rh immunization and placenta previa. A case report and review of the literature. Acta Obstet Gynecol Scand 1997;76(9):890–2.
38. O'Donnell JS. Severe factor V deficiency and pregnancy - a role for solvent-detergent plasma? Haemophilia 2005;11(4):422–3.
39. Bhavnani M, Evans DI. Carriers of factor VII deficiency are not always asymptomatic. Clin Lab Haematol 1984;6(4):363–8.
40. Castoldi E, Govers-Riemslag JW, Pinotti M, et al. Coinheritance of factor V (FV) Leiden enhances thrombin formation and is associated with a mild bleeding phenotype in patients homozygous for the FVII 9726+5G>A (FVII Lazio) mutation. Blood 2003;102(12):4014–20.
41. Kario K, Narita N, Matsuo T, et al. Genetic determinants of plasma factor VII activity in the Japanese. Thromb Haemost 1995;73(4):617–22.
42. Giansily-Blaizot M, Biron-Andreani C, Aguilar-Martinez P, et al. Inherited factor VII deficiency and surgery: clinical data are the best criteria to predict the risk of bleeding. Br J Haematol 2002;117(1):172–5.
43. Robertson LE, Wasserstrum N, Banez E, et al. Hereditary factor VII deficiency in pregnancy: peripartum treatment with factor VII concentrate. Am J Hematol 1992;40(1):38–41.
44. Fadel HE, Krauss JS. Factor VII deficiency and pregnancy. Obstet Gynecol 1989;73(3 Pt 2):453–4.
45. Dalaker K, Prydz H. The coagulation factor VII in pregnancy. Br J Haematol 1984;56:233–41.
46. Eskandari N, Feldman N, Greenspoon JS. Factor VII deficiency in pregnancy treated with recombinant factor VIIa. Obstet Gynecol 2002;99(5 Pt 2):935–7.
47. Kulkarni AA, Lee CA, Kadir RA. Pregnancy in women with congenital factor VII deficiency. Haemophilia 2006;12(4):413–6.
48. Pehlivanov B, Milchev N, Kroumov G. Factor VII deficiency and its treatment in delivery with recombinant factor VII. Eur J Obstet Gynecol Reprod Biol 2004; 116(2):237–8.
49. Muleo G, Santoro R, Iannaccaro PG, et al. The use of recombinant activated factor VII in congenital and acquired factor VII deficiencies. Blood Coagul Fibrinolysis 1998;9(4):389–90.

50. Jimenez-Yuste V, Villar A, Morado M, et al. Continuous infusion of recombinant activated factor VII during caesarean section delivery in a patient with congenital factor VII deficiency. Haemophilia 2000;6(5):588–90.
51. Mannucci PM, Tuddenham EG. The hemophilias–from royal genes to gene therapy. N Engl J Med 2001;344(23):1773–9.
52. Lyon MF. Sex chromatin and gene action in the mammalian X-chromosome. Am J Hum Genet 1962;14:135–48.
53. Lusher JM, McMillan CW. Severe factor VIII and factor IX deficiency in females. Am J Med 1978;65(4):637–48.
54. Greer IA, Lowe GD, Walker JJ, et al. Haemorrhagic problems in obstetrics and gynaecology in patients with congenital coagulopathies. Br J Obstet Gynaecol 1991;98(9):909–18.
55. Knol HM, Voskuilen MA, Holterman F, et al. Reproductive choices and obstetrical experience in Dutch carriers of haemophilia A and B. Haemophilia 2010 [Epub ahead of print]. DOI:10.1111/j.1365-2516.2010.02351.x.
56. Kadir RA, Economides DL, Braithwaite J, et al. The obstetric experience of carriers of haemophilia. Br J Obstet Gynaecol 1997;104(7):803–10.
57. Santacroce R, Vecchione G, Tomaiyolo M, et al. Identification of fetal gender in maternal blood is a helpful tool in the prenatal diagnosis of haemophilia. Haemophilia 2006;12:417–22.
58. Ljung R, Lindgren AC, Petrini P, et al. Normal vaginal delivery is to be recommended for haemophilia carrier gravidae. Acta Paediatr 1994;83(6):609–11.
59. El-Refaey H, Rodeck C. Post-partum haemorrhage: definitions, medical and surgical management. A time for change. Br Med Bull 2003;67:205–17.
60. Hoveyda F, MacKenzie IZ. Secondary postpartum haemorrhage: incidence, morbidity and current management. BJOG 2001;108(9):927–30.
61. Kulkarni R, Lusher JM. Intracranial and extracranial hemorrhages in newborns with hemophilia: a review of the literature. J Pediatr Hematol Oncol 1999;21(4):289–95.
62. Uprichard J, Perry DJ. Factor X deficiency. Blood Rev 2002;16(2):97–110.
63. Graham J, Barrow EM, Hougie C. Stuart clotting defect. II. Genetic aspects of a 'new' hemorrhagic state. J Clin Invest 1957;36(3):497–503.
64. Menegatti M, Peyvandi F. Factor X deficiency. Semin Thromb Hemost 2009; 35(4):407–15.
65. Peyvandi F, Mannucci PM, Lak M, et al. Congenital factor X deficiency: spectrum of bleeding symptoms in 32 Iranian patients. Br J Haematol 1998;102(2):626–8.
66. Brown DL, Kouides PA. Diagnosis and treatment of inherited factor X deficiency. Haemophilia 2008;14(6):1176–82.
67. Knight RD, Barr CF, Alving BM. Replacement therapy for congenital factor X deficiency. Transfusion 1985;25(1):78–80.
68. Condie RG. A serial study of coagulation factors XII, XI and X in plasma in normal pregnancy and in pregnancy complicated by pre-eclampsia. Br J Obstet Gynaecol 1976;83(8):636–9.
69. Mamopoulos A, Vakalopoulou S, Lefkou E, et al. Pregnancy in a patient with severe factor X deficiency. Haemophilia 2009;15(6):1351–3.
70. Arai S. Mycoplasma. Rinsho Biseibutshu Jinsoku Shindan Kenkyukai Shi 2001; 12(1):1–7 [in Japanese].
71. Beksac MS, Atak Z, Ozlu T. Severe factor X deficiency in a twin pregnancy. Arch Gynecol Obstet 2010;281:151–2.
72. van Veen JJ, Hampton KK, Maclean R, et al. Blood product support for delivery in severe factor X deficiency: the use of thrombin generation to guide therapy. Blood Transfus 2007;5(4):204–9.

73. Chiossi G, Spero JA, Esaka EJ, et al. Plasma exchange in a case of severe factor X deficiency in pregnancy: critical review of the literature. Am J Perinatol 2008;25(3):189–92.
74. Girolami A, Lazzarin M, Scarpa R, et al. Further studies on the abnormal factor X (factor X Friuli) coagulation disorder: a report of another family. Blood 1971; 37(5):534–41.
75. de Sousa C, Clark T, Bradshaw A. Antenatally diagnosed subdural haemorrhage in congenital factor X deficiency. Arch Dis Child 1988;63(10 Spec No): 1168–70.
76. Konje JC, Murphy P, de Chazal R, et al. Severe factor X deficiency and successful pregnancy. Br J Obstet Gynaecol 1994;101(10):910–1.
77. Larrain C. Congenital blood coagulation factor X deficiency. [Successful result of the use prothrombin concentrated complex in the control of ++cesarean section hemorrhage in 2 pregnancies]. Rev Med Chil 1994;122(10):1178–83 [in Spanish].
78. Kumar M, Mehta P. Congenital coagulopathies and pregnancy: report of four pregnancies in a factor X-deficient woman. Am J Hematol 1994;46(3):241–4.
79. Bofill JA, Young RA, Perry KG Jr. Successful pregnancy in a woman with severe factor X deficiency. Obstet Gynecol 1996;88(4 Pt 2):723.
80. Rezig K, Diar N, Benabidallah D, et al. [Factor X deficiency and pregnancy]. Ann Fr Anesth Reanim 2002;21(6):521–4 [in French].
81. Romagnolo C, Burati S, Ciaffoni S, et al. Severe factor X deficiency in pregnancy: case report and review of the literature. Haemophilia 2004;10(5):665–8.
82. Asakai R, Davie EW, Chung DW. Organization of the gene for human factor XI. Biochemistry 1987;26(23):7221–8.
83. Seligsohn U. High gene frequency of factor XI (PTA) deficiency in Ashkenazi Jews. Blood 1978;51(6):1223–8.
84. Peyvandi F, Lak M, Mannucci PM. Factor XI deficiency in Iranians: its clinical manifestations in comparison with those of classic hemophilia. Haematologica 2002;87(5):512–4.
85. Rapaport SI, Proctor RR, Patch MJ, et al. The mode of inheritance of PTA deficiency: evidence for the existence of major PTA deficiency and minor PTA deficiency. Blood 1961;18:149–65.
86. Leiba H, Ramot B, Many A. Heredity and coagulation studies in ten families with factor XI (plasma thromboplastin antecedent) deficiency. Br J Haematol 1965; 11(6):654–65.
87. Bolton-Maggs PH, Young Wan-Yin B, McCraw AH, et al. Inheritance and bleeding in factor XI deficiency. Br J Haematol 1988;69(4):521–8.
88. Gomez K, Bolton-Maggs P. Factor XI deficiency. Haemophilia 2008;14(6): 1183–9.
89. Bolton-Maggs PH, Patterson DA, Wensley RT, et al. Definition of the bleeding tendency in factor XI-deficient kindreds–a clinical and laboratory study. Thromb Haemost 1995;73(2):194–202.
90. Ragni MV, Sinha D, Seaman F, et al. Comparison of bleeding tendency, factor XI coagulant activity, and factor XI antigen in 25 factor XI-deficient kindreds. Blood 1985;65(3):719–24.
91. Kadir RA, Lee CA, Sabin CA, et al. Pregnancy in women with von Willebrand's disease or factor XI deficiency. Br J Obstet Gynaecol 1998;105(3):314–21.
92. Myers B, Pavord S, Kean L, et al. Pregnancy outcome in factor XI deficiency: incidence of miscarriage, antenatal and postnatal haemorrhage in 33 women with factor XI deficiency. BJOG 2007;114:643–6.

93. Chi C, Kulkarni A, Lee CA, et al. The obstetric experience of women with factor XI deficiency. Acta Obstet Gynecol Scand 2009;88:1095–100.
94. Salomon O, Steinberg DM, Tamarin I, et al. Plasma replacement therapy during labor is not mandatory for women with severe factor XI deficiency. Blood Coagul Fibrinolysis 2005;16:37–41.
95. Mannucci PM, Bauer KA, Santagostino E, et al. Activation of the coagulation cascade after infusion of a factor XI concentrate in congenitally deficient patients. Blood 1994;84:1314–9.
96. Bolton-Maggs PH, Colvin BT, Satchi BT, et al. Thrombogenic potential of factor XI concentrate. Lancet 1994;344(8924):748–9.
97. Bolton-Maggs PH, Wensley RT, Kernoff PB, et al. Production and therapeutic use of a factor XI concentrate from plasma. Thromb Haemost 1992;67(3):314–9.
98. Bern MM, Sahud M, Zhukov O, et al. Treatment of factor XI inhibitor using re-combinant activated factor VIIa. Haemophilia 2005;11(1):20–5.
99. Lawler P, White B, Pye S, et al. Successful use of recombinant factor VIIa in a patient with inhibitor secondary to severe factor XI deficiency. Haemophilia 2002;8(2):145–8.
100. Board PG, Losowsky MS, Miloszewski KJ. Factor XIII: inherited and acquired deficiency. Blood Rev 1993;7(4):229–42.
101. Asahina T, Kobayashi T, Okada Y, et al. Maternal blood coagulation factor XIII is associated with the development of cytotrophoblastic shell. Placenta 2000; 21(4):388–93.
102. Koseki-Kuno S, Yamakawa M, Dickneite G, et al. Factor XIII A subunit-deficient mice developed severe uterine bleeding events and subsequent spontaneous miscarriages. Blood 2003;102(13):4410–2.
103. Asahina T, Kobayashi T, Takeuchi K, et al. Congenital blood coagulation factor XIII deficiency and successful deliveries: a review of the literature. Obstet Gyne-col Surv 2007;62:255–60.
104. Ichinose A. Physiopathology and regulation of factor XIII. Thromb Haemost 2001;86:57–65.
105. Kobayashi T, Terao T, Kojima T, et al. Congenital factor XIII deficiency with treat-ment of factor XIII concentrate and normal vaginal delivery. Gynecol Obstet Invest 1990;29:235–8.
106. Kobayashi T, Asahina T, Okada Y, et al. Studies on the localisation of adhesive proteins associated with the development of extravillous cytotrophoblast. Troph Res 1999;13:35–53.
107. Burrows RF, Ray JG, Burrows EA. Bleeding risk and reproductive capacity among patients with factor XIII deficiency: a case presentation and review of the literature. Obstet Gynecol Surv 2000;55(2):103–8.
108. Fukue H, Arai M. Factor XIIIA subunit deficiency. Jpn J Thromb Hemost 2001;12: 66–73.
109. Giddings JC, Seligsohn U, Bloom AL. Immunological studies in combined factor V and factor VIII deficiency. Br J Haematol 1977;37(2):257–64.
110. Nichols WC, Seligsohn U, Zivelin A, et al. Mutations in the ER-Golgi intermediate compartment protein ERGIC-53 cause combined deficiency of coagulation factors V and VIII. Cell 1998;93(1):61–70.
111. Zhang B, McGee B, Yamaoka JS, et al. Combined deficiency of factor V and factor VIII is due to mutations in either LMAN1 or MCFD2. Blood 2006;107(5): 1903–7.
112. Spreafico M, Peyvandi F. Combined FV and FVIII deficiency. Haemophilia 2008; 14:1201–8.

113. Rost S, Fregin A, Ivaskevicius V, et al. Mutations in VKORC1 cause warfarin resistance and multiple coagulation factor deficiency type 2. Nature 2004; 427(6974):537–41.

114. Brenner B, Sanchez-Vega B, Wu SM, et al. A missense mutation in gamma-glutamyl carboxylase gene causes combined deficiency of all vitamin K-dependent blood coagulation factors. Blood 1998;92(12):4554–9.

115. Oldenburg J, von Brederlow B, Fregin A, et al. Congenital deficiency of vitamin K dependent coagulation factors in two families presents as a genetic defect of the vitamin K-epoxide-reductase-complex. Thromb Haemost 2000;84(6): 937–41.

116. McMahon MJ, James AH. Combined deficiency of factors II, VII, IX, and X (Borgschulte-Grigsby deficiency) in pregnancy. Obstet Gynecol 2001;97(5 Pt 2):808–9.

117. Mousallem M, Spronk HM, Sacy R, et al. Congenital combined deficiencies of all vitamin K-dependent coagulation factors. Thromb Haemost 2001;86(5):1334–6.

118. Johnson CA, Chung KS, McGrath KM, et al. Characterization of a variant prothrombin in a patient congenitally deficient in factors II, VII, IX and X. Br J Haematol 1980;44(3):461–9.

119. Vicente V, Maia R, Alberca I, et al. Congenital deficiency of vitamin K-dependent coagulation factors and protein C. Thromb Haemost 1984;51(3):343–6.

120. Lindley CM, Sawyer WT, Macik BG, et al. Pharmacokinetics and pharmacodynamics of recombinant factor VIIa. Clin Pharmacol Ther 1994;55(6):638–48.

Treating Venous Thromboembolism in Pregnancy

Annemarie E. Fogerty, MD[a,b], Jean M. Connors, MD[b,c],*

KEYWORDS

- Venous thromboembolism • Pregnancy • Diagnostic testing
- Heparin

INCIDENCE

The likelihood for venous thromboembolism (VTE) in pregnancy is increased fourfold to fivefold, with an estimated incidence of 0.76 to 1.72 per 1000 pregnancies.[1,2] Two thirds of deep vein thromboses (DVT) occur antepartum and are distributed evenly between trimesters, while approximately 50% of pulmonary emboli (PE) occur postpartum.[2–5] Estimates of death for PE are 1.1 to 1.5 per 100,000 deliveries in the United Sates and Europe.[2,6] While there is decreased blood flow velocity in the distal legs as pregnancy progresses, the fact that DVTs are evenly distributed between trimesters argues that hormonal or coagulation changes inherent to pregnancy are the primary drivers of increased VTE risk.

COAGULATION CHANGES DURING PREGNANCY

Changes during normal pregnancy promote coagulation, decrease anticoagulation, and inhibit fibrinolysis.[7,8] Specifically there is a marked increase in coagulation factors II, VII, VIII, IX, and X, as well as von Willebrand factor. There is also a decrease of physiologic anticoagulants, with protein S levels falling to 40% to 60%, starting in the first trimester and remaining decreased for 3 months postpartum. This change is attributable to an estrogen-induced decrease in total protein S and an increase in C4b, which binds protein S. The combined impact of decreased protein S and increased Factor VIII leads to increased resistance to activated protein C.

[a] Department of Hematology/Oncology, Massachusetts General Hospital Cancer Center, 55 Fruit Street, Yawkey 7B, Boston, MA 02114, USA
[b] Harvard Medical School, Boston, MA, USA
[c] Division of Hematology, Department of Medicine, Brigham and Women's Hospital and Dana Farber Cancer Institute, 75 Francis Street, Boston, MA 02115, USA
* Corresponding author. Division of Hematology, Department of Medicine, Brigham and Women's Hospital, 75 Francis Street, Boston, MA 02115, USA.
E-mail address: jconnors@partners.org

Hematol Oncol Clin N Am 25 (2011) 379–391
doi:10.1016/j.hoc.2011.02.004
0889-8588/11/$ – see front matter © 2011 Published by Elsevier Inc.

DIAGNOSIS: LABORATORY ANALYSIS

As pregnant women are at increased risk, clinicians should exercise a heightened suspicion for VTE. Making the diagnosis, however, can be complicated by the fact that reasonable alternatives to VTE also exist at higher frequencies in pregnant women. The traditional signs of VTE, such as an edematous or tender extremity, chest wall pain, shortness of breath, tachypnea, or tachycardia can occur in healthy pregnancies. To complicate matters further, the D-dimer test, which is commonly used in nonpregnant patients to indicate VTE probability, is often elevated in healthy pregnancies. Therefore, as highlighted in the following two studies, the D-dimer is not a reliable marker for determining the likelihood of gestational VTE.

In a prospective study of 800 women,[9] who had 391 with uncomplicated pregnancies, vaginal deliveries and uneventful postpartum periods were analyzed. The D-dimer concentration increased progressively throughout gestation, peaking on postpartum day 1 and decreasing starting on postpartum day 2. A D-dimer level of 0.5 mg/L or greater is the generally accepted threshold for determining high probability versus low probability for VTE in nonpregnant patients. Between gestational weeks 13 and 20, however, more than 25% of included pregnant patients had D-dimer levels that exceeded 0.5 mg/L. After week 36, virtually all pregnant patients had D-dimer levels greater than 0.5 mg/L. These patients had no complaints consistent with symptoms of VTE.

Similar findings were seen by Kovac and colleagues,[10] who collected D-dimer values prospectively in 89 healthy pregnancies and compared these with the D-dimer values of 12 pregnant women clinically suspected to have VTE. Among the women with healthy pregnancies, 84% had normal D-dimer levels in the first trimester. The number of women with normal D-dimer values decreased to 33% in the second trimester and was only 1% in the third trimester. Women with positive ultrasound findings for VTE, however, had a statistically significant elevation in the D-dimer level compared with controls. Thus, the investigators proposed new values for D-dimer thresholds in pregnancy that should vary with trimesters: 286, 457, and 644 ng/mL in the first, second, and third trimesters, respectively. This increased D-dimer threshold is intended to reflect the natural increase in D-dimer during gestation. This approach has not yet been validated.

DIAGNOSIS: RADIOLOGIC STUDIES

Given the lack of reliability in pregnancy, D-dimer levels should not be used independently to diagnose or exclude VTE. The clinician therefore must also be aware of the risks and sensitivity of radiographic studies used to assess VTE in pregnancy.

Compression duplex ultrasonography of the legs is noninvasive and considered safe in pregnancy. Given the safety profile, it should be the first test obtained for any pregnant woman presenting with symptoms suggestive of VTE. Its limitations are that efficacy has not been clearly defined in the pregnant population. In addition, pregnant women may also develop iliac vein thrombosis, which would not be detected on traditional compression duplex ultrasonography. These women typically present with back pain and swelling of the entire lower limb. If a DVT is diagnosed, treatment with therapeutic anticoagulation should be started. If clinical suspicion is high for DVT but the initial ultrasound result is negative, the ultrasound scan should be repeated in 1 week. Ultrasonography should also be repeated in 1 week if a superficial thrombosis is present but the ultrasonogram is negative for DVT. If there is concern for iliac vein thrombosis, magnetic resonance venography or pulsed Doppler study is recommended.

If a PE is suspected clinically, examination of the lower extremities with duplex ultrasonography should still be the first diagnostic test performed. A definitive DVT is treated with the same intensity and duration of anticoagulation as a PE, and therefore radiologic confirmation of a PE is not required. Alternatively, if a PE is suspected but the ultrasonogram is negative for DVT, further testing is required.

The majority of trials establishing the use of radionuclide imaging to diagnose PE excluded pregnant subjects. One small study[11] examined 120 pregnant patients with ventilation perfusion scans (VQ scans) to evaluate symptoms suggestive of PE. Eight of these women were already receiving anticoagulation at the time of the study. Of the remaining cases, 73.5% of the VQ scans were normal, 24.8% were nondiagnostic, and 1.8% were of high probability for PE. Images were evaluated by 2 independent experts. The women with normal or nondiagnostic images were not treated with anticoagulation, and the patients were followed for a mean of 20.6 months. During this follow-up interval, there was no subsequent diagnosis of PE.

This study[11] also examined pregnancy outcomes in the women who had undergone VQ scanning. A low number of adverse pregnancy outcomes such as early or late pregnancy loss were reported for all stages of pregnancy. A low incidence of congenital structural anomalies and developmental disorders in early childhood were noted. None of these were felt to be attributable to exposure from VQ scanning. There were no childhood cancers or leukemia reported in this small study. Therefore, use of VQ scanning in these pregnant subjects was not associated with any increased risk of poor fetal outcome.

While VQ scanning has an acceptable safety profile in pregnancy, this same study highlights that one-fourth of cases will be nondiagnostic. In fact, VQ scans are known to be negative in 73% to 92% of pregnant women suspected to have PE.[12,13] When a VQ scan is nondiagnostic a computed tomography (CT) scan is often required, which ultimately exposes the patient to more total radiation than if the CT scan was the first diagnostic test performed. Another advantage of the CT scan is that unlike the VQ scan, CT provides alternative diagnostic information, such as evidence of pneumonia, pulmonary edema, or aortic dissection, when PE is not confirmed. Therefore, the CT scan is the preferred tool for evaluating respiratory complaints or diagnosing PE in pregnancy.

One noninferiority randomized trial[14] directly compared CT and VQ scans in assessing patients with high clinical suspicion for PE, based on the Wells Clinical Criteria and a positive D-dimer test. Patients with high clinical suspicion for PE but with negative or nondiagnostic images also underwent ultrasound evaluation of the legs. Although pregnant women were excluded, these data demonstrate that CT is not inferior to VQ scanning for ruling out PE. Of the 701 patients randomized to undergo CT, 19.2% were diagnosed with PE or DVT, versus 14.2% of the 716 patients randomized to the VQ arm. The difference in the percentage of VTE diagnosis was statistically significant between the two groups, raising some concern that the CT scan may be diagnosing clinically insignificant events. The primary outcome of this study was the subsequent development of symptomatic PE or proximal DVT among the patients with an initial negative image and an excluded PE diagnosis. Of these patients, 1.0% of the VQ scan patients versus 0.4% of the CT scan patients were ultimately diagnosed with VTE in the 3-month follow-up period, including one fatal PE in the VQ scan group. This difference was not statistically significant. Of note, 54.2% of patients in the VQ scan arm had nondiagnostic images. Among this group, 7.0% were ultimately diagnosed with VTE after further testing (initial ultrasound scans of the lower extremities, CT scan, or conventional pulmonary angiography), suggesting that clinicians in the study lacked confidence in a nondiagnostic VQ scan when there was high clinical suspicion of PE. Alternatively, in only 3 cases was a VQ scan ordered following a negative CT scan in a patient with high clinical suspicion of PE; in all of these cases, the VQ scan was also negative.[14] Although these results support that fact that the VQ scan and CT scan are equivalent in diagnosing PE in the appropriate high-risk clinical group, the assignment of high risk was determined based on D-dimer testing and the Wells Clinical Criteria for PE. As previously described, these two metrics are different in the pregnant and nonpregnant populations, and therefore the authors' recommendation favoring CT over VQ scan when chest imaging is required to assess for PE in pregnancy.

Despite this recommendation, there are no published data documenting the specificity and sensitivity of diagnosing PE by CT in pregnant patients. There is also theoretical concern that the hyperdynamic circulation and increased plasma volume of pregnancy may decrease the sensitivity. In addition, there is concern that ionizing radiation may increase the risk of fetal malignancy or other birth defects; therefore, appropriate radiation reduction strategies should be exercised. There are insufficient data on the safety of gadolinium in pregnant patients to recommend magnetic resonance angiographic techniques in assessing gestational VTE.

Despite the theoretical concern of using ionizing radiation in pregnant women, the 2004 American Congress of Obstetricians and Gynecologists (ACOG) committee guidelines state that fetal risks from radiation exposure are negligible when doses are less than 0.05 Gy. Doses of 0.1 Gy and higher were determined to result in a combined increased risk of organ malformation or childhood cancers of approximately 1%. The guidelines further estimate that the combined radiation from chest radiography, CT, and pulmonary angiography expose the fetus to around 1.5 mGy of radiation, which is well below the 0.05 Gy dose recommendation.[15]

Other published estimates of fetal exposure from maternal CT scanning when dose reduction methods are employed confirm that the overall dose is low.[16,17] Most of the literature on childhood cancers and in utero radiation exposure is case reports. These reports were reviewed by Ginsberg and colleagues[18] who found a small, but statistically significant increased relative risk of childhood cancer when exposed to 0.05 Gy. In the cases reviewed, however, there was no increase in pregnancy loss or growth retardation.

Another study measured the amount of radiation to which a fetus would be exposed during CT pulmonary angiography scans by using an anthropomorphic phantom to represent the chest and gravid abdomen of a woman in late gestation. Three different helical scanners were studied, and estimated fetal doses ranged from 60 to 230 mGy. Strategies for reducing fetal exposure were variably effective: milliampere modulation, shielding with a lead coat, and using a 5-cm shorter scan length. These strategies reduced fetal exposure by 10%, 35%, and 56% respectively.[19] Decreasing scan length by 5 cm excludes the bases of the lungs and therefore prevents examination of the subsegmental arteries. This strategy is predicated on the notion that thrombosis of the subsegmental vessels is associated with less morbidity and mortality.

In a 2009 quality initiatives report, The Radiological Society of North America lists methods to reduce the radiation dose of the maternal breasts and fetus at CT pulmonary angiography (CTA).[20] These methods include lead shielding, a thin-layer bismuth breast shield, reduction in tube current and voltage, increase in pitch, increase in detector collimation thickness, reduction of Z-axis, oral barium preparation, elimination of lateral scout image, fixed injection timing rather than test run, and elimination of any additional CT sequences. Although there is less breast radiation exposure during VQ scans than with CTA, as discussed earlier VQ scans yield more nondiagnostic results. Using VQ scans as the initial diagnostic approach may therefore necessitate a second diagnostic scan using CTA, which results in more overall radiation. The chest CTA results in 0.02 to 0.06 Gy breast radiation, which can be reduced by 50% with use of breast shields.[21,22] There have been no studies that document whether the breast tissue in pregnant women is more vulnerable to radiation damage than in nonpregnant women of the same age.

In summary, the risk of an undiagnosed and therefore untreated VTE in pregnancy is much higher than the risk introduced by using appropriate diagnostic tools in the pregnant patient. Clinical judgment is of chief importance and, when necessary, appropriate expert consultation should be sought to evaluate a pregnant woman presenting with signs suggestive of VTE. Obvious care should be taken to minimize the risks and exposure involved in diagnostic testing. Pregnant women suspected to have VTE should first undergo compression ultrasonography of the lower extremities to assess for DVT. If the ultrasonogram is negative in a patient with suspected DVT or superficial thrombophlebitis, the ultrasound scan should be repeated in 1 week. If the ultrasonogram is negative for DVT and PE is suspected, pulmonary imaging with CTA should be performed with radiation-minimizing practices. If VTE is diagnosed by positive extremity ultrasonogram but respiratory symptoms persist after appropriate treatment with anticoagulation, diagnostic chest imaging should be performed to investigate for alternative diagnoses. Our strategy for evaluation of symptoms suggestive of VTE in a pregnant patient is summarized in **Fig. 1**.

TREATMENT GUIDELINES

The most recent guidelines from the American College of Chest Physicians (ACCP)[23] and the *American Journal of Obstetrics and Gynecology* Consensus Report[24] outline treatment recommendations for VTE in pregnancy. Women who develop VTE at any point during gestation require anticoagulation for the remainder of the pregnancy and for 6 to 8 weeks postpartum. Treatment should be continued beyond 2 months

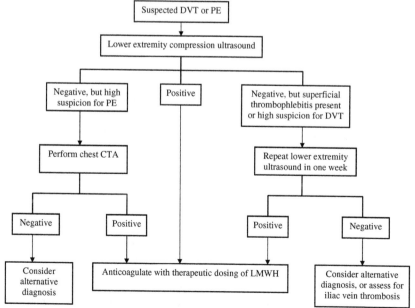

Fig. 1. Approach to diagnosis of suspected VTE in pregnancy.

postpartum if necessary to complete a minimum of 6 months' total anticoagulation. Treatment for VTE is full-intensity anticoagulation, usually with low molecular weight heparin (LMWH), adjusted for weight changes throughout pregnancy. Fondaparinux, a pentasaccharide anticoagulant, has also been used in pregnancy, although the published case reports are limited[25,26] to a small number of women unable to tolerate LMWH. Although there have been no adverse outcomes, more data are needed to document safety and efficacy of fondaparinux in pregnancy. Direct thrombin inhibitors have been demonstrated to cross the placenta in animal models, albeit with low transference, and therefore are not used in pregnant humans.[27] Similarly, the new oral Xa inhibitor agents available for use in treating VTE in Europe and Canada have not been used in pregnant women.

The majority of pregnant patients with VTE can be safely treated at home. Their weight needs to be regularly monitored and the LMWH dose should be adjusted accordingly. The pharmacokinetics of LMWH have not been clearly defined in pregnancy, and may be variable between women. The half-life of LMWH has been demonstrated to be shorter in pregnancy, likely due to increased renal clearance.[28] Routine monitoring of anti-Xa levels, however, is not usually performed. Exceptions are made for patients with renal insufficiency or obesity. In such patients anti-Xa levels should be checked for each dose change, change in creatinine clearance, or other parameters affecting levels, and at least once each trimester to ensure that the patient is in the desired therapeutic range.[29] Additional information on treatment in patients with renal insufficiency is given later in a separate section. Compression stockings are recommended to prevent postphlebitic syndrome in any DVT diagnosis.

While many studies have supported the safety of both unfractionated heparin (UFH) and LMWH in pregnancy, LMWH is preferred because it requires less monitoring and is associated with less bone loss, and there have been no documented cases of heparin-induced thrombocytopenia when used in pregnancy.[30]

Warfarin

Women receiving warfarin for VTE diagnosed before pregnancy should be transitioned to a heparin product once pregnancy is confirmed. Women receiving warfarin for reasons other than VTE (such as mechanical heart valves) are outside the scope of this review and are not necessarily transitioned to heparin for the entire pregnancy. Warfarin is not used for treatment of VTE in pregnancy because birth defects have been reported in 5% to 10% of children exposed to warfarin in utero between weeks 6 and 12. Warfarin also crosses the placenta and may therefore anticoagulate the fetus, posing the potential risk of fetal intracranial hemorrhage during delivery.[23,31,32] Women taking warfarin for VTE who desire pregnancy should be advised to check pregnancy tests frequently, and contact their medical team with a positive test to discontinue warfarin and start heparin at that time. These women do not require transitioning from warfarin to heparin prior to a confirmed pregnancy. Women can safely receive warfarin postpartum.

LMWH Versus Heparin: Osteopenia

Long-term use of UFH at treatment doses is known to cause osteopenia. There is less risk associated with use of LMWH. One study[33] examined bone health in 184 pregnant women who received long-term subcutaneous prophylaxis with UFH twice daily because of increased risk of VTE. The mean heparin dose was 19,100 IU in a 24-hour period, and the average duration of exposure was 25 weeks. Symptomatic osteoporotic fractures of the spine occurred in 4 women postpartum, which represented 2.2% of the total group studied. The mean heparin dose for these 4 women was 24,500 IU in 24 hours.

It is possible that the osteopenia secondary to UFH is reversible. In one study,[34] 70 pregnant women received UFH subcutaneously for either treatment of or thromboprophylaxis against VTE. Sixty-eight of these women underwent spine and hip radiographs in the first week postpartum. Twelve of these women (17%) had osteopenia; 2 (3%) had multiple fractures. Reexamination 6 to 12 months later showed that the osteopenia was reversed in most cases. A second part of this study repeated the radiographs 3 years after gestational UFH exposure. Among the 18 women included in this delayed investigation, there was no osteopenia documented.

There is less concern for osteopenia when using LMWH as compared with UFH. One larger study[35] undertaken to determine the effectiveness of antepartum LMWH on pregnancy outcomes included a substudy of 77 patients to evaluate the rate of osteoporosis associated with gestational LMWH exposure. The women received dalteparin and underwent bone mineral density testing. In total, 62 patients were analyzed. The intervention group received dalteparin antepartum and postpartum (mean of 212 total days); the control group received dalteparin only postpartum (mean of 38 days). There was no difference in mean bone mineral densities between the groups. Similar findings were seen in a trial of 44 pregnant women randomized to receive LMWH (dalteparin) once daily or UFH twice daily because of history of previous or current VTE.[36] Bone mineral density was collected from each group, as well as from pregnant women who did not receive any anticoagulation. The mean bone mineral density was significantly lower in the UFH group than in the LMWH and non-anticoagulated groups. A large meta-analysis[30] including 64 studies and 2777 total pregnancies in which LMWH was used reported one case of documented osteoporosis and postpartum vertebral fracture. This woman had received high-dose dalteparin for 36 weeks.

Bleeding

The more commonly cited concern for use of heparin products in pregnancy is bleeding. Neither UFH[37] nor LMWH cross the placenta. Anti-Xa levels have been measured in fetal blood from mothers receiving LMWH, and showed no activity.[38,39] A meta-analysis frequently cited in support of thromboprophylaxis[30] included 64 studies and 2777 total pregnancies in which LMWH was used, for both treatment and prophylaxis. The prophylaxis group had widely variable indications for use, but in total there was a reported VTE rate of 0.84%. Given the heterogeneous diagnoses of included women, this study does not support the efficacy of LMWH for prophylaxis; however, it can be used to assess the safety profile of LMWH in pregnancy. The overall hemorrhage rate was 1.99%: 0.42% antenatal, 0.92% postpartum, and 0.65% wound hematomas.

Thrombolytic Therapy

As in nonpregnant patients, the use of thrombolytic drugs in pregnancy should be reserved for treatment of those patients with significant hemodynamic instability or compromise. In a review of 28 cases using thrombolysis in pregnancy,[40] 7 women received treatment for PE and 3 women for DVT. The complication rate was similar to that of nonpregnant patients. Another publication[41] reviewed use of thrombolytic medications in 172 pregnant women, with varied indications. In total there were 1.2% maternal deaths, 5.8% pregnancy losses, and 8.1% hemorrhagic complications. It has yet to be determined whether the observed pregnancy specific complications such as preterm labor, pregnancy loss, or placental abruption were caused by underlying PE, thrombolytic therapy, both, or neither.

Special Circumstances: Renal Insufficiency and Obesity

Pregnant women with renal insufficiency require close monitoring with anti-Xa levels when using either UFH or LMWH. The trough anti-Xa level should be collected just before the next dose is administered. Once a stable dosing schedule is determined by this method, anti-Xa levels should be repeated for any change in weight, anticoagulant dose, or creatinine clearance.

Anti-Xa level is preferred over partial thromboplastin time (PTT), as the PTT in pregnancy is influenced by factors other than anticoagulation alone. PTT can be attenuated by increased fibrinogen and Factor VIII activity. Thus, a pregnant patient would require a higher heparin dose to achieve the same PTT level, which may result in overdosing. This process was demonstrated in one study[42] where known concentrations of UFH were added to the in vitro plasma samples of 13 pregnant women in their third trimesters and compared with plasma samples of 15 nonpregnant women. The PTT and anti-Xa activities were measured at increasing UFH concentrations. The anti-Xa levels more accurately correlated with change in heparin concentrations. Therefore, the anti-Xa level is preferred for monitoring UFH.

PERIPARTUM MANAGEMENT

Balancing the bleeding risks of delivery and associated procedures with the risk of recurrent VTE is most difficult during the peripartum time period, as the timing of onset of spontaneous labor is unpredictable. Anticoagulation therapy is usually altered during the last weeks of pregnancy to minimize bleeding risks and allow for neuraxial anesthesia if desired or necessary. Collaboration between obstetricians, hematologists, and anesthesiologists is required to determine optimal management of anticoagulation at the time of labor and delivery, and the use of regional anesthesia in a pregnant woman with VTE.

For pregnant women with VTE diagnosed longer than 4 weeks before estimated delivery, LMWH anticoagulation should be held 24 hours before scheduled delivery and restarted immediately after hemostasis is assured. While there is obvious concern about excessive maternal bleeding, studies do not necessarily support this concern. One small study[43] reviewed 41 total pregnancies managed with LMWH, where 87.5% of included subjects received only prophylactic dosing of 40 mg enoxaparin daily. Women received LMWH throughout gestation, labor, and delivery, and immediately postpartum. There were no reports of excessive bleeding in these patients, including the small number of therapeutically anticoagulated mothers. There were no cases of intraventricular hemorrhage in the neonates. For most women on full-intensity anticoagulation, simply holding the LMWH for 24 hours is sufficient if scheduled induction or cesarean section is planned for obstetric purposes.

In the immediate 2- to 4-week period after VTE diagnosis, there is a high rate of mortality if therapeutic anticoagulation is stopped or actively reversed. Therefore, it is unfavorable for women diagnosed with VTE within 4 weeks of expected delivery to have therapeutic anticoagulation held for 24 hours for the purposes of labor and delivery. In this circumstance, use of continuous intravenous UFH and should be considered. The intravenous UFH can be stopped 4 to 6 hours before delivery or when the patient goes into labor, with the PTT and anti-Xa levels used to monitor the coagulation status. In patients with extensive DVT or PE, consideration for scheduled induction of labor or cesarean delivery should be considered to minimize the duration of time without anticoagulation.

Use of inferior vena cava (IVC) filters in patients with DVT to permit reversal of anti-coagulation for labor is controversial and is generally not advised, as the data for nonpregnant patients suggests that IVC filters have limited efficacy in preventing PE. In particular, one review cataloged the complications involved in IVC filter placement,[44] with the most significant early complication being insertion site thrombosis at 8.5%. However, over a course of 15 months of follow-up, the risk for recurrent DVT was 21%, recurrent PE 3%, IVC thrombosis 2% to 10%, and postthrombotic syndrome 15% to 40%. Another retrospective study[45] showed that IVC filter placement in a patient who can tolerate anticoagulation offers no benefit in recurrent DVT, PE, or mortality. Given the potential complications of IVC filter placement and risk for long-term sequelae if the filter is unable to be removed, the overall low risk for bleeding even in fully anticoaugulated mothers, and the option of limiting the time without anticoagulation to several hours, the authors do not recommend routine use of IVC filters.

UFH has a shorter half life than LMWH: 1.5 hours for UFH versus 3 to 6 hours after a single dose of LMWH.[46,47] The half-life of enoxaparin may increase to 7 hours after repeated dosing. This feature is the rationale behind the common practice of transitioning a woman from LMWH to UFH at approximately 36 weeks' gestation. There is also the perceived appeal of being able to use protamine to reverse UFH for a laboring mother who is anticoagulated. However, the impact of protamine on the fetus has not been widely studied. There is one case report[48] of significant respiratory depression in a neonate born at 39.5 weeks where the mother received 25 mg of protamine. Therefore, the use of protamine should be reserved for cases of significant bleeding and not reflexively given to all anticoagulated mothers receiving heparin.

Recently the American Society of Regional Anesthesia and Pain Medicine (ASRAPM) published evidence-based guidelines for use of regional anesthesia in patients receiving antithrombotic therapy.[49] There is limited literature specific to the use of regional anesthesia in pregnant patients and, as such, the obstetric guidelines are based on data adopted from other surgical literature. This publication notes that there have been no published case reports of spinal hematoma in a pregnant patient receiving antithrombotic therapy at the time of delivery, with or without the use of neuraxial blockade. These guidelines advocate the use of UFH or LMWH by gestational week 36 for the rare patient managed with oral anticoagulants. The guidelines further suggest discontinuing LMWH at least 36 hours before induction of labor or cesarean section, and substituting UFH (either intravenously or subcutaneously) if needed. If intravenous heparin is instituted, it should be held 4 to 6 hours before anticipated delivery with PTT monitoring to ensure acceptable range. Based on this recommendation, many practitioners choose to transition a pregnant patient from LMWH to UFH at 36 weeks, particularly in cases of anticipated spontaneous labor. For scheduled induction of labor and cesarean sections, however, use of LMWH can be continued beyond 36 weeks.

The ASRAPM guidelines also present recommendations for the timing of neuraxial anesthesia when a patient is receiving prophylactic UFH or LMWH. In general, guidelines recommend delaying needle placement until 4 to 12 hours after the last dose of UFH, and waiting at least 1 hour after catheter removal before resuming heparin. For women receiving therapeutic dosing of LMWH, the guidelines recommend delaying needle placement until 24 hours after the last administered dose. There is no single rule regarding the safety of using epidural anesthesia and the exact timing of discontinuation of anticoagulation for all pregnant women, and decisions must be made in collaboration with hematologists, obstetricians, and anesthesiologists in the best interest of the individual patient.

POSTPARTUM MANAGEMENT

After hemostasis is assured and epidural catheters safely removed, women should be restarted on anticoagulation. Treatment should be continued for a minimum of 6 weeks following a vaginal delivery and 8 weeks following a cesarean delivery, but extended as needed to complete a total of 6 months of anticoagulation from the date of the VTE diagnosis. Therapeutic anticoagulation with either heparin or warfarin is safe in nursing mothers.

SUMMARY

Clinicians should exercise a heightened level of suspicion for VTE in pregnant women, as they are at increased risk for VTE but can present with symptoms that can have multiple etiological factors. Although the D-dimer assay has limited diagnostic value in pregnancy, the use of compression ultrasonography, VQ, and pulmonary CT can be used safely. The authors' preferred diagnostic approach is to start with a lower extremity ultrasonogram in women with suspected VTE, reserving use of pulmonary CT for negative ultrasound results or persistent pulmonary complaint after starting anticoagulation in women with documented DVT. Treatment is full-intensity anticoagulation with a heparin product for the remainder of pregnancy and 6 to 8 weeks postpartum, to complete a minimum of 6 months. LMWH has been documented to be safe in pregnancy, with minimal side effects. The most difficult aspect of treating VTE in pregnancy is planning the interruption of anticoagulation for labor and delivery. Decisions on the exact plan for management of anticoagulation in preparation for labor and delivery should be made on an individual case basis with input from all members of a multidisciplinary team involving obstetricians, hematologists, and anesthesiologists.

REFERENCES

1. Heit JA, Kobbervig CE, James AH, et al. Trends in the incidence of venous thromboembolism during pregnancy or postpartum: a 30-year population-based study. Ann Intern Med 2005;143(10):697–706.
2. James AH, Jamison MG, Brancazio LR, et al. Venous thromboembolism during pregnancy and the postpartum period: incidence, risk factors, and mortality. Am J Obstet Gynecol 2006;194(5):1311–5.
3. Ray JG, Chan WS. Deep vein thrombosis during pregnancy and the puerperium: a meta-analysis of the period of risk and the leg of presentation. Obstet Gynecol Surv 1999;54(4):265–71.
4. Simpson EL, Lawrenson RA, Nightingale AL, et al. Venous thromboembolism in pregnancy and the puerperium: incidence and additional risk factors from a London perinatal database. BJOG 2001;108(1):56–60.
5. James AH, Tapson VF, Goldhaber SZ. Thrombosis during pregnancy and the postpartum period. Am J Obstet Gynecol 2005;193(1):216–9.
6. Weindling AM. The confidential enquiry into maternal and child health (CEMACH). Arch Dis Child 2003;88(12):1034–7.
7. Lockwood CJ. Pregnancy-associated changes in the hemostatic system. Clin Obstet Gynecol 2006;49(4):836–43.
8. Hellgren M. Hemostasis during normal pregnancy and puerperium. Semin Thromb Hemost 2003;29(2):125–30.

9. Szecsi PB, Jorgensen M, Klajnbard A, et al. Haemostatic reference intervals in pregnancy. Thromb Haemost 2010;103(4):718–27.
10. Kovac M, Mikovic Z, Rakicevic L, et al. The use of D-dimer with new cutoff can be useful in diagnosis of venous thromboembolism in pregnancy. Eur J Obstet Gynecol Reprod Biol 2010;148(1):27–30.
11. Chan WS, Ray JG, Murray S, et al. Suspected pulmonary embolism in pregnancy: clinical presentation, results of lung scanning, and subsequent maternal and pediatric outcomes. Arch Intern Med 2002;162(10):1170–5.
12. Scarsbrook AF, Bradley KM, Gleeson FV. Perfusion scintigraphy: diagnostic utility in pregnant women with suspected pulmonary embolic disease. Eur Radiol 2007; 17(10):2554–60.
13. Scarsbrook AF, Evans AL, Owen AR, et al. Diagnosis of suspected venous thromboembolic disease in pregnancy. Clin Radiol 2006;61(1):1–12.
14. Anderson DR, Kahn SR, Rodger MA, et al. Computed tomographic pulmonary angiography vs ventilation-perfusion lung scanning in patients with suspected pulmonary embolism: a randomized controlled trial. JAMA 2007;298(23):2743–53.
15. ACOG Committee on Obstetric Practice. ACOG Committee Opinion. Number 299, September 2004 (replaces No. 158, September 1995). Guidelines for diagnostic imaging during pregnancy. Obstet Gynecol 2004;104(3):647–51.
16. Le Gal G, Righini M. More on: diagnosing pulmonary embolism in pregnancy: rationalizing fetal radiation exposure in radiological procedures. J Thromb Haemost 2005;3(4):813–4 [author reply: 814–5].
17. Nijkeuter M, Geleijns J, De Roos A, et al. Diagnosing pulmonary embolism in pregnancy: rationalizing fetal radiation exposure in radiological procedures. J Thromb Haemost 2004;2(10):1857–8.
18. Ginsberg JS, Hirsh J, Rainbow AJ, et al. Risks to the fetus of radiologic procedures used in the diagnosis of maternal venous thromboembolic disease. Thromb Haemost 1989;61(2):189–96.
19. Doshi SK, Negus IS, Oduko JM. Fetal radiation dose from CT pulmonary angiography in late pregnancy: a phantom study. Br J Radiol 2008;81(968):653–8.
20. Pahade JK, Litmanovich D, Pedrosa I, et al. Quality initiatives: imaging pregnant patients with suspected pulmonary embolism: what the radiologist needs to know. Radiographics 2009;29(3):639–54.
21. Hurwitz LM, Yoshizumi TT, Reiman RE, et al. Radiation dose to the female breast from 16-MDCT body protocols. AJR Am J Roentgenol 2006;186(6): 1718–22.
22. Hopper KD, King SH, Lobell ME, et al. The breast: in-plane x-ray protection during diagnostic thoracic CT—shielding with bismuth radioprotective garments. Radiology 1997;205(3):853–8.
23. Bates SM, Greer IA, Pabinger I, et al. Venous thromboembolism, thrombophilia, antithrombotic therapy, and pregnancy: American College of Chest Physicians evidence-based clinical practice guidelines (8th edition). Chest 2008;133(Suppl 6):844S–86S.
24. Duhl AJ, Paidas MJ, Ural SH, et al. Antithrombotic therapy and pregnancy: consensus report and recommendations for prevention and treatment of venous thromboembolism and adverse pregnancy outcomes. Am J Obstet Gynecol 2007;197(5):457, e1–21.
25. Dempfle CE. Minor transplacental passage of fondaparinux in vivo. N Engl J Med 2004;350(18):1914–5.
26. Mazzolai L, Hohlfeld P, Spertini F, et al. Fondaparinux is a safe alternative in case of heparin intolerance during pregnancy. Blood 2006;108(5):1569–70.

27. Markwardt F, Fink G, Kaiser B, et al. Pharmacological survey of recombinant hirudin. Pharmazie 1988;43(3):202–7.
28. Sephton V, Farquharson RG, Topping J, et al. A longitudinal study of maternal dose response to low molecular weight heparin in pregnancy. Obstet Gynecol 2003;101(6):1307–11.
29. Laposata M, Green D, Van Cott EM, et al. College of American Pathologists Conference XXXI on laboratory monitoring of anticoagulant therapy: the clinical use and laboratory monitoring of low-molecular-weight heparin, danaparoid, hirudin and related compounds, and argatroban. Arch Pathol Lab Med 1998;122(9): 799–807.
30. Greer IA, Nelson-Piercy C. Low-molecular-weight heparins for thromboprophylaxis and treatment of venous thromboembolism in pregnancy: a systematic review of safety and efficacy. Blood 2005;106(2):401–7.
31. Chan WS, Anand S, Ginsberg JS. Anticoagulation of pregnant women with mechanical heart valves: a systematic review of the literature. Arch Intern Med 2000;160(2):191–6.
32. Hall JG, Pauli RM, Wilson KM. Maternal and fetal sequelae of anticoagulation during pregnancy. Am J Med 1980;68(1):122–40.
33. Dahlman TC. Osteoporotic fractures and the recurrence of thromboembolism during pregnancy and the puerperium in 184 women undergoing thromboprophylaxis with heparin. Am J Obstet Gynecol 1993;168(4):1265–70.
34. Dahlman T, Lindvall N, Hellgren M. Osteopenia in pregnancy during long-term heparin treatment: a radiological study post partum. Br J Obstet Gynaecol 1990;97(3):221–8.
35. Rodger MA, Kahn SR, Cranney A, et al. Long-term dalteparin in pregnancy not associated with a decrease in bone mineral density: substudy of a randomized controlled trial. J Thromb Haemost 2007;5(8):1600–6.
36. Pettila V, Leinonen P, Markkola A, et al. Postpartum bone mineral density in women treated for thromboprophylaxis with unfractionated heparin or LMW heparin. Thromb Haemost 2002;87(2):182–6.
37. Flessa HC, Kapstrom AB, Glueck HI, et al. Placental transport of heparin. Am J Obstet Gynecol 1965;93(4):570–3.
38. Forestier F, Daffos F, Rainaut M, et al. Low molecular weight heparin (CY 216) does not cross the placenta during the third trimester of pregnancy. Thromb Haemost 1987;57(2):234.
39. Forestier F, Daffos F, Capella-Pavlovsky M. Low molecular weight heparin (PK 10169) does not cross the placenta during the second trimester of pregnancy study by direct fetal blood sampling under ultrasound. Thromb Res 1984;34(6): 557–60.
40. Leonhardt G, Gaul C, Nietsch HH, et al. Thrombolytic therapy in pregnancy. J Thromb Thrombolysis 2006;21(3):271–6.
41. Turrentine MA, Braems G, Ramirez MM. Use of thrombolytics for the treatment of thromboembolic disease during pregnancy. Obstet Gynecol Surv 1995;50(7): 534–41.
42. Chunilal SD, Young E, Johnston MA, et al. The APTT response of pregnant plasma to unfractionated heparin. Thromb Haemost 2002;87(1):92–7.
43. Dulitzki M, Pauzner R, Langevitz P, et al. Low-molecular-weight heparin during pregnancy and delivery: preliminary experience with 41 pregnancies. Obstet Gynecol 1996;87(3):380–3.
44. Hann CL, Streiff MB. The role of vena caval filters in the management of venous thromboembolism. Blood Rev 2005;19(4):179–202.

45. Billett HH, Jacobs LG, Madsen EM, et al. Efficacy of inferior vena cava filters in anticoagulated patients. J Thromb Haemost 2007;5(9):1848–53.
46. Estes JW, Poulin PF. Pharmacokinetics of heparin. Distribution and elimination. Thromb Diath Haemorrh 1975;33(1):26–37.
47. Weitz JI. Low-molecular-weight heparins. N Engl J Med 1997;337(10):688–98.
48. Wittmaack FM, Greer FR, FitzSimmons J. Neonatal depression after a protamine sulfate injection. A case report. J Reprod Med 1994;39(8):655–6.
49. Horlocker TT, Wedel DJ, Rowlingson JC, et al. Regional anesthesia in the patient receiving antithrombotic or thrombolytic therapy: American Society of Regional Anesthesia and Pain Medicine evidence-based guidelines (third edition). Reg Anesth Pain Med 2010;35(1):64–101.

Transfusion Medicine and the Pregnant Patient

Alfred Ian Lee, MD, PhD[a], Richard M. Kaufman, MD[b],*

KEYWORDS

- Hemolytic disease of the fetus and newborn
- Fetomaternal hemorrhage
- Fetal and neonatal alloimmune thrombocytopenia
- Postpartum hemorrhage • Obstetric hemorrhage
- Disseminated intravascular coagulation
- Recombinant factor VIIa • Parvovirus B19

In 1901, Landsteiner[1] proposed the existence of defined blood groups based on the observation that cross-mixing of red blood cells and sera from different healthy individuals sometimes led to red blood cell agglutination. Landsteiner's finding of reproducible isoagglutination patterns among healthy individuals led to the elucidation of the ABO blood group, eventually allowing the development of safe and routine blood transfusions. Since the discovery of the ABO system, 30 other blood groups encompassing 308 blood group antigens have been identified.[2]

A blood group system is defined as the set of red cell antigens produced by the alleles of a single genetic locus. The blood group antigens represent a heterogeneous collection of red cell surface molecules with diverse functions in membrane structure and physiology. Blood group antigens exert influence over a variety of human diseases, from thrombophilia to malarial infection.[3] Clinically, the most significant property of blood group antigens is their immunogenicity, with alloimmunization occurring in antigen-negative recipients of allogeneic blood product transfusions and in pregnant women following exposure to fetal antigens. The major blood groups are those whose antigens have the most potent immunogenicity; in humans, these are ABO and Rh.

Pregnancy poses a special immunologic challenge in that maternal immunity offers fetal protection, yet the fetus itself represents an alloantigen from the perspective of

The authors have nothing to disclose.

[a] Department of Medical Oncology, Dana-Farber Cancer Institute, Harvard Medical School, 44 Binney Street, Smith 353, Boston, MA 02118, USA

[b] Department of Pathology, Brigham and Women's Hospital, Harvard Medical School, 75 Francis Street, Boston, MA 02115, USA

* Corresponding author.

E-mail address: rmkaufman@partners.org

the maternal adaptive immune system.[4] Maternal IgG antibodies, but not other isotypes, cross the placental barrier, and confer immunity to the fetus throughout fetal life and for the first few months postpartum. To mitigate the potential immunologic risks associated with maternal IgG antibodies bearing specificity against fetal antigens, the fetus uses several protective mechanisms, including expression of non-classic human leukocyte antigen (HLA) molecules with limited polymorphism, creation of a "placental sink" to trap detrimental maternal antibodies via fetal trophoblastic Fcg receptors, modulation of placental complement activity, and suppression cytotoxic Th1-type responses in favor of humoral Th2-type responses within the placental milieu. The maternal/fetal immunologic relationship may endure beyond birth, as microchimerisms containing fetal DNA remain detectable in maternal blood for years.[5]

Alloimmunity in pregnancy is the basis for two of the major complications of pregnancy in transfusion medicine: hemolytic disease of the fetus and newborn (HDFN) and fetal and neonatal alloimmune thrombocytopenia (FNAIT). Other roles for transfusion medicine in pregnancy include management of obstetric hemorrhage, parvovirus B19 infection, hemoglobinopathies, and aplastic anemia.

HEMOLYTIC DISEASE OF THE FETUS AND NEWBORN

HDFN (formerly erythroblastosis fetalis) encompasses a spectrum of fetal and neonatal disease, characterized by jaundice, hepatosplenomegaly, hemolytic anemia, and hydrops (fetal anasarca). In the early part of the twentieth century, the biologic basis for HDFN was postulated to be maternal alloantibodies against unidentified fetal antigens.[6] In 1939 Levine and Stetson reported the landmark case of a 25-year-old G_2P_1 female who developed preeclampsia, delivered a macerated fetus at 33 weeks' gestation, and sustained a profound hemolytic anemia following transfusion of her husband's ABO-matched blood for postpartum hemorrhage.[7] Similar isoagglutination reactions involving ABO-matched donor/recipient pairings had been reported earlier in recipients of multiple blood transfusions. Work by Landsteiner, Wiener, and colleagues ultimately established Rh incompatibility as the biologic basis both for ABO-independent isoagglutination and for HDFN via inappropriate exposure of paternally derived fetal Rh antigens to an Rh-negative mother as a result of complications during pregnancy or delivery.

Rh Proteins and Rh(D) Phenotypes

The Rh blood group is the most polymorphic of the human blood groups, with 50 distinct blood group antigens.[8] The 5 major Rh antigens—C, c, E, e, and D—represent the products of two genes on chromosome 1p, *RHCE* and *RHD*, which encode the 30 kDa RhCE and RhD transmembrane proteins, respectively. RhCE and RhD are expressed on the red cell surface as part of a 170 kDa complex that includes the related RhAG (Rh-associated glycoprotein) protein encoded by *RHAG* on chromosome 6p. The Rh and RhAG proteins function as ammonia transporters.

While maternal/fetal incompatibility in many different blood groups can lead to HDFN, antibodies to Rh(D) remain the most significant cause due to the unique immunogenicity of the Rh(D) protein. Several Rh(D) phenotypes have been characterized.[8] *D+* corresponds to the wild-type *RHD* gene sequence, although silent polymorphisms have been reported. *D-negative* corresponds to mutations that eliminate RhD production, including regulatory defects in *RHD* expression, deletions in *RHD*, or deletions of the entire *RHCE-RHD* locus ("Rh null disease"). *Weak D* arises from mutations encoding amino acid substitutions in transmembrane or intracytoplasmic portions of the

RhD protein, generating reduced levels of RhD that retain the immunogenicity of the most critical extracellular epitopes. *Partial D* arises from mutations that encode amino acid substitutions on or near the red cell extracellular surface, where most of the immunogenic epitopes lie, resulting in impaired immunogenicity. Approximately 85% of the United States population is D+, including 83% of whites, 93% of blacks, 93% of Hispanics, 96% of Native Americans, and 98% of Asians.[9] Less than 1% of the population harbors a weak or partial D phenotype.[10]

Pathogenesis, Clinical Features, and Epidemiology of HDFN

Paternally derived fetal Rh(D) is synthesized in fetal red blood cells as early as 5 to 12 weeks' gestation. Due to the immunologic privilege afforded by the placental barrier, maternal Rh(D) alloimmunization requires direct exposure of Rh(D) to the maternal circulation via one of the following mechanisms.

Fetomaternal hemorrhage (FMH, transplacental hemorrhage, or fetomaternal transplacental hemorrhage)

FMH is defined as entry of fetal blood cells into the maternal circulation before or during delivery. Minute hemorrhagic volumes of less than 0.5 mL fetal red cells are capable of inducing maternal alloimmunization.[11] The risk of FMH increases over the course of pregnancy and is greatest at delivery, with 70% to 100% of postpartum mothers having detectable circulating fetal cells after birth, albeit usually at concentrations insufficient to induce clinically significant alloantibody production.[12,13]

Transfusion of D+ blood into a D-negative mother

The risk of alloantibody formation following transfusion of Rh(D)-incompatible blood is directly proportional to the inoculating donor red cell dose. In transfusion studies of D-negative men injected with different volumes of D+ red cells, more than 40% developed anti-D antibodies following inoculation of 5 to 20 mL of cells, compared with more than 90% with inoculation volumes of 200 to 500 mL.[14]

HDFN primarily affects second or later pregnancies. Initial exposure of fetal Rh(D) to a D-negative mother generates a primary, IgM-mediated antibody response, whereas reexposure produces a secondary (anamnestic), IgG-predominant response. Following Rh(D) alloimmunization and reexposure, maternal anti-D IgG antibodies enter the fetal circulation and bind to D+ fetal red cells. As the opsonized cells migrate through the fetal circulation, they are recognized by Fcg receptors on fetal hepatic and splenic macrophages, inducing erythrophagocytosis. Extravascular hemolysis ensues, leading to jaundice, kernicterus, hepatosplenomegaly (from extramedullary hematopoiesis), reticulocytosis, and hydrops (from hypoalbuminemia due to liver dysfunction and shifts in cardiac output due to impaired tissue oxygenation).

Prior to the introduction of Rh(D) immune globulin, clinically significant maternal anti-D alloantibodies developed in 13% to 16% of cases of maternal/fetal Rh(D) phenotypic incompatibility.[15] Factors affecting the likelihood of maternal anti-D IgG antibody production and severity of HDFN include the following.

Maternal/fetal ABO incompatibility

In studies before the era of Rh(D) immune globulin, 2% of D-negative mothers with D+ fetuses and concurrent maternal/fetal ABO incompatibility became immunized to Rh (D), compared with 16% for ABO-compatible pairings.[15] The protective effect of ABO-incompatibility in this setting is attributed to antigen clearance by maternal anti-A or anti-B IgM antibodies, leading to complement-mediated removal of opsonized A+ or B+ fetal red cells from the maternal circulation.

IgG subclass

HDFN can be caused by anti-D alloantibodies of either IgG1 or IgG3 subclass. IgG1 antibodies penetrate the placental barrier earlier than IgG3 antibodies, resulting in higher fetal concentrations and more severe fetal disease.[16]

Weak or partial D phenotypes

Due to the preservation of immunogenic Rh(D) epitopes in mutations that give rise to weak D phenotypes, weak D mothers are usually tolerant to Rh(D), whereas partial D mothers are typically unsensitized. In practice, the risk of HDFN in D+ fetuses conceived in weak or partial D mothers is variable, although cases of HDFN have been reported.[17,18]

Maternal anti-D IgG alloantibody titer

In 62% of cases, maternal anti-D alloantibody titer predicts onset and severity of HDFN.[19]

In the era before Rh(D) immune globulin, HDFN was fatal in up to one-third of neonates. The advent of Rh(D) immune globulin as effective prophylaxis dramatically reduced the incidence of HDFN, from 45.1 cases per 10,000 live births in the United States in 1970 to 14.3 in 1983.[20] With the addition of universal antenatal screening and use of intrauterine transfusion in cases of severe HDFN, D+ neonates born to D-negative, sensitized mothers in the modern era rarely display the full breadth of disease manifestations of HDFN. In a seminal epidemiologic study of HDFN conducted in 1986,[20] jaundice was observed in 77% of cases and hydrops fetalis in only 4%; less than 1% of cases resulted in death. Fourteen percent of neonates were premature and 17% had low birth weights. A little over half of cases represented a second or third pregnancy. Only 16% occurred during a first pregnancy. Per 10,000 live births, Hispanics comprised 12.4 cases; whites, 10.5; blacks, 8.1; and Asians, 2.2.

Rh(D) Typing: Anti-D and Antihuman Globulin Tests

Two diagnostic tests are routinely used in Rh(D) typing. The anti-D test is a hemagglutinin-based assay that detects the presence of Rh(D) antigen on red blood cells. Anti-D antibody-containing reagent is incubated with a patient's red cells. Agglutination occurs if Rh(D) is present, allowing for classification of the red cells as D+ or D-negative. The direct antiglobulin test (DAT, or "direct Coombs test") detects the presence of anti-D IgG antibodies on the surfaces of red blood cells. Antihuman globulin (AHG) with specificity against the Fcg portion of IgG is added to donor red cells. Agglutination occurs if the red cells contain minute amounts of Rh(D)/anti-D IgG complexes.

Blood donors identified as D-negative by the anti-D test are routinely tested for weak expression of D by DAT. Donors who are negative by both the anti-D test and by DAT are classified as D-negative, whereas donors who are negative by the anti-D test and positive by DAT are classified as weak D. Classification of donor cells as D+, D-negative, or weak D ensures that red cells that are even weakly positive for D will not be transfused to D-negative recipients. By contrast, at many institutions transfusion recipients are typed for D using only the anti-D test, and further testing for weak D is not performed. This practice ensures that weak or partial D recipients will be typed as D-negative and will receive only D-negative blood, thereby reducing the risk that a woman with a partial D phenotype will become sensitized to Rh(D) and develop anti-D alloantibodies. Using similar reasoning, the AABB (formerly the American Association of Blood Banks) does not recommend routine maternal typing for weak or partial D phenotypes in pregnancy,[19] although hospital practice in this regard varies considerably.[21] On the other hand, a neonate born to a D-negative mother should be typed for weak D, to ensure appropriate Rh(D) immune globulin prophylaxis of the mother.

Diagnosis of HDFN and Determination of Maternal and Fetal Rh(D) Phenotypes

The diagnostic criteria for HDFN require maternal/fetal Rh(D) phenotypic incompatibility between a D-negative mother and a D+ fetus, and a positive fetal or neonatal DAT for the presence of anti-D IgG antibodies on fetal or neonatal red blood cells.[20] Maternal Rh(D) phenotyping is performed using the anti-D test. The fetal Rh(D) phenotype is determined noninvasively if possible, beginning with paternal Rh(D) genotyping for *RHD* zygosity. Alternatively, the fetal *RHD* genotype can be analyzed by polymerase chain reaction (PCR) of maternal blood during the second trimester.[22] In cases of uncertainty, the gold standard for fetal Rh(D) typing is amniocentesis, which can be performed at 16 to 18 weeks' gestation, with analysis of amniotic fluid by PCR using primers for fetal *RHD*.[23] Fetal red cell destruction may be assessed by spectrophotometry, which measures spectral absorption at 450 nm as a marker of amniotic fluid bilirubin and fetal hemolysis.[24] Fetal blood may be obtained directly for Rh(D) phenotyping using chorionic villus sampling as early as 9 to 12 weeks' gestation or, less commonly, cordocentesis, although the risks of FMH and fetal loss are higher with these procedures than with amniocentesis.[23] Following delivery, a DAT is routinely performed on neonatal umbilical cord blood.

Evaluation of HDFN

Pregnancies complicated by maternal/fetal Rh(D) incompatibility should undergo surveillance for high-risk clinical, laboratory, and radiographic features that may increase the likelihood of HDFN or that may indicate development of HDFN.

FMH

Any number of invasive procedures or complications of pregnancy should prompt evaluation for FMH, including trauma, amniocentesis, chorionic villus sampling, cordocentesis, abortion, miscarriage, hydrops, fetal or neonatal anemia, or a documented or perceived decrease in fetal movements (the most common prenatal presentation of FMH).[25] The *rosette test* is a rapid, qualitative screening assay for FMH, in which maternal blood is mixed with anti-D–containing reagent. After excess anti-D is washed away, D+ "indicator" red cells are added, which will form rosettes around antibody-coated, D+ fetal red cells. If the rosette test is positive, a *Kleihauer-Betke test* is typically performed to quantify FMH volume. The Kleihauer-Betke test identifies fetal red cells based on staining with erythrosin B, which binds fetal hemoglobin F (HbF). Adequate Kleihauer-Betke testing requires manual examination of 10,000 red cells, rendering the test highly labor intensive. The Kleihauer-Betke test may also overestimate the number of fetal red cells in patients with certain hemoglobinopathies (eg, sickle cell disease or β-thalassemia) in which endogenous HbF levels are increased. *Flow cytometry*, using fluorescent antibodies against HbF or other fetal red cell antigens, demonstrates superior efficiency and reproducibility over Kleihauer-Betke testing, and is increasingly being used at many academic centers for accurate quantitation of fetal red cells and approximation of FMH volumes.

Antibody titers in HDFN

Baseline maternal anti-D IgG antibody titers are measured early in pregnancy and at recurring intervals of 2 to 4 weeks beginning at 18 weeks' gestation, with anti-D titers above 16 to 32 (the "critical titer" at most institutions) prompting initiation of more intensive fetal monitoring for HDFN.[19]

Intensive fetal monitoring for HDFN

Techniques for measuring fetal anemia in HDFN include amniotic fluid spectrophotometry,[24,26] fetal cordocentesis,[27] fetal ultrasound (allowing for visualization of fetal size and organomegaly), and Doppler ultrasonography of fetal middle cerebral artery peak systolic velocity (which correlates with fetal hemoglobin).[28]

Prevention of HDFN: The Role of Prophylactic Rh(D) Immune Globulin

Prophylactic use of exogenous anti-D antibodies was initially developed on the basis of the protective effect of ABO mismatch in opsonizing and clearing D+ fetal red cells from the maternal circulation.[12] In early clinical trials, the source of anti-D was whole serum from Rh(D)-immunized donors who had high titers of anti-D antibodies. Subsequent studies made use of anti-D immunoglobulin ("Rh(D) immune globulin") harvested from pooled plasma.[11,29] The approval of Rh(D) immune globulin in 1968 for widespread use in the United States and the United Kingdom heralded a marked decline in the incidence of maternal Rh(D) alloimmunization, HDFN, and fetal/neonatal morbidity.[20,30]

Indications for Rh(D) immune globulin

Guidelines from the AABB, the US Preventive Service Task Force, the American Congress of Obstetricians and Gynecologists, and the Society of Obstetricians and Gynaecologists of Canada (SOGC) recommend that D-negative (or partial D) mothers receive Rh(D) immune globulin postpartum within 72 hours of delivery, unless postpartum Rh(D) typing of neonatal umbilical cord blood by the anti-D test and by DAT reveals the infant to be D-negative.[19] Antepartum, Rh(D) immune globulin may additionally be administered at 28 weeks' gestation in D-negative mothers with no detectable anti-D antibodies. Rh(D) immune globulin is indicated following abortion, amniocentesis, chorionic villus sampling, cordocentesis, ectopic pregnancy, molar pregnancy, or any other conditions associated with FMH. Partial efficacy may be seen with Rh(D) immune globulin administered up to 2 weeks after delivery.[31]

Dosing of Rh(D) immune globulin

Administration of 20 µg Rh(D) immune globulin results in removal of approximately 1 mL of D+ fetal red cells from the maternal circulation.[14] In North America the standard dose is 300 µg, with larger doses used when greater volumes of FMH are suspected. In the United Kingdom, Rh(D) immune globulin is given antenatally at 28 and 34 weeks at a dose of 100 µg, and within 72 hours postpartum at a dose of 100 µg. For sensitizing events before 20 weeks' gestation, a 50-µg dose is given, whereas sensitizing events beyond 20 weeks are treated with a dose of 100 µg. In Australia, Rh(D) immune globulin is given antenatally at 28 and 34 weeks at a dose of 125 µg, and within 72 hours postpartum at a dose of 125 µg; for sensitizing events in the first trimester, a 50-µg dose is given, whereas sensitizing events in the third trimester are treated with a dose of 125 µg.

Complications of Rh(D) immune globulin

Rh(D) immune globulin has been linked to two prior outbreaks of hepatitis C transmission, and is no longer produced in the United Kingdom because of epidemiologic concerns regarding prion disease.[32] Current formulations of Rh(D) immune globulin, however, undergo multiple viral inactivation steps and are considered to be extremely safe. While the predominant antibody isotype in Rh(D) immune globulin is IgG, small amounts of IgA and/or IgM may be present, and occasionally cause systemic reactions. Rh(D) immune globulin can cross the placental barrier, although the risk of fetal complications from this is small.

Possible mechanisms underlying the efficacy of Rh(D) immune globulin include macrophage clearance of anti-D IgG-opsonized fetal red cells, inhibition of T cells required for development of endogenous anti-D antibodies, inhibition of B-cell function, sequestration of Rh(D) epitopes through binding of exogenous anti-D antibodies (a phenomenon known as steric hindrance), and alteration of processing and presentation of Rh(D) in the adaptive immune response.[33] Monoclonal anti-D antibodies, produced from human or murine cells, have been developed but have not been as effective as Rh(D) immune globulin in multiple clinical trials, possibly because of post-translational modifications including aberrant glycosylation.[34]

Treatment of HDFN

Rh(D) immune globulin is ineffective in cases where maternal anti-D alloantibodies have already formed. In such instances, intensive monitoring for the onset and progression of HDFN is indicated, with therapy directed at specific disease manifestations.

Neonatal hyperbilirubinemia

The major risks of fetal or neonatal hyperbilirubinemia are neurotoxicity and kernicterus.[35] First-line treatment is neonatal phototherapy. Maternal injection of phenobarbital, which stimulates hepatic bilirubin conjugation, has also been used. In severe cases, postpartum neonatal exchange transfusion is effective at reducing neonatal bilirubin levels, although procedure-associated complications are seen in approximately 10% of patients (eg, bradycardia from calcium infusion, portal vein and other thromboses, infection, and necrotizing enterocolitis).[36] Due to the immaturity of the neonatal immune system, neonatal transfusions carry a risk of transfusion-associated graft-versus-host disease (TA-GVHD).[37] The use of irradiated red cells is therefore mandatory in this setting to destroy contaminating donor leukocytes. In light of these risks, the American Academy of Pediatrics recommends exchange transfusion only for neonates with severe hyperbilirubinemia or acute kernicterus.

Fetal anemia

Intrauterine transfusion (IUT) has significantly advanced the care of fetuses with severe HDFN, yielding fetal and neonatal survival rates of over 70% to 90%.[38] IUT is indicated at 18 to 35 weeks' gestation in fetuses with HDFN and severe anemia (defined as fetal hematocrit of less than 25% at 18–26 weeks' gestation, or less than 30% after 26 weeks), with a target posttransfusion hematocrit of 35% to 40%. Two infusion routes are used: intraperitoneal (IPT), in which blood is injected into the fetal intraperitoneal space, or intravascular (IVT), in which blood is transfused directly into the fetal umbilical circulation.[39,40] IVT is generally preferred over IPT based on data from case-control studies.[41] IUT carries a risk of TA-GVHD, particularly in infants who undergo both IUT and postpartum neonatal exchange.[37] IUT has also been associated with maternal alloantibody formation against donor and fetal antigens, even with adequate cross-matching.[42] Donor blood must be O-negative, D-negative, CMV seronegative, and irradiated. Packed red cells are used to reduce transfusion volume. Alternative approaches to IUT include the use of autologous blood from maternal donors, which may be more effective than allogeneic blood at stabilizing fetal hemoglobin levels but carries a higher risk of TA-GVHD due to maternal/fetal HLA haploidentity,[43] and intrauterine exchange transfusion via percutaneous umbilical cord sampling.[44]

Maternal alloantibody titers

Plasmapheresis of maternal blood was historically used in severe cases of HDFN to reduce alloantibody titers, although this technique largely disappeared from use following the advent of IUT. Maternal administration of intravenous immunoglobulin (IVIG), with or without plasmapheresis, may also reduce maternal alloantibody titers and postpartum exchange transfusion requirements.[45,46]

HDFN from Alleles Other than Rh(D)

Maternal/fetal phenotypic incompatibility in K antigen (of the Kell blood group) represents 10% of all cases of HDFN; incompatibility in Rh(c) represents 3.5%.[47] Up to 40% of K-sensitized pregnancies develop HDFN, typically with severe disease manifestations.[48] While fetal anemia is severe in anti-K HDFN, neonatal hyperbilirubinemia and fetal reticulocytosis are not as profound as in classic anti-D HDFN, suggesting that suppression of erythropoiesis rather than hemolysis may underlie the pathology of anti-K HDFN.[49] Rarely, severe HDFN can also be seen with phenotypic incompatibility in Rh(E), Rh(c), or Colton antigens. Mismatches in Rh(C), Rh(e), and other antigens of the MNS, Duffy, Kidd, and Sciana blood groups are unlikely to cause HDFN, owing to reduced immunogenicity and antigenic frequency. Incompatibility in Le^a or Le^b of the Lewis group, or P1 of the P group, leads to a predominantly IgM response and does not cause HDFN. Finally, maternal/fetal ABO mismatch, while reducing the risk of HDFN from Rh(D) incompatibility, can itself cause HDFN. Such disease is usually mild, although severe forms have been reported.[50]

FETAL AND NEONATAL ALLOIMMUNE THROMBOCYTOPENIA

More than 60 years ago, a rare condition of "congenital thrombocytopenic purpura" or "thrombocytopenic purpura in the newborn" was first reported, characterized by neonatal petechiae, purpura, gastrointestinal bleeding, and neurologic abnormalities, occurring hours to days after birth.[51] Studies of the related adult condition of post-transfusion purpura, in the context of the evolving model of HDFN, led to the identification of maternal antiplatelet alloantibodies with specificity against paternally derived fetal platelet antigens as the cause of neonatal thrombocytopenia without maternal thrombocytopenia (renamed "fetal/neonatal alloimmune thrombocytopenia," or FNAIT). Large-scale studies have since established FNAIT as the single most common cause of neonatal thrombocytopenia, representing approximately 20% to 70% of all documented cases, with an incidence in the general population of 1 in 1000 to 1 in 3000 live births.[52–56]

Pathogenesis of FNAIT

Following occult exposure of fetal platelets to the maternal circulation, maternal allo-antibodies are generated against paternally derived fetal platelet antigens that are absent in the maternal host. Such antigens are expressed by the fetus as early as 16 weeks' gestation and reach adult levels by 18 to 26 weeks.[57] That the severity of FNAIT appears to increase with subsequent pregnancies suggests that a primary antibody response results from the initial platelet antigen exposure, followed by an anamnestic response on antigen reexposure.[58–60] Maternal IgG antibodies against fetal platelet antigens cross the placental barrier, leading to complement-mediated destruction of fetal platelets. The fetal/neonatal Fc receptor (FcRn) has been suggested in murine models to mediate transplacental transfer of maternal antibodies in FNAIT and possibly other alloimmune or autoimmune diseases, including HDFN, lupus, and immune thrombocytopenia (ITP).[61]

FNAIT differs from HDFN in several important respects. Whereas HDFN is predominantly a disease of second or later pregnancies, 25% to 60% of cases of FNAIT occur during first pregnancy.[62,63] Fetal platelet antigens induce higher rates of maternal alloimmunization than Rh or other red cell antigens. Among first-time pregnancies with maternal/fetal platelet antigen incompatibility, maternal antiplatelet antibodies can be detected in up to 50%,[64] although most antiplatelet alloantibodies that arise during pregnancy will not lead to FNAIT, as transient alloantibodies are frequently observed.[54] Whereas initial maternal Rh immunization usually occurs at the time of delivery, maternal antibodies directed against fetal platelet antigens can be detected as early as 20 weeks' gestation in a first-time pregnancy, or several weeks earlier for a second or later pregnancy.[54,58,59]

Biology of Platelet Antigens in FNAIT: the GP Ia/IIa, GP Ib/IX/V, and GP IIb/IIIa Receptors

Twenty-four human platelet antigens (HPA) have been recognized by the International Society of Blood Transfusion (ISBT) and the International Society on Thrombosis and Haemostasis (ISTH).[65] Eleven encode polymorphisms in surface glycoprotein (GP) IIIa, while 9 represent variants of GP Ia, GP Ib, or GP IIb. These glycoproteins constitute critical components of platelet cell surface receptors, whose interactions form the basis for platelet hemostatic function.[66] Mutations in GP Ia, GP Ib, or GP IIIa associated with FNAIT are thought to disrupt areas of the proteins corresponding to key epitopes recognized by the adaptive immune response, as illustrated by biochemical and crystallographic studies of HPA-1a in complex with the major histocompatibility (MHC) Class I molecule HLA-DRB3*0101.[67] The HPAs are numbered according to the order of their discovery; 12 are classified into 6 "biphenotypic" systems, each comprising one of two distinct antigenic phenotypes (eg, HPA-1a/1b, HPA-2a/2b, HPA-3a/3b, HPA-4a/4b, HPA-5a/5b, HPA-15a/15b). Such biphenotypic allelism is a central component of the pathogenesis of FNAIT, as the appearance of one allele in an individual leads to host antibodies directed against the other allele. Hence, most cases of FNAIT are associated with antigenic mismatch in 1 of the 6 biphenotypic HPAs, although many exceptions have been reported.[68]

Among Caucasians, the HPA-1b allele is uncommon, occurring in only 2%. Approximately three-quarters of FNAIT cases in Caucasians arise as a consequence of maternal anti–HPA-1a alloantibodies in HPA-1b mothers carrying HPA-1a fetuses.[62,63,69,70] Coexistence of maternal HPA-1a antibodies with the MHC Class I allele phenotype HLA-DRB3*0101 appears to be a prerequisite for development of anti-HPA-1a–mediated FNAIT.[54] Such allelic restriction is thought to arise from binding interactions between HPA-1a peptides and HLA-DRB3*0101 within the antigen/MHC Class I complex that serve to enhance antigenicity of HPA-1a epitopes.

Phenotypic incompatibility in several other platelet antigens beyond HPA-1 can give rise to FNAIT, although disease penetrance and severity vary considerably across different populations.[62,69,71–80] Among Caucasians and Asians, alloantibodies to HPA-5b are the most common maternal antibodies in pregnancy yet only rarely cause FNAIT. When FNAIT has been reported in association with anti–HPA-5b, the disease has been severe.[81–83] The vast majority of FNAIT in Japan and east Asia is caused by antibodies to HPA-4b[84]; paradoxically, HPA-4a is the most prevalent allele in the Japanese population. Anti-HPA/MHC restrictions have been observed with some, but not all, of the other HPAs implicated in FNAIT.[83] Finally, there have been multiple reports of FNAIT from anti-HLA antibodies arising in the context of maternal/fetal HLA incompatibility, although it remains controversial whether anti-HLA antibodies play a direct role in the pathogenesis of FNAIT, in part due to the ubiquity of the HLA antigens in contrast to the specificity of platelet effects seen in FNAIT.[85]

Clinical Features of FNAIT

Petechiae, purpura, and ecchymoses may be seen in up to 90% of newborns with FNAIT. Neonatal platelet counts are less than 50×10^9/L in 50% to 90% of cases.[64,70]

A minority of affected neonates have mucosal bleeding. The most feared complication is intracranial hemorrhage (ICH), occurring in approximately 10% to 20% of cases, and fatal in up to one-third. Most instances of ICH develop in utero, some as early as 16 to 20 weeks' gestation. Major risk factors for ICH include severe neonatal thrombocytopenia (defined as a platelet count of $<20 \times 10^9$/L), multiparity, and history of fetal/neonatal ICH in prior pregnancies complicated by FNAIT.[58–60]

Diagnosis of FNAIT

The diagnosis of FNAIT requires a fetal or neonatal platelet count less than 50×10^9/L, maternal/fetal HPA incompatibility, and maternal antiplatelet alloantibodies with specificity against fetal platelet antigens.[64] HPA typing is performed using enzyme-linked immunosorbent assay (ELISA) and other fluorescence-based assays. Paternal HPA testing can suffice for fetal testing in many cases. Antiplatelet alloantibodies are detected using the monoclonal antibody-specific immobilization of platelet antigens (MAIPA) test, an ELISA-based assay that uses preformed monoclonal antibodies against specific platelet antigens to determine host antiplatelet alloantibody specificity.[86] To establish a diagnosis of FNAIT, other conditions associated with fetal or neonatal thrombocytopenia must be excluded, including congenital TORCH (Toxoplasmosis/Other/Rubella/Cytomegalovirus/Herpes simplex) and perinatal infections (eg, *Escherichia coli*, Group B *Streptococcus*, and *Haemophilus influenzae*), autoimmune diseases (eg, lupus and ITP associated with maternal thrombocytopenia), severe HDFN, thrombosis, leukemia and other malignancies, aneuploidy (eg, trisomies in 13, 18, and 21), Wiskott-Aldrich syndrome, vascular anomalies (eg, Kassabach-Merritt and Klipel-Trenaunay-Weber syndromes), congenital thrombocytopenia syndromes, and fetal emergencies (eg, preeclampsia and HELLP syndrome [Hemolysis, Elevated Liver enzyme, Low Platelet]).[87]

Prevention of FNAIT

Two large-scale studies in Scotland and Norway, encompassing more than 25,000 and 100,000 births, respectively, explored the feasibility of population-wide screening for HPA-1a.[55,56] In both studies, pregnant women were screened for the HPA-1a allele; those negative for HPA-1a were additionally screened for the presence of serum anti–HPA-1a antibodies and subjected to further interventions if anti–HPA-1a antibodies were detected (eg, cesarean section to avoid the trauma of vaginal delivery, in the Norwegian study). From a cost perspective, the results were not entirely supportive of universal screening. However, a marked reduction in morbidity in comparison with historical controls was seen among severe cases of FNAIT in the Norwegian study ($\sim$5% vs $\sim$20%). At present, efforts are under way to evaluate vaccination as a means of FNAIT prevention.[88]

Therapies for FNAIT and Natural History After Delivery

First-line treatment for FNAIT is maternal infusion of IVIG at a dose of 1 g/kg per week, beginning at 12 to 20 weeks' gestation, and continuing until delivery. Response rates to IVIG are 25% to 60%.[89–94] For high-risk neonates (defined as those with severe thrombocytopenia or with a family history of a previous sibling with fetal ICH), either IVIG 1 g/kg/d plus a steroid (prednisone 0.5–1 mg/kg/d or methylprednisolone 1 mg every 8 hours) or IVIG at a dose of 2 g/kg/d is used, although the specific role of steroids is uncertain. A risk-adapted approach for high-risk neonates has also been reported, incorporating escalating doses of IVIG and steroids based on the gestational age at which prior siblings developed ICH.[64] In cases of HPA-1a–associated FNAIT refractory to IVIG and steroids, IUT into the fetal umbilical vein may be performed, with a fetal mortality rate of 15%. IUT in treatment of high-risk FNAIT uses either HPA-1a–negative or maternal platelets that have been washed to remove alloantibodies prior to transfusion.[63,94] Following any of these interventions, cordocentesis is performed to monitor fetal platelet counts, with a target platelet count of 100 $\times$ 10^9/L. After delivery, neonatal thrombocytopenia may persist for up to several weeks, treatment of which is typically IVIG (1 g/kg) with or without steroids, with a target platelet count of 30 $\times$ 10^9/L.

OBSTETRIC HEMORRHAGE

Across the globe an estimated 13,795,000 cases of postpartum hemorrhage (PPH) occur each year. PPH is responsible for more than 100,000 maternal deaths annually, and is the most common cause of maternal death worldwide.[95] In North America, PPH is defined as hemorrhage of at least 500 mL following vaginal delivery, or at least 1000 mL following cesarean section; in Australia, the respective volumes are 500 mL and 750 mL. Alternative diagnostic criteria include a drop in postpartum hematocrit of at least 10%, or any maternal requirement for blood product transfusion following delivery. The vast majority of PPH occurs within the first 24 hours after delivery and is designated as primary PPH. Cases occurring 24 hours to 2 weeks after delivery are classified as secondary PPH.

Traditionally, the major causes of PPH have been categorized into 4 groups, called the "4 Ts": uterine atony ("tone"), retained placenta and other products of conception ("tissue"), uterine or cervical injury ("trauma"), and disseminated intravascular coagulation (DIC, or "thrombin").[96] Retained placenta and an abnormal third stage of labor are the risk factors with the highest odds ratios for predicting severe PPH.[97,98] Primary PPH and retained placenta are each associated with development of secondary PPH.[99]

Hemostasis During Pregnancy: Pathogenesis of PPH and DIC

During pregnancy, several hemostatic mechanisms act in concert to reduce the risk and complications of hemorrhage, particularly at the time of delivery. Maternal cardiac output and blood volume increase to 20% to 100% above baseline by the third trimester. Expansion of plasma volume exceeds that of overall red cell mass, forming the basis for the physiologic anemia of pregnancy Within the placenta local thrombosis is favored, and fibrinolytic activity mildly suppressed, due to placental expression of tissue factor (TF) and plasminogen activator inhibitors 1 and 2.[100] Systemically, levels of multiple coagulation factors (I, V, VII, VIII, IX, X, and thrombin), von Willebrand factor (vWF), and fibrinogen levels increase as tissue plasminogen activator and protein S levels decrease, promoting thrombogenesis.[101] As a compensatory measure, antithrombin III levels increase. Antithrombin III binds thrombin, forming thrombin:antithrombin III (TAT) complexes. With labor and delivery, D-dimer levels increase.[102] Uterine retraction controls hemorrhage via compression of uterine vessels in the myometrium. In the days following delivery, coagulation factors, D-dimer, and vWF levels return to normal, and fibrinolysis is restored.

DIC, whether obstetric or nonobstetric, occurs as a consequence of concurrent hyperactivation of coagulation and fibrinolytic cascades.[103] Five features characterize DIC[104]: thrombocytopenia (observed in nearly all cases), elevated prothrombin time (PT) and/or activated partial thromboplastin time (aPTT) (observed in most cases), hypofibrinogenemia (sensitivity ~30%), fibrin degradation products (sensitivity $\geq$90%), and schistocytes on peripheral blood smear (with schistocytes comprising more than 1% of red blood cells, or at least 2 schistocytes per 100$\times$ oil immersion field, considered pathologic[105]). The International Society for Thrombosis and Haemostasis has created a DIC scoring system composed of platelet count, fibrin degradation products, prolonged PT, and fibrinogen level, although its use is currently limited to research protocols.[106]

The relationship between PPH and DIC is complex. In a seminal prospective study, women with severe PPH (defined as a drop in hemoglobin of >4 g/dL, a need for invasive hemostatic interventions, or death, all within 24 hours of onset of PPH) had lower levels of fibrinogen, Factor V, antithrombin, and protein C, and higher levels of aPTT, D-dimer, and TAT than those with nonsevere disease.[107] In multivariate analyses, fibrinogen level was the sole coagulation parameter significantly associated with severe hemorrhage, with a 2.63-fold increase in severity of PPH for every 100 mg/dL decrease in fibrinogen.

Prevention and Obstetric Management of PPH

Consensus statements from the World Health Organization, International Confederation of Midwives, International Federation of Gynaecologists and Obstetricians, and the SOGC support a prophylactic role for active management in the third stage of labor to prevent PPH. Core components of active management include administration of uterotonic agents (preferably oxytocin, although ergot alkaloids and misoprostol are acceptable), controlled cord traction, and uterine massage for placental delivery. Side effects of active management include nausea, vomiting, and hypertension partly from ergot alkaloid use. Tranexamic acid, an antifibrinolytic agent that inhibits conversion of plasminogen to plasmin, has been shown in a few trials to have efficacy in prophylaxis for PPH.[108] In cases where PPH has already developed, obstetric interventions include uterine balloon tamponade, uterine arterial embolization, iliac or uterine artery ligation, or, when all other measures have failed, hysterectomy.

Blood Product Transfusion in PPH

First-line medical management of patients with obstetric hemorrhage, or massive hemorrhage from any other cause, involves adequate fluid resuscitation to maintain mean arterial pressure, accompanied by transfusion of blood products to maintain tissue oxygenation and achieve hemostasis. Large-volume transfusion of blood products can produce several acute complications, the most significant being dilutional coagulopathy as a consequence of volume expansion. Other side effects include metabolic acidosis, hypocalcemia, hyperkalemia, and hypothermia.[109] Patients receiving massive transfusions should have frequent monitoring (eg, every 1–4 hours) of electrolytes, complete blood count, coagulation studies, and fibrinogen levels, with correction as needed.

Few transfusion studies have been conducted in patients with obstetric hemorrhage. Transfusion guidelines for PPH and obstetric DIC are adapted from those for massive blood loss in other clinical settings. Recommended target parameters are hemoglobin greater than 8 g/dL, a platelet count of at least 50 to 75 $\times$ 10^9/L, PT/ aPTT 1.5 times the institutional lower limit of normal or less, and fibrinogen greater than 100 mg/dL.[109] Before standardization of blood separation techniques, whole blood was used in PPH in an effort to rapidly restore circulatory volume and prevent dilutional coagulopathy. Observational studies of PPH patients transfused with whole blood showed reduced rates of acute tubular necrosis, acute respiratory distress syndrome, hypofibrinogenemia, intensive care hospitalization, and maternal death, but increased cases of pulmonary edema, compared with combinations of individual blood products.[110] Retrospective studies of trauma patients from the United States military and other trauma centers reported reduced mortality with transfusion of packed red blood cells, platelets, and fresh frozen plasma (FFP) in approximately 1:1:1 ratios, suggesting a central role for FFP in initial resuscitative efforts.[111] However, these studies all had significant methodologic limitations, and it has been argued that the observed mortality benefit may be largely a result of survivorship bias.[112–114] At present, there is no high-quality evidence to inform decisions regarding optimal ratios of blood product transfusions in patients with obstetric hemorrhage. Data from well-designed prospective trials are needed.

Recombinant Factor VIIa in PPH

In cases of obstetric hemorrhage where large volume transfusion fails to promote hemostasis and a definite cause of surgical bleeding is not identified, recombinant Factor VIIa (rFVIIa) may be considered for use. Human rFVII is produced from transfected baby hamster kidney cells; purification with murine monoclonal antibodies induces spontaneous activation. In vitro studies demonstrate dependence of rFVIIa activity on temperature and pH, with optimal activity observed at physiologic values of both.[115] rFVIIa was approved in 1999 by the Food and Drug Administration (FDA) for treatment of bleeding in hemophilia patients with acquired inhibitors to Factors VIII or IX. In contrast to endogenous Factor VIIa, which acts exclusively in concert with TF, rFVIIa induces thrombosis through tissue TF-dependent and TF-independent pathways, generating a stronger thrombus than that produced by endogenous Factor VII.[116]

Beyond its FDA-approved use in hemophilia, rFVIIa has been tried as a hemostatic agent in several other settings, including ICH, surgery, and trauma. Off-label, rFVIIa has been reported to be clinically effective in many case reports and uncontrolled series of patients with severe bleeding. In randomized controlled trials, however, clinical outcomes of off-label rFVIIa have been mixed, with several trials in several different clinical settings failing to demonstrate either reduced blood product use or improved survival with rFVIIa over placebo.[117–124] In retrospective studies of PPH, rFVIIa has been reported to be effective or partially effective in achieving hemostasis in approximately 70% to 90% of cases.[125–135] Efficacy is dependent on correction of coagulation parameters, particularly fibrinogen, which should be repleted before rFVIIa administration.[128,136] Off-label use of rFVIIa is traditionally discouraged in DIC because of concerns regarding uncontrolled propagation of DIC and increased risk of thrombosis.[137] Among published case series of PPH, thromboses occurred in 2.5% of patients who received rFVIIa, with venous thromboembolism occurring more commonly than arterial thrombosis.[138] By contrast, in nonobstetric conditions the thrombotic risk of off-label rFVIIA use is 1% to 2%, with an increase in arterial but not venous thromboembolism.[139]

OTHER INDICATIONS FOR TRANSFUSION IN PREGNANCY

Transfusion medicine is central to the management of pregnancies complicated by hemoglobinopathies or aplastic anemia. The role of simple transfusions, exchange transfusions, IUT, and fetal hematopoietic stem cell transplantation in these conditions is discussed separately (see the article by Lee and Okam elsewhere in this issue for further exploration of this topic).

Parvovirus B19 Infection

Parvovirus B19 is a single-stranded DNA virus that causes a range of infections in different hosts. In pregnant women, the major concern is fetal infection, leading to fetal anemia, hydrops fetalis, spontaneous abortion, or, in infants who survive, congenital abnormalities.[140–142] The risk of maternal to fetal transmission is approximately one-third, with fetal complications seen in 3% of infected women. Earlier maternal infection, particularly infection before 20 weeks of gestation, increases the risk of fetal complications. Hydrops fetalis occurs 2 to 4 weeks after fetal infection. In serologic tests, maternal positivity to IgG antibodies against parvovirus denotes immunity and carries no fetal risks, whereas IgG negativity with IgM positivity is diagnostic for parvovirus infection. For infected mothers a comprehensive prenatal program is advised, incorporating fetal Doppler ultrasonography of middle cerebral artery peak systolic velocity, amniocentesis and/or cordocentesis to measure viral titers, and, for infected fetuses, IUT, the latter of which is the only effective therapy other than delivery.

SUMMARY

In summary, transfusion medicine is integral to several diseases of pregnancy, from immunologic processes such as HDFN and FNAIT governed by maternal/fetal antigenic compatibility, to management of obstetric hemorrhage and various hematologic disorders. While the use of Rh(D) immune globulin has revolutionized the clinical course of Rh(D)-incompatible pregnancies, comparable advances other than blood product transfusions are lacking in FNAIT, although large-scale population screening for HPA alleles and HPA vaccinations may hold promise. Treatment of obstetric hemorrhage involves adequate fluid resuscitation and appropriate blood product transfusions, with repletion of coagulation factors particularly in the setting of dilutional coagulopathy. In select cases of refractory bleeding, administration of rFVIIa may be effective in achieving hemostasis, although the benefits and safety of off-label rFVIIa use are uncertain. For severe fetal anemia such as seen with HDFN and various hemoglobinopathies, IUT has demonstrable efficacy, and fetal allogeneic stem cell transplantation has been successfully performed in some cases. The clinical applications of transfusion medicine in pregnancy are therefore very broad and will continue to expand with our growing understanding of the principles of immunology, coagulation, and thrombosis in pregnancy.

REFERENCES

1. Landsteiner K. On agglutination of normal human blood. Transfusion 1961;1: 5–8.
2. Daniels G, Reid ME. Blood groups: the past 50 years. Transfusion 2010;50(2): 281–9.
3. Anstee DJ. The relationship between blood groups and disease. Blood 2010; 115(23):4635–43.
4. Poole JA, Claman HN. Immunology of pregnancy. Implications for the mother. Clin Rev Allergy Immunol 2004;26(3):161–70.
5. Nelson JL. Microchimerism in human health and disease. Autoimmunity 2003; 36(1):5–9.
6. Darrow RR. Icterus gravis (erythroblastosis) neonatorum. Arch Pathol 1938;25: 378–417.
7. Levine P, Stetson RE. Landmark article July 8, 1939. An unusual case of intragroup agglutination. By Philip Levine and Rufus E Stetson. JAMA 1984; 251(10):1316–7.
8. Westhoff CM. The structure and function of the Rh antigen complex. Semin Hematol 2007;44(1):42–50.
9. Garratty G. Advances in red blood cell immunology 1960 to 2009. Transfusion 2010;50(3):526–35.

10. Denomme GA, Wagner FF, Fernandes BJ, et al. Partial D, weak D types, and novel RHD alleles among 33,864 multiethnic patients: implications for anti-D alloimmunization and prevention. Transfusion 2005;45(10):1554–60.
11. Prevention of Rh-haemolytic disease: results of the clinical trial. A combined study from centres in England and Baltimore. Br Med J 1966;2(5519):907–14.
12. Finn R, Clarke CA, Donohoe WT, et al. Experimental studies on the prevention of Rh haemolytic disease. Br Med J 1961;1(5238):1486–90.
13. Medearis AL, Hensleigh PA, Parks DR, et al. Detection of fetal erythrocytes in maternal blood post partum with the fluorescence-activated cell sorter. Am J Obstet Gynecol 1984;148(3):290–5.
14. Pollack W, Ascari WQ, Kochesky RJ, et al. Studies on Rh prophylaxis. 1. Relationship between doses of anti-Rh and size of antigenic stimulus. Transfusion 1971;11(6):333–9.
15. Bowman J. Thirty-five years of Rh prophylaxis. Transfusion 2003;43(12):1661–6.
16. Lambin P, Debbia M, Puillandre P, et al. IgG1 and IgG3 anti-D in maternal serum and on the RBCs of infants suffering from HDN: relationship with the severity of the disease. Transfusion 2002;42(12):1537–46.
17. Lacey PA, Caskey CR, Werner DJ, et al. Fatal hemolytic disease of a newborn due to anti-D in an Rh-positive Du variant mother. Transfusion 1983;23(2):91–4.
18. Cannon M, Pierce R, Taber EB, et al. Fatal hydrops fetalis caused by anti-D in a mother with partial D. Obstet Gynecol 2003;102(5 Pt 2):1143–5.
19. Judd WJ. Practice guidelines for prenatal and perinatal immunohematology, revisited. Transfusion 2001;41(11):1445–52.
20. Chavez GF, Mulinare J, Edmonds LD. Epidemiology of Rh hemolytic disease of the newborn in the United States. JAMA 1991;265(24):3270–4.
21. Domen RE. Policies and procedures related to weak D phenotype testing and Rh immune globulin administration. Results from supplementary questions to the Comprehensive Transfusion Medicine Survey of the College of American Pathologists. Arch Pathol Lab Med 2000;124(8):1118–21.
22. Lo YM, Hjelm NM, Fidler C, et al. Prenatal diagnosis of fetal RhD status by molecular analysis of maternal plasma. N Engl J Med 1998;339(24):1734–8.
23. Bennett PR, Le Van Kim C, Colin Y, et al. Prenatal determination of fetal RhD type by DNA amplification. N Engl J Med 1993;329(9):607–10.
24. Bowman JM, Pollock JM. Amniotic fluid spectrophotometry and early delivery in the management of erythroblastosis fetalis. Pediatrics 1965;35:815–35.
25. Wylie BJ, D'Alton ME. Fetomaternal hemorrhage. Obstet Gynecol 2010;115(5):1039–51.
26. Liley AW. Liquor amnil analysis in the management of the pregnancy complicated by rhesus sensitization. Am J Obstet Gynecol 1961;82:1359–70.
27. Weiner CP, Williamson RA, Wenstrom KD, et al. Management of fetal hemolytic disease by cordocentesis. I. Prediction of fetal anemia. Am J Obstet Gynecol 1991;165(3):546–53.
28. Mari G, Deter RL, Carpenter RL, et al. Noninvasive diagnosis by Doppler ultrasonography of fetal anemia due to maternal red-cell alloimmunization. Collaborative group for Doppler assessment of the blood velocity in anemic fetuses. N Engl J Med 2000;342(1):9–14.
29. Freda VJ, Gorman JG, Pollack W. Rh factor: prevention of isoimmunization and clinical trial on mothers. Science 1966;151(3712):828–30.
30. Clarke CA, Whitfield AG, Mollison PL. Deaths from Rh haemolytic disease in England and Wales in 1984 and 1985. Br Med J (Clin Res Ed) 1987;294(6578):1001.

31. Samson D, Mollison PL. Effect on primary Rh immunization of delayed administration of anti-Rh. Immunology 1975;28(2):349–57.
32. Smith DB, Lawlor E, Power J, et al. A second outbreak of hepatitis C virus infection from anti-D immunoglobulin in Ireland. Vox Sang 1999;76(3):175–80.
33. Brinc D, Lazarus AH. Mechanisms of anti-D action in the prevention of hemolytic disease of the fetus and newborn. Hematology Am Soc Hematol Educ Program 2009;185–91.
34. Kumpel BM. Efficacy of RhD monoclonal antibodies in clinical trials as replacement therapy for prophylactic anti-D immunoglobulin: more questions than answers. Vox Sang 2007;93(2):99–111.
35. Dennery PA, Seidman DS, Stevenson DK. Neonatal hyperbilirubinemia. N Engl J Med 2001;344(8):581–90.
36. Keenan WJ, Novak KK, Sutherland JM, et al. Morbidity and mortality associated with exchange transfusion. Pediatrics 1985;75(2 Pt 2):417–21.
37. Ruhl H, Bein G, Sachs UJ. Transfusion-associated graft-versus-host disease. Transfus Med Rev 2009;23(1):62–71.
38. Schumacher B, Moise KJ Jr. Fetal transfusion for red blood cell alloimmunization in pregnancy. Obstet Gynecol 1996;88(1):137–50.
39. Liley AW. Intrauterine transfusion of foetus in haemolytic disease. Br Med J 1963;2(5365):1107–9.
40. Rodeck CH, Kemp JR, Holman CA, et al. Direct intravascular fetal blood transfusion by fetoscopy in severe Rhesus isoimmunisation. Lancet 1981;1(8221):625–7.
41. Harman CR, Bowman JM, Manning FA, et al. Intrauterine transfusion—intraperitoneal versus intravascular approach: a case-control comparison. Am J Obstet Gynecol 1990;162(4):1053–9.
42. Schonewille H, Klumper FJ, van de Watering LM, et al. High additional maternal red cell alloimmunization after Rhesus- and K-matched intrauterine intravascular transfusions for hemolytic disease of the fetus. Am J Obstet Gynecol 2007;196(2):143, e1–6.
43. el-Azeem SA, Samuels P, Rose RL, et al. The effect of the source of transfused blood on the rate of consumption of transfused red blood cells in pregnancies affected by red blood cell alloimmunization. Am J Obstet Gynecol 1997;177(4):753–7.
44. Grannum PA, Copel JA, Plaxe SC, et al. In utero exchange transfusion by direct intravascular injection in severe erythroblastosis fetalis. N Engl J Med 1986;314(22):1431–4.
45. Gottstein R, Cooke RW. Systematic review of intravenous immunoglobulin in haemolytic disease of the newborn. Arch Dis Child Fetal Neonatal Ed 2003;88(1):F6–10.
46. Ruma MS, Moise KJ Jr, Kim E, et al. Combined plasmapheresis and intravenous immune globulin for the treatment of severe maternal red cell alloimmunization. Am J Obstet Gynecol 2007;196(2):138, e1–6.
47. Poole J, Daniels G. Blood group antibodies and their significance in transfusion medicine. Transfus Med Rev 2007;21(1):58–71.
48. Caine ME, Mueller-Heubach E. Kell sensitization in pregnancy. Am J Obstet Gynecol 1986;154(1):85–90.
49. Weiner CP, Widness JA. Decreased fetal erythropoiesis and hemolysis in Kell hemolytic anemia. Am J Obstet Gynecol 1996;174(2):547–51.
50. Desjardins L, Blajchman MA, Chintu C, et al. The spectrum of ABO hemolytic disease of the newborn infant. J Pediatr 1979;95(3):447–9.

51. Patterson WB. Thrombocytopenic purpura in pregnancy and in the newborn. J Am Med Assoc 1946;130:700–2.
52. Hohlfeld P, Forestier F, Kaplan C, et al. Fetal thrombocytopenia: a retrospective survey of 5,194 fetal blood samplings. Blood 1994;84(6):1851–6.
53. Dreyfus M, Kaplan C, Verdy E, et al. Frequency of immune thrombocytopenia in newborns: a prospective study. Immune Thrombocytopenia Working Group. Blood 1997;89(12):4402–6.
54. Williamson LM, Hackett G, Rennie J, et al. The natural history of fetomaternal alloimmunization to the platelet-specific antigen HPA-1a (PIA1, Zwa) as determined by antenatal screening. Blood 1998;92(7):2280–7.
55. Turner ML, Bessos H, Fagge T, et al. Prospective epidemiologic study of the outcome and cost-effectiveness of antenatal screening to detect neonatal alloimmune thrombocytopenia due to anti-HPA-1a. Transfusion 2005;45(12):1945–56.
56. Kjeldsen-Kragh J, Killie MK, Tomter G, et al. A screening and intervention program aimed to reduce mortality and serious morbidity associated with severe neonatal alloimmune thrombocytopenia. Blood 2007;110(3):833–9.
57. Gruel Y, Boizard B, Daffos F, et al. Determination of platelet antigens and glycoproteins in the human fetus. Blood 1986;68(2):488–92.
58. Giovangrandi Y, Daffos F, Kaplan C, et al. Very early intracranial haemorrhage in alloimmune fetal thrombocytopenia. Lancet 1990;336(8710):310.
59. Murphy MF, Metcalfe P, Waters AH, et al. Antenatal management of severe fetomaternal alloimmune thrombocytopenia: HLA incompatibility may affect responses to fetal platelet transfusions. Blood 1993;81(8):2174–9.
60. Bussel JB, Zabusky MR, Berkowitz RL, et al. Fetal alloimmune thrombocytopenia. N Engl J Med 1997;337(1):22–6.
61. Chen P, Li C, Lang S, Zhu G, et al. Animal model of fetal and neonatal immune thrombocytopenia: role of neonatal Fc receptor in the pathogenesis and therapy. Blood 2010;116(18):3660–8.
62. Mueller-Eckhardt C, Kiefel V, Grubert A, et al. 348 cases of suspected neonatal alloimmune thrombocytopenia. Lancet 1989;1(8634):363–6.
63. Ghevaert C, Campbell K, Walton J, et al. Management and outcome of 200 cases of fetomaternal alloimmune thrombocytopenia. Transfusion 2007;47(5):901–10.
64. Bussel JB, Primiani A. Fetal and neonatal alloimmune thrombocytopenia: progress and ongoing debates. Blood Rev 2008;22(1):33–52.
65. Metcalfe P, Watkins NA, Ouwehand WH, et al. Nomenclature of human platelet antigens. Vox Sang 2003;85(3):240–5.
66. Coller BS, Shattil SJ. The GPIIb/IIIa (integrin alphaIIbbeta3) odyssey: a technology-driven saga of a receptor with twists, turns, and even a bend. Blood 2008;112(8):3011–25.
67. Parry CS, Gorski J, Stern LJ. Crystallographic structure of the human leukocyte antigen DRA, DRB3*0101: models of a directional alloimmune response and autoimmunity. J Mol Biol 2007;371(2):435–46.
68. Peterson JA, Balthazor SM, Curtis BR, et al. Maternal alloimmunization against the rare platelet-specific antigen HPA-9b (Max a) is an important cause of neonatal alloimmune thrombocytopenia. Transfusion 2005;45(9):1487–95.
69. Davoren A, Curtis BR, Aster RH, et al. Human platelet antigen-specific alloantibodies implicated in 1162 cases of neonatal alloimmune thrombocytopenia. Transfusion 2004;44(8):1220–5.
70. Serrarens-Janssen VM, Semmekrot BA, Novotny VM, et al. Fetal/neonatal alloimmune thrombocytopenia (FNAIT): past, present, and future. Obstet Gynecol Surv 2008;63(4):239–52.

71. von dem Borne AE, von Riesz E, Verheugt FW, et al. Baka, a new platelet-specific antigen involved in neonatal allo-immune thrombocytopenia. Vox Sang 1980;39(2):113–20.
72. Friedman JM, Aster RH. Neonatal alloimmune thrombocytopenic purpura and congenital porencephaly in two siblings associated with a "new" maternal anti-platelet antibody. Blood 1985;65(6):1412–5.
73. Maslanka K, Lucas GF, Gronkowska A, et al. A second case of neonatal alloimmune thrombocytopenia associated with anti-PlA2 (Zwb) antibodies. Haematologia (Budap) 1989;22(2):109–13.
74. Kuijpers RW, van den Anker JN, Baerts W, et al. A case of severe neonatal thrombocytopenia with schizencephaly associated with anti-HPA-1b and anti-HPA-2a. Br J Haematol 1994;87(3):576–9.
75. Mercier P, Chicheportiche C, Reviron D, et al. Neonatal thrombocytopenia in HLA-DR, -DQ, -DP-typed mother due to rare anti-HPA-1b (PLA2) (Zwb) fetomaternal immunization. Vox Sang 1994;67(1):46–51.
76. Van den Anker JN, Huiskes E, Porcelein L, et al. Anti-HPA-1b really causes neonatal thrombocytopenia. Br J Haematol 1995;89(2):428.
77. Winters JL, Jennings CD, Desai NS, et al. Neonatal alloimmune thrombocytopenia due to anti-HPA-1b (PLA2) (Zwb). A case report and review. Vox Sang 1998;74(4):256–9.
78. Glade-Bender J, McFarland JG, Kaplan C, et al. Anti-HPA-3A induces severe neonatal alloimmune thrombocytopenia. J Pediatr 2001;138(6):862–7.
79. Koh Y, Taniue A, Ishii H, et al. Neonatal alloimmune thrombocytopenia caused by an antibody specific for a newly identified allele of human platelet antigen-7. Transfusion 2010;50(6):1276–84.
80. Matsuhashi M, Tsuno NH, Kawabata M, et al. The first case of alloantibody against human platelet antigen-15b in Japan: possible alloimmunization by a hydatidiform mole. Transfusion 2010;50(5):1126–30.
81. Kaplan C, Morel-Kopp MC, Kroll H, et al. HPA-5b (Br(a)) neonatal alloimmune thrombocytopenia: clinical and immunological analysis of 39 cases. Br J Haematol 1991;78(3):425–9.
82. Ohto H, Yamaguchi T, Takeuchi C, et al. Anti-HPA-5b-induced neonatal alloimmune thrombocytopenia: antibody titre as a predictor. Collaborative Study Group. Br J Haematol 2000;110(1):223–7.
83. Panzer S, Auerbach L, Cechova E, et al. Maternal alloimmunization against fetal platelet antigens: a prospective study. Br J Haematol 1995;90(3):655–60.
84. Shibata Y, Matsuda I, Miyaji T, et al. Yuka, a new platelet antigen involved in two cases of neonatal alloimmune thrombocytopenia. Vox Sang 1986;50(3):177–80.
85. Taaning E. HLA antibodies and fetomaternal alloimmune thrombocytopenia: myth or meaningful? Transfus Med Rev 2000;14(3):275–80.
86. Kiefel V, Santoso S, Weisheit M, et al. Monoclonal antibody-specific immobilization of platelet antigens (MAIPA): a new tool for the identification of platelet-reactive antibodies. Blood 1987;70(6):1722–6.
87. Roberts I, Stanworth S, Murray NA. Thrombocytopenia in the neonate. Blood Rev 2008;22(4):173–86.
88. Husebekk A, Killie MK, Kjeldsen-Kragh J, et al. Is it time to implement HPA-1 screening in pregnancy? Curr Opin Hematol 2009;16(6):497–502.
89. Bussel JB, Berkowitz RL, Lynch L, et al. Antenatal management of alloimmune thrombocytopenia with intravenous gamma-globulin: a randomized trial of the addition of low-dose steroid to intravenous gamma-globulin. Am J Obstet Gynecol 1996;174(5):1414–23.

90. Kaplan C, Murphy MF, Kroll H, et al. Feto-maternal alloimmune thrombocytopenia: antenatal therapy with IvIgG and steroids—more questions than answers. European Working Group on FMAIT. Br J Haematol 1998;100(1):62–5.

91. Berkowitz RL, Kolb EA, McFarland JG, et al. Parallel randomized trials of risk-based therapy for fetal alloimmune thrombocytopenia. Obstet Gynecol 2006; 107(1):91–6.

92. Berkowitz RL, Lesser ML, McFarland JG, et al. Antepartum treatment without early cordocentesis for standard-risk alloimmune thrombocytopenia: a randomized controlled trial. Obstet Gynecol 2007;110(2 Pt 1):249–55.

93. Bussel JB, Berkowitz RL, McFarland JG, et al. Antenatal treatment of neonatal alloimmune thrombocytopenia. N Engl J Med 1988;319(21):1374–8.

94. Daffos F, Forestier F, Muller JY, et al. Prenatal treatment of alloimmune thrombocytopenia. Lancet 1984;2(8403):632.

95. Khan KS, Wojdyla D, Say L, et al. WHO analysis of causes of maternal death: a systematic review. Lancet 2006;367(9516):1066–74.

96. Anderson JM, Etches D. Prevention and management of postpartum hemorrhage. Am Fam Physician 2007;75(6):875–82.

97. Bais JM, Eskes M, Pel M, et al. Postpartum haemorrhage in nulliparous women: incidence and risk factors in low and high risk women. A Dutch population-based cohort study on standard (> or = 500 ml) and severe (> or = 1000 ml) postpartum haemorrhage. Eur J Obstet Gynecol Reprod Biol 2004;115(2): 166–72.

98. Sosa CG, Althabe F, Belizán JM, et al. Risk factors for postpartum hemorrhage in vaginal deliveries in a Latin-American population. Obstet Gynecol 2009; 113(6):1313–9.

99. Hoveyda F, MacKenzie IZ. Secondary postpartum haemorrhage: incidence, morbidity and current management. BJOG 2001;108(9):927–30.

100. Brenner B. Haemostatic changes in pregnancy. Thromb Res 2004;114(5/6): 409–14.

101. Andersson T, Lorentzen B, Hogdahl H, et al. Thrombin-inhibitor complexes in the blood during and after delivery. Thromb Res 1996;82(2):109–17.

102. Epiney M, Boehlen F, Boulvain M, et al. D-dimer levels during delivery and the postpartum. J Thromb Haemost 2005;3(2):268–71.

103. Levi M. Current understanding of disseminated intravascular coagulation. Br J Haematol 2004;124(5):567–76.

104. Levi M, Toh CH, Thachil J, et al. Guidelines for the diagnosis and management of disseminated intravascular coagulation. British Committee for Standards in Haematology. Br J Haematol 2009;145(1):24–33.

105. Burns ER, Lou Y, Pathak A. Morphologic diagnosis of thrombotic thrombocytopenic purpura. Am J Hematol 2004;75(1):18–21.

106. Taylor FB Jr, Toh CH, Hoots WK, et al. Towards definition, clinical and laboratory criteria, and a scoring system for disseminated intravascular coagulation. Thromb Haemost 2001;86(5):1327–30.

107. Charbit B, Mandelbrot L, Samain E, et al. The decrease of fibrinogen is an early predictor of the severity of postpartum hemorrhage. J Thromb Haemost 2007; 5(2):266–73.

108. Novikova N, Hofmeyr GJ. Tranexamic acid for preventing postpartum haemorrhage. Cochrane Database Syst Rev 2010;7:CD007872.

109. British Committee for Standards in Haematology, Stainsby D, MacLennan S, Thomas D, et al. Guidelines on the management of massive blood loss. Br J Haematol 2006;135(5):634–41.

110. Alexander JM, Sarode R, McIntire DD, et al. Whole blood in the management of hypovolemia due to obstetric hemorrhage. Obstet Gynecol 2009;113(6):1320–6.

111. Holcomb JB. Optimal use of blood products in severely injured trauma patients. Hematology Am Soc Hematol Educ Program 2010;2010:465–9.

112. Scalea TM, Bochicchio KM, Lumpkins K, et al. Early aggressive use of fresh frozen plasma does not improve outcome in critically injured trauma patients. Ann Surg 2008;248(4):578–84.

113. Snyder CW, Weinberg JA, McGwin G Jr, et al. The relationship of blood product ratio to mortality: survival benefit or survival bias? J Trauma 2009;66(2):358–62 [discussion: 362–4].

114. Johansson PI, Stensballe J. Hemostatic resuscitation for massive bleeding: the paradigm of plasma and platelets—a review of the current literature. Transfusion 2010;50(3):701–10.

115. Meng ZH, Wolberg AS, Monroe DM 3rd, et al. The effect of temperature and pH on the activity of factor VIIa: implications for the efficacy of high-dose factor VIIa in hypothermic and acidotic patients. J Trauma 2003;55(5):886–91.

116. Lisman T, De Groot PG. Mechanism of action of recombinant factor VIIa. J Thromb Haemost 2003;1(6):1138–9.

117. Friederich PW, Henny CP, Messelink EJ, et al. Effect of recombinant activated factor VII on perioperative blood loss in patients undergoing retropubic prostatectomy: a double-blind placebo-controlled randomised trial. Lancet 2003; 361(9353):201–5.

118. Boffard KD, Riou B, Warren B, et al. Recombinant factor VIIa as adjunctive therapy for bleeding control in severely injured trauma patients: two parallel randomized, placebo-controlled, double-blind clinical trials. J Trauma 2005; 59(1):8–15 [discussion: 15–8].

119. Lodge JP, Jonas S, Jones RM, et al. Efficacy and safety of repeated perioperative doses of recombinant factor VIIa in liver transplantation. Liver Transpl 2005; 11(8):973–9.

120. Pihusch M, Bacigalupo A, Szer J, et al. Recombinant activated factor VII in treatment of bleeding complications following hematopoietic stem cell transplantation. J Thromb Haemost 2005;3(9):1935–44.

121. Bosch J, Thabut D, Albillos A, et al. Recombinant factor VIIa for variceal bleeding in patients with advanced cirrhosis: a randomized, controlled trial. Hepatology 2008; 47(5):1604–14.

122. Sachs B, Delacy D, Green J, et al. Recombinant activated factor VII in spinal surgery: a multicenter, randomized, double-blind, placebo-controlled, dose-escalation trial. Spine (Phila Pa 1976) 2007;32(21):2285–93.

123. Mayer SA, Brun NC, Begtrup K, et al. Efficacy and safety of recombinant activated factor VII for acute intracerebral hemorrhage. N Engl J Med 2008; 358(20):2127–37.

124. Gill R, Herbertson M, Vuylsteke A, et al. Safety and efficacy of recombinant activated factor VII: a randomized placebo-controlled trial in the setting of bleeding after cardiac surgery. Circulation 2009;120(1):21–7.

125. Moscardó F, Pérez F, de la Rubia J, et al. Successful treatment of severe intra-abdominal bleeding associated with disseminated intravascular coagulation using recombinant activated factor VII. Br J Haematol 2001;114(1):174–6.

126. Bouwmeester FW, Jonkhoff AR, Verheijen RH, et al. Successful treatment of life-threatening postpartum hemorrhage with recombinant activated factor VII. Obstet Gynecol 2003;101(6):1174–6.

127. Boehlen F, Morales MA, Fontana P, et al. Prolonged treatment of massive post-partum haemorrhage with recombinant factor VIIa: case report and review of the literature. BJOG 2004;111(3):284–7.
128. Segal S, Shemesh IY, Blumental R, et al. The use of recombinant factor VIIa in severe postpartum hemorrhage. Acta Obstet Gynecol Scand 2004;83(8):771–2.
129. Ahonen J, Jokela R. Recombinant factor VIIa for life-threatening post-partum haemorrhage. Br J Anaesth 2005;94(5):592–5.
130. Pepas LP, Arif-Adib M, Kadir RA. Factor VIIa in puerperal hemorrhage with disseminated intravascular coagulation. Obstet Gynecol 2006;108(3 Pt 2):757–61.
131. Sobieszczyk S, Breborowicz GH, Platicanov V, et al. Recombinant factor VIIa in the management of postpartum bleeds: an audit of clinical use. Acta Obstet Gynecol Scand 2006;85(10):1239–47.
132. Alfirevic Z, Elbourne D, Pavord S, et al. Use of recombinant activated factor VII in primary postpartum hemorrhage: the Northern European registry 2000–2004. Obstet Gynecol 2007;110(6):1270–8.
133. Haynes J, Laffan M, Plaat F. Use of recombinant activated factor VII in massive obstetric haemorrhage. Int J Obstet Anesth 2007;16(1):40–9.
134. Franchini M, Franchi M, Bergamini V, et al. A critical review on the use of recombinant factor VIIa in life-threatening obstetric postpartum hemorrhage. Semin Thromb Hemost 2008;34(1):104–12.
135. Isbister J, Phillips L, Dunkley S, et al. Recombinant activated factor VII in critical bleeding: experience from the Australian and New Zealand Haemostasis Register. Intern Med J 2008;38(3):156–65.
136. Lewis NR, Brunker P, Lemire SJ, et al. Failure of recombinant factor VIIa to correct the coagulopathy in a case of severe postpartum hemorrhage. Transfusion 2009;49(4):689–95.
137. Franchini M, Manzato F, Salvagno GL, et al. Potential role of recombinant activated factor VII for the treatment of severe bleeding associated with disseminated intravascular coagulation: a systematic review. Blood Coagul Fibrinolysis 2007;18(7):589–93.
138. Franchini M, Franchi M, Bergamini V, et al. The use of recombinant activated FVII in postpartum hemorrhage. Clin Obstet Gynecol 2010;53(1):219–27.
139. Levi M, Levy JH, Andersen HF, et al. Safety of recombinant activated factor VII in randomized clinical trials. N Engl J Med 2010;363(19):1791–800.
140. Nagel HT, de Haan TR, Vandenbussche FP, et al. Long-term outcome after fetal transfusion for hydrops associated with parvovirus B19 infection. Obstet Gynecol 2007;109(1):42–7.
141. Oepkes D, Adama van Scheltema P. Intrauterine fetal transfusions in the management of fetal anemia and fetal thrombocytopenia. Semin Fetal Neonatal Med 2007;12(6):432–8.
142. Staroselsky A, Klieger-Grossmann C, Garcia-Bournissen F, et al. Exposure to fifth disease in pregnancy. Can Fam Physician 2009;55(12):1195–8.

Hematologic Disease in Pregnancy: The Obstetrician's Perspective

Nicole A. Smith, MD, MPH*, Katherine E. Economy, MD, MPH

KEYWORDS

- Pregnancy • Hematology • Delivery planning

Hematologic disease is common among reproductive age women and therefore hematologic conditions are seen frequently in pregnancy. Most disorders can be safely managed through parturition, with the result of a healthy mother and child. Although the risks of pregnancy and impact of disease will differ based on the condition present, the general approach to the gravid patient remains the same. The care plan should address how pregnancy affects her disease, and how the disease affects pregnancy. Discussions with the pregnant woman should include the impact of her condition on common obstetric complications, medication concerns, labor and delivery management, and risks of heritability.

HOW THE DISEASE AFFECTS PREGNANCY

The effect of hematologic disease on pregnancy varies by trimester. Most women with medical conditions should be advised that they will have increased maternal and fetal surveillance during their pregnancies. This may involve increased visits, laboratory draws, or fetal evaluation. In addition, there may be extensive planning for labor and delivery.

The First Trimester

Women with bleeding disorders are at increased risk for obstetric complications in the first trimester of pregnancy. Embryo implantation, miscarriage, molar and ectopic pregnancy are all associated with bleeding. Miscarriage (loss before 24 weeks' gestation) complicates 10% to 15% of pregnancies.[1] Bleeding associated with miscarriage may be heavy, depending on the gestational age at the time of loss. Some women

---

The authors have nothing to disclose.

Division of Maternal Fetal Medicine, Department of Obstetrics and Gynecology, Brigham and Women's Hospital and Harvard Medical School, 75 Francis Street, Boston, MA 02115, USA

* Corresponding author.

E-mail address: nasmith@partners.org

Hematol Oncol Clin N Am 25 (2011) 415–423

doi:10.1016/j.hoc.2011.01.002

choose to pass early pregnancies at home, whereas others prefer to have surgical evacuations by vacuum aspiration or dilation and curettage. Because they are at increased risk of uncontrolled hemorrhage, women with bleeding disorders are typically best served by a surgical evacuation, which requires careful surgical planning. Molar pregnancies are rare, occurring in approximately 0.1% of pregnancies.[2] Bleeding is a hallmark of molar pregnancy, and surgical evacuation is required.

The Second Trimester

Women with hematologic disorders may desire invasive testing for aneuploidy in the second trimester. Options include chorionic villus sampling (CVS) and amniocentesis. In CVS, a biopsy of the placenta is taken between 11 and 14 weeks' gestation. This procedure may entail more risk for women with bleeding disorders and special precautions such as pretreating with desmopressin acetate (DDAVP), or blood products should be considered. Amniocentesis is associated with a lower risk for bleeding; however, the risks and benefits of the procedure should still be addressed with the patient and her obstetrician. Prophylactic anticoagulation is often held for 1 day before either procedure, particularly CVS, depending on provider preference.

The Third Trimester

A small number of women experience complications that put their health, or the health of their fetus, at risk. These typically occur in the third trimester. Three of the most common, and those most likely to be affected by hematologic disease, are placental abruption, placenta previa, and preterm labor. A careful obstetric history may help to stratify the risks, because complications frequently recur. These complications are often unpreventable and of sudden onset, a carefully documented emergency management plan is essential.

Placental abruption

Placental abruption is defined as a separation of the placental bed from the uterine wall. An abruption may be characterized by light bleeding, or by major obstetric hemorrhage requiring emergent delivery. Rates of abruption vary by population from 0.7%[3] to 1.4%.[4] The incidence is higher in women with risk factors such as smoking, hypertension, or prior abruption. Bleeding disorders and anticoagulation may substantially increase the risk to both mother and fetus in this setting. All pregnant women with bleeding disorders should have a plan in place that outlines how to manage unexpected bleeding.

Abnormal placentation

Placenta previa describes the situation in which the placenta is implanted close to, or overlying, the uterine cervix, whereas placenta accreta describes invasion of the placenta into the uterine wall. The risks of placenta previa and accreta increase with greater numbers of cesarean deliveries or uterine surgeries. Previa is associated with a risk of bleeding from unprotected placental vessels, which often leads to hospitalization and preterm birth. For most women without a prior cesarean delivery, a placenta previa seen early in pregnancy spontaneously resolves as the uterus grows during gestation. Placenta accreta almost universally necessitates hysterectomy at the time of delivery.

Preterm labor

Preterm labor affects approximately 13% of the population, with more than 70% of these babies born between 34 and 36 weeks' gestation.[5] Preterm contractions without labor are even more common. The diagnosis of preterm labor is often challenging to make. Although some women presents in labor and subsequently deliver within a few hours, others report contractions without cervical change for several days before cervical dilation. The unpredictable nature of obstetrics makes the management of patients with significant hematologic disease challenging. For example, for women maintained on therapeutic anticoagulation, there may be inadequate time for anticoagulation to be reversed, preventing the patient from getting regional anesthesia in labor, and increasing the risks of bleeding at delivery. Conversely, women with idiopathic thrombocytopenic purpura (ITP), who are often not treated until later in the pregnancy, may miss the opportunity for therapy before delivery, increasing their risks of bleeding.

Tocolytic medications including nifedipine, terbutaline, indomethicin, and magnesium sulfate are often given in an effort to halt preterm labor. Tocolysis is controversial, although many believe that it may arrest labor for 48 hours, the time period in which steroids are given to induce fetal lung maturity. For all of these reasons, it is important to make careful delivery plans early in gestation. These plans may be complex, making the accurate diagnosis and management of preterm labor critical.

Labor and Delivery: Specific Concerns

Many women who pass easily through their pregnancies are surprised at the level of planning and risk that delivery entails. Coordination between multiple teams is often required, including obstetrics (generally maternal fetal medicine specialists, if available), hematology, anesthesia, blood bank, and nursing, and it is never too early to start planning. As discussed earlier, many women have unexpected pregnancy complications, including bleeding and preterm labor, and a carefully laid plan can prevent substantial maternal and fetal morbidity.

A detailed labor and delivery plan should discuss mode of delivery, anesthesia concerns, and specific risks to the mother or fetus related to the hematologic disorder in question. In specific cases, it may also be helpful to provide the patient with a copy of her delivery plan, particularly if she lives at distance from the hospital or is planning to travel.

Pregnant women with medical disease are often advised to schedule delivery either by induction of labor or cesarean section, to optimize safety surrounding the delivery or to allow postpartum therapies that are contraindicated during pregnancy. Most of these deliveries can be undertaken in the 39th week, when fetal outcomes are optimized, but before many women have entered into spontaneous labor. There are some cases in which delivery before 39 weeks is indicated, most notably when maternal medical needs outweigh the small risks of late preterm birth to the fetus. The earlier in gestation that induction of labor is undertaken, the more likely that the uterine cervix is unfavorable, which increases the duration of the induction.

Both induction of labor and cesarean delivery carry significant risks. There are few strict indications for cesarean section. Inarguable maternal indications include a history of several different types of uterine surgery or abnormal placentation (placenta previa or accreta). Women may also have uncommon medical or physical conditions for which cesarean delivery is preferred, such as an inability to obtain lithotomy position, or pelvic contractures. Strict fetal indications include malpresentation (the presenting fetus is persistently breech or transverse) and some fetal anomalies, for example neural tube defect. Cesarean delivery is also commonly performed for several other reasons, including maternal request and suspected fetal macrosomia. Indications for cesarean delivery must be individualized, but most women are candidates for vaginal birth.

Induction of labor is achieved through use of vaginal prostaglandins, mechanical dilation, and intravenous (IV) oxytocin. During the period of cervical ripening, most women are not yet in labor, and may not be for another 24 hours or longer. For those with a prior vaginal birth, delivery may be attained in under one day. Without a prior vaginal birth, induction is less predictable and may take several days, depending on provider and patient tolerance. Some women experience minor bleeding during cervical dilation; however, most bleeding occurs around delivery. Bleeding continues until vaginal lacerations are repaired and uterine tone is achieved, typically within 40 minutes after the infant's birth. Typical blood loss for vaginal birth is less than 500 mL.

Cesarean section accounts for more than 30% of deliveries.[5] The operation is typically performed through a transverse lower abdominal skin incision, and transverse uterine incision. The duration of surgery is commonly 30 to 60 minutes, with blood loss under 1000 mL. The procedure can be scheduled at the convenience of the obstetric and medical teams, often making it an appealing option. Nonetheless, cesarean delivery carries greater maternal risks of hemorrhage and infection than does vaginal delivery, and increases the chance of abnormal placentation in a future pregnancy. With each surgery, these risks rise. Incidence of thromboembolic disease is also increased for 6 weeks postpartum. For all of these reasons, cesarean delivery should only be performed with appropriate indications.

For both vaginal birth and cesarean delivery, careful consideration must be given to the management timeline. At any point during a labor induction, an emergent delivery might become necessary. Anticoagulation is held during labor for all but the most critical indications (eg, artificial heart valves, severe prothrombotic states). For that reason, some would recommend a cesarean delivery to limit the time off anticoagulation; however, surgery increases the risk of postpartum clot formation compared with vaginal delivery. In addition, vaginal delivery is less likely to be complicated by postdelivery bleeding that would be worsened by anticoagulation. In a carefully monitored setting, with appropriate anesthesia and blood bank support, women may be anticoagulated during labor, with anticoagulation held at delivery and in the immediate postpartum period. This strategy should be reserved for the most critically ill patients who have a life-threatening risk of thrombosis.

A woman who requires platelet or other transfusion support would have a different scenario. For that patient, consideration must to given to frequency of laboratory evaluation, and timing and indications for transfusion. If the patient is to be induced, should transfusions begin on admission, in the active phase of labor, or when delivery is imminent? For the patient requiring platelets, should transfusions be initiated if platelets decline, or when they reach a certain threshold? Every patient should also have an emergency backup plan, in case of complications such as a transfusion reaction or the need for an unscheduled cesarean delivery.

The importance of communication among various members of the team cannot be overstated. Before delivery, it is helpful to have a detailed discussion regarding what complications from the pregnancy and disease may be anticipated, as well as any known complications of therapy. In addition, definition of critical laboratory values and an algorithm with which to treat them are essential. If an induction is planned, clear communication with the blood bank to ensure adequate stocking of the appropriate products and preparation of medications is also of key importance. If adequate products cannot be assured, consideration should be given to transfer of the patient to a facility with appropriate resources.

Anesthesia

Anesthesia is an important component of labor and delivery planning. Many women undergoing spontaneous or induced labor request epidural anesthesia, and most uncomplicated cesarean deliveries are performed under spinal anesthesia. There is controversy in the anesthesia literature regarding safe platelet levels for regional anesthesia. Although some sources suggest platelets greater than 100,000 minimize the risk of epidural hematoma,[6] others[7,8] report safe placement with platelets as low as 69,000. At our institution, platelets of 70,000 are required for both regional anesthesia placement and removal of the epidural catheter.[9] Additional options for pain control during a vaginal birth include intravenous or intramuscular narcotics, and for cesarean delivery, general anesthesia. General anesthesia increases the likelihood of need for neonatal resuscitation, including intubation.

Postpartum hemorrhage

Postpartum hemorrhage (PPH) is defined as blood loss greater than 500 mL for a vaginal delivery or 1000 mL for a cesarean delivery. Rates of PPH vary by study, but have been reported to be as high as 19% in a low-risk European population.[10,11] Many healthy young women tolerate the increased blood loss well. Almost all hemorrhages occur within 24 hours of delivery (early PPH), with a small minority occurring 24 hours to 6 weeks after delivery (late PPH). Bleeding may be brisk, because between 500 and 800 mL of blood pass through the term uterus each minute. Given the frequency of PPH, the unique risks hemorrhage may hold for the patient with hematologic disease need to be considered, as well as parameters for transfusion or medication therapy.

Fetal Concerns

An important consideration when caring for pregnant women with medical disease is the risk that the fetus will either inherit the disease in question, or be affected by the mother's condition. Any woman with a potentially heritable disorder should be offered genetic counseling before pregnancy or early in gestation, because genetic testing for the fetus may be possible. Understanding fetal risk is also essential for delivery planning. If the fetus has a known or suspected bleeding disorder, or, as in ITP, there is concern for neonatal thrombocytopenia, operative vaginal delivery (forceps or vacuum-assisted delivery) is contraindicated, as is fetal monitoring using a scalp electrode. In these infants, profound thrombocytopenia may develop in the first days of life, therefore communication with the pediatric team is essential.

HOW PREGNANCY AFFECTS THE DISEASE

Pregnancy may impact medical disease in several ways. It may affect the ability to diagnose or treat disease, or it may change the course of disease. The goal of medical treatment in pregnancy should be to achieve the same level of care that would be seen in the absence of pregnancy.

Diagnosis

Many diagnostic procedures are considered low risk, and should be used if they can improve maternal outcomes. Nonionizing radiation is considered safe in pregnancy. With regard to ionizing radiation, studies have shown that with exposure of less than 5 rad at any point in pregnancy, noncancer health effects are not detectable. Exposure of 5 to 50 rad before 15 weeks may be associated with an increased incidence of major malformations and growth restriction, reduction in intelligence quotient, and increase in severe mental retardation. These risks are seen with exposure to more than 50 rad at any point in pregnancy.[12,13]

Ionizing radiation raises the risk of childhood cancers, and may increase the lifetime risk for solid tumors. Exposure of less than 5 rad is associated with a 0.3% to 1% incidence of childhood cancers, particularly leukemia, in comparison with a background risk of 0.3%. The incidence of childhood cancers increases to 6% with exposure of greater than 50 rad. Radiation exposure from a typical computed tomography (CT) scan of the abdomen is less than 2.6 rad, whereas from a CT head it is less than 0.5 rad. Fetal radiation exposure in an abdominal radiograph is less than 0.3 rad.[12,13]

In practice, many obstetricians counsel patients that appropriately indicated radiologic studies should be performed, with an effort made to avoid ionizing radiation exposure in the first trimester if possible.

Pregnant women can also safely undergo many procedures, including bone marrow biopsies. Surgery such as splenectomy can be performed during gestation if necessary, optimally in the second trimester.

Medication Use

Commonly used medications include steroids, anticoagulants, narcotics, erythropoietin, DDAVP, and intravenous immunoglobulin (IVIG). In most cases, the benefits of these medications outweigh the low risk to the fetus. Many chemotherapeutic agents can also be used safely in pregnancy.

Medication use is most restricted in the first trimester because of concerns for teratogenicity and pregnancy loss. Many women with nausea and vomiting in the first months of pregnancy find it difficult to tolerate pills and do best with intravenous or per rectum administration. Later in gestation, some medications can be associated with growth restriction of the fetus. In this case, we recommend serial ultrasound surveillance of fetal growth. The specific risks of some commonly used medications are outlined later.

A large number of medications are also compatible with lactation. Unlike guidelines for medication use in pregnancy, those for use in lactation differ depending on the reference used. The most current information can be obtained from a free National Institutes of Health–sponsored Web site called LactMed (toxnet.nlm.nih.gov).

Commonly Used Medications in Pregnancy and Lactation

Prednisone: US Food and Drug Administration category B or C, compatible with breastfeeding

Prednisone is converted in the liver into its active metabolite prednisolone, which can be expected to cross the placenta. Prednisone and other glucocorticoids are associated with oral clefting in animals. That relationship has not been proved in humans; however, a recent review suggests that a relationship with oral clefting cannot be excluded.[14] Prednisone use has been associated with fetal growth restriction, although growth restriction may be more highly correlated with the underlying condition. Most obstetricians are comfortable using prednisone during pregnancy, avoiding use during organogenesis if possible, and with appropriate surveillance for fetal growth.

The American Academy of Pediatrics has classified prednisone and prednisolone as compatible with breastfeeding, despite the secretion of small amounts of the medication into breast milk.[15]

Heparin (category C) and low molecular weight heparins (category B): both compatible with breastfeeding

Because of the large size of these molecules, heparin and low molecular weight heparins do not cross the placenta or enter breast milk.[16]

Fondaparinux: category B, probably compatible with breastfeeding
No human studies exist to define the risk of malformations with the use of fondaparinux during organogenesis. Animal models have not shown increased risk. Small amounts of fondaparinux cross the placenta, with newborn blood concentrations approximately 10% of those in the mother.[17]

Despite the high molecular weight of this molecule, excretion in milk of lactating rats has been described, therefore excretion into human milk can be expected. The potential effects on the fetus are unknown, but likely clinically insignificant.[18]

Epoetin alfa: category C, compatible with breastfeeding
Epoetin alfa does not seem to cross the placenta. Presence alfa in human milk has not been studied; however, erythropoietin is a normal component of breast milk.[19]

DDAVP: category B, compatible with breastfeeding
Anecdotal reports of congenital anomalies exist, but no causal relationship has been established. There is a theoretic risk of DDAVP causing uterine contractions; however, it is highly specific to the V2 receptor, and seems to have little effect on the smooth muscle V1 receptor. Use of DDAVP is therefore safe in pregnancy, because it does not lead to increased uterine activity.[20] There is minimal excretion of DDAVP into breast milk, and oral absorption by the infant is poor.[21]

Iron
> *Iron dextran: category C, compatible with breastfeeding*
> *Iron sucrose: category B, compatible with breastfeeding*
> *Sodium ferric gluconate: category B, compatible with breastfeeding.*

Iron dextran has been shown to be teratogenic and embryocidal to animals when given in 3 times the maximum human dose. Studies regarding placental transfer have been inconclusive. Some iron dextran does seem to reach the fetus, but it is unknown in what form. In practice, iron dextran is given when indicated to pregnant women. Neither iron sucrose nor sodium ferric gluconate have been shown to be teratogenic in animals, and no human studies exist.[22–24]

Traces of unmetabolized iron dextran are present in human milk. An oral agent may be preferred because of limited experience in lactation. If this drug is required, breastfeeding should not be discontinued. Iron sucrose does not appear to increase breast milk iron. It is unknown whether sodium ferric gluconate is excreted in breast milk, but use is considered compatible with breastfeeding.[25–27]

The Course of Disease

In some cases, pregnancy affects the course of disease, either by increasing the progression of illness or by increasing the likelihood of complications. For example, pregnancy is a hypercoagulable state, and therefore associated with an increased risk of thrombosis in women with thrombophilias. Although outcomes for pregnant women with sickle cell disease have improved, pregnancy is associated with an increase in both morbidity and mortality in affected women.[28] This is an important component of counseling because it may affect a woman's choice to conceive or continue a pregnancy.

SUMMARY

Pregnancy can be a time of significantly increased morbidity and mortality in women with hematologic disease; however, with careful planning and preparation, most women can be cared for safely, resulting in a healthy mother and healthy child.

ACKNOWLEDGMENTS

The authors wish to thank Bhavani Kodali, MD, Louise Wilkins-Haug, MD, PhD, and Meaghan Muir, MLIS, for assistance in the preparation of this manuscript.

REFERENCES

1. Neilson JP, Gyte GM, Hickey M, et al. Medical treatments for incomplete miscarriage (less than 24 weeks). Cochrane Database Syst Rev 2010;1:CD007223.
2. Lurain JR. Gestational trophoblastic disease I: epidemiology, pathology, clinical presentation and diagnosis of gestational trophoblastic disease, and management of hydatidiform mole. Am J Obstet Gynecol 2010;203(6):531–9.
3. Ananth CV, Wilcox AJ. Placental abruption and perinatal mortality in the United States. Am J Epidemiol 2001;153(4):332–7.
4. Ananth CV, Oyelese Y, Yeo L, et al. Placental abruption in the United States, 1979 through 2001: temporal trends and potential determinants. Am J Obstet Gynecol 2005;192(1):191–8.
5. Hamilton BE, Martin JA, Ventura SJ, et al. Births: final data for 2007. Natl Vital Stat Rep 2010;28(24). Available at: http://www.cdc.gov/nchs/data/nvsr/nvsr58/nvsr58_24.pdf. Accessed October 4, 2010.
6. Bromage PR. Neurologic complications of regional anesthesia for obstetrics. In: Schnider SM, Levinson G, editors. Anesthesia for obstetrics. 3rd edition. Baltimore (MD): Williams & Wilkins; 1993. p. 443–4.
7. Beilin Y, Zahn J, Comerford M. Safe epidural analgesia in thirty parturients with platelet counts between 69,000 and 98,000 mm(-3). Anesth Analg 1997;85(2):385–8.
8. Rolbin SH, Abbott D, Musclow E, et al. Epidural anesthesia in pregnant patients with low platelet counts. Obstet Gynecol 1988;71:918–20.
9. Datta S, Kodali BS, Segal S. Obstetric anesthesia handbook. New York (NY): Springer; 2010. p. 326–9.
10. Rossen J, Okland I, Nilsen OB, et al. Is there an increase of postpartum hemorrhage, and is severe hemorrhage associated with more frequent use of obstetric interventions? Acta Obstet Gynecol Scand 2010;89(10):1248–55.
11. Bais JM, Eskes M, Pel M, et al. Postpartum haemorrhage in nulliparous women: incidence and risk factors in low and high risk women. A Dutch population-based cohort study on standard (> or = 500 ml) and severe (> or = 1000 ml) postpartum haemorrhage. Eur J Obstet Gynecol Reprod Biol 2004;115(2):166–72.
12. Radiation and pregnancy: a fact sheet for clinicians. Centers for disease control and prevention web site. 2005. Available at: http://www.bt.cdc.gov/radiation/prenatalphysician.asp. Accessed October 4, 2010.
13. Williams PM, Fletcher S. Health effects of prenatal radiation exposure. Am Fam Physician 2010;82(5):488–93.
14. van Runnard Heimel PJ, Schobben AF, Huisjes AJ, et al. The transplacental passage of prednisolone in pregnancies complicated by early-onset HELLP syndrome. Placenta 2005;26:842–5.
15. Committee on Drugs. American academy of pediatrics. The transfer of drugs and other chemicals into human breast milk. Pediatrics 2001;108:776–87.
16. Reprotox [database]. Heparin. Chevy Chase (MD): Reproductive Toxicology Center; 2010. Available at: http://www.reprotox.org. Accessed October 25, 2010.
17. Dempfle CE. Minor transplacental passage of fondaparinux in vivo. N Engl J Med 2004;350:1914–5.

18. Briggs GG, Freeman RK, Yaffe SJ. Drugs in pregnancy and lactation. Philadelphia: Lippincott Williams & Wilkins; 2005.
19. Reprotox [database]. Epoetin alfa. Chevy Chase (MD): Reproductive Toxicology Center; 2010. Available at: http://www.reprotox.org. Accessed October 25, 2010.
20. Kitchens CS, Alving BM, Kessler CM. Consultative hemostasis and thrombosis. Philadelphia: WB Saunders; 2002. p. 440.
21. Drugs and Lactation Database (LactMed). Desmopressin CASRN: 16679-58-6. Bethesda (MD): National Library of Medicine; 2007. Available at: http://toxnet. nlm.nih.gov/cgi-bin/sis/search/f?./temp/~1kMFyc:1. Accessed October 25, 2010.
22. Center for Drug Evaluation and Research, US Food and Drug Administration. INFeD NDA 017441 final printed labeling. 2009. Available at: http://www. accessdata.fda.gov/drugsatfda_docs/label/2009/017441s171lbl.pdf. Accessed October 25, 2010.
23. Center for Drug Evaluation and Research, US Food and Drug Administration. Venofer NDA 021135 final printed labeling. 2007. Available at: http://www. accessdata.fda.gov/drugsatfda_docs/nda/2000/21135_Venofer_prntlbl.pdf. Accessed October 25, 2010.
24. Center for Drug Evaluation and Research, US Food and Drug Administration. Ferrlecit NDA 020955 final printed labeling. 2006. Available at: http://www. accessdata.fda.gov/drugsatfda_docs/label/2006/020955s010lbl.pdf. Accessed October 25, 2010.
25. Drugs and Lactation Database (LactMed). Iron sucrose CASRN: 8047-67-4. Bethesda (MD): National Library of Medicine; 2007. Available at: http://toxnet. nlm.nih.gov/cgi-bin/sis/search/f?./temp/~1iksqV:1. Accessed October 25, 2010.
26. Reprotox [database]. Iron dextran. Chevy Chase (MD): Reproductive Toxicology Center; 2010. Available at: http://www.reprotox.org. Accessed October 25, 2010.
27. Drugdex [database]. Sodium ferric gluconate. Greenwood Village (CO): Thomson Reuters (Healthcare); October 19, 2010. Available at: http://www. thomsonhc.com. Accessed October 25, 2010.
28. Rogers DT, Molokie R. Sickle cell disease in pregnancy. Obstet Gynecol Clin North Am 2010;37(2):223–37.

Anesthesia in the Pregnant Patient with Hematologic Disorders

Lorraine Chow, MD, FRCPC, Michaela K. Farber, MD,
William R. Camann, MD*

KEYWORDS

- Anesthesia • Pregnancy • Hematology • Epidural
- Coagulopathy • Anticoagulation

OVERVIEW OF OBSTETRIC ANESTHESIA

Introduction

Anesthetic management of the obstetric patient with hematologic disease requires establishing a plan for anesthesia that incorporates the patient's specific hematologic problem, the comorbidities, and the obstetric situation. The increasing popularity of regional anesthesia in the last several decades has greatly changed the experience of labor. Whereas the use of regional anesthesia has aided in decreasing maternal morbidity and mortality, a new dimension to the evaluation of hematologic issues and the increased awareness of maternal thrombophilias has led to the present widespread use of various anticoagulant medications in the pregnant population. Moreover, the increasing rate of cesarean delivery has resulted in an increased incidence of placental implantation abnormalities with resultant maternal hemorrhage concerns. This discussion briefly reviews the common principles of anesthesia for obstetric patients, provides an obstetric anesthesiologist's perspective on the implications of regional anesthesia in obstetrics, and enhances communication between the specialties.

Principles of General Anesthesia for Cesarean Delivery

When general anesthesia is required for cesarean delivery, a rapid sequence technique is typically used whereby an intravenous induction agent (most commonly sodium thiopental [Pentothal] or propofol) and the paralytic agent succinylcholine

The authors have nothing to disclose.
Department of Anesthesiology, Perioperative and Pain Medicine, Harvard Medical School, Brigham and Women's Hospital, 75 Francis Street, CWN L1, Boston, MA 02115, USA
* Corresponding author.
E-mail address: wcamann@partners.org

Hematol Oncol Clin N Am 25 (2011) 425–443
doi:10.1016/j.hoc.2011.01.003   hemonc.theclinics.com
0889-8588/11/$ – see front matter © 2011 Elsevier Inc. All rights reserved.

are given in quick succession, followed by endotracheal intubation using cricoid pressure to prevent passive regurgitation of the stomach contents. Anesthesia is maintained using a volatile inhalation anesthetic agent, with the addition of nitrous oxide after umbilical cord clamping to minimize the concentration of volatile agent and the risk of uterine atony and postpartum bleeding.[1] Parenteral opioid boluses or intravenous opioid patient-controlled analgesia (PCA) are used for postoperative pain management.[1]

The incidence of cesarean deliveries has increased in the past decade and accounts for almost 40% of all deliveries in some countries.[2] The relative risk of maternal mortality is greater with general anesthesia compared with neuraxial anesthesia because general anesthesia is more commonly performed in the presence of underlying comorbidities or obstetric complications.[2] Approximately 25% of cesarean deliveries are done in an urgent or emergent manner for maternal or fetal indications.[2] In these situations, general anesthesia may still be required to achieve rapid anesthetic depth for surgery and to prevent maternal or fetal compromise. The presence of uncorrected coagulopathy or the use of anticoagulant or antithrombotic medications may also necessitate the use of general anesthesia. Major concerns of general anesthesia include difficult airway management, risk of maternal awareness, depressant effects of inhalation anesthetics on uterine tone and the ensuing postpartum hemorrhage, and drug effects on early fetal alertness and later fetal neuronal development.[2]

Maternal mortality has decreased dramatically in the last 50 years, due in large part to the widespread adoption of neuraxial anesthetic techniques.[3] The regional anesthesia use for cesarean delivery was 55% in 1981 compared with 84% in 1992.[3] This change in practice has paralleled the decline in maternal mortality related to anesthesia. An analysis of the liability claims between the years 1990 and 2003 compared with claims pre-1990 showed that respiratory causes of injuries decreased from 21% to 4%. During this time, the claims for maternal nerve injury and maternal back pain increased significantly.[4,5] The incidence of failed tracheal intubation in the pregnant population is 8 times higher than in the nonpregnant population (up to 1 in 250) and can be unexpected.[6–9] Pilkington and colleagues[10] examined the maternal airway and found a 34% increase in the incidence of the most difficult airway classification (Mallampati 4, Samsoon modification) when comparing their airways at 12 and 38 weeks' gestation. These changes have been attributed to pregnancy-related fluid retention, weight gain, and breast enlargement. The process of labor and delivery can further worsen airway edema, making airway instrumentation even more difficult (**Fig. 1**).[11] Coupled with the pregnancy-related increase in oxygen consumption and decrease in functional residual capacity, these patients are at a high risk of arterial oxygen desaturation during apneic episodes. This risk is exaggerated even further in morbidly obese patients and those with preeclampsia and multiple gestations.[2]

Although gastric emptying of liquids does not seem to decline during pregnancy and labor,[12,13] the reduction in lower esophageal sphincter tone and cephalad displacement of the stomach by the gravid uterus increases the risk of gastroesophageal reflux disease during pregnancy.[14] According to the American Society of Anesthesiologists (ASA) task force on preoperative fasting guidelines, the ingestion of clear fluids is allowed throughout labor and up to 2 hours before a scheduled surgical procedure but oral intake of solids should cease at least 6 hours before elective cesarean delivery.[15,16]

Principles of Regional Anesthesia

Neuraxial techniques such as spinal, epidural, and combined spinal-epidural (CSE) can be used both for pain relief during labor as well as surgical anesthesia during cesarean delivery. The choice of technique depends on patient factors, the need for

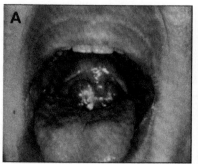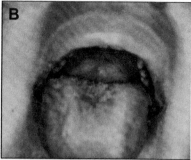

Fig. 1. Airway changes during labor (*A*) Airway before labor (Samsoon modification of Mallampati class 1 airway). (*B*) Airway of the same patient after labor (Samsoon modification of Mallampati class 3 airway). (*Reproduced from* Kodali BS, Chandrasekha S, Bulich LN, et al. Airway changes during labor and delivery. Anesthesiology 2008;108:360; with permission.)

speed and reliability of onset, the ability to titrate and redose via a catheter-based technique, and individual preference. Spinal anesthesia relies on the deposition of local anesthetic (usually in combination with an opioid) into the cerebrospinal fluid. This technique is quick, reliable, provides excellent surgical anesthesia, and uses a small gauge (25 gauge) pencil-point needle for administration.[1] The disadvantages of spinal anesthetics are the risk of hypotension from rapid onset of sympathectomy and vasodilation, as well as a limited duration of action (typically 1–2 hours). Epidural anesthesia is performed by placing a catheter in the epidural space, with the option for continual infusion or intermittent boluses through the catheter (**Fig. 2**A). Epidural anesthesia is slower in onset and associated with less hemodynamic instability compared with spinal anesthesia. The presence of a catheter allows for titration of medication dose as well as readministration of local anesthetic for the duration of labor and for prolonged surgical procedures. The catheter can also be left in place for postoperative pain management or when the risk of bleeding requiring reoperation is a concern. The disadvantages of this technique include occasional inadequate spread of the anesthetic and the increased risk of venous injury and epidural hematoma formation with the use of a larger-gauge needle (17 gauge or 18 gauge).[17] The use of neuraxial techniques in a parturient with hematologic disease may be precluded by uncorrected coagulopathy or when the risk of epidural hematoma outweighs the benefit.

Physiologic Changes of Pregnancy: Epidural Vein Dilation

The epidural space contains a venous plexus that becomes distended during pregnancy, labor, and delivery.[18] During routine spinal and epidural placement, puncture of this plexus can lead to venous bleeding. The accumulation of blood in the epidural space can lead to compression of spinal cord and spinal nerves, with potential for permanent neurologic deficits if the compression is not relieved within 6 to 12 hours.

Regional Anesthesia for Cesarean Delivery

Neuraxial technique is the most common method of anesthesia for cesarean delivery.[19] For most elective cesarean deliveries, a single injection of local anesthetic and opioid is given through a pencil-point spinal needle (eg, 25-gauge Whitacre needle) with a typical duration of anesthesia of 1 to 2 hours depending on the drug and dose. If a longer surgical procedure is anticipated (ie, previous abdominal surgeries and risk of adhesions, abnormal placental implantation, maternal obesity), a CSE

428

A Epidural Analgesia

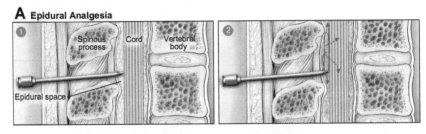

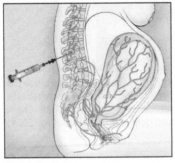

B Combined Spinal–Epidural Analgesia

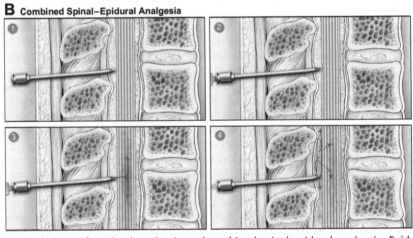

Fig. 2. Technique of epidural analgesia and combined spinal-epidural analgesia. Epidural analgesia (A) is achieved by placing a catheter into the lumbar epidural space (1). After the desired intervertebral space (eg, between L3 and L4) has been identified and infiltrated with local anesthetic, a hollow epidural needle is placed in the intervertebral ligaments. These ligaments are characterized by a high degree of resistance to penetration. A syringe connected to the epidural needle allows the anesthesiologist to confirm the resistance of these ligaments. In contrast, the epidural space has a low degree of resistance. When anesthesiologists slowly advance the needle while feeling for resistance, they recognize the epidural space by a sudden loss of resistance as the epidural needle enters the epidural space (2). Next, an epidural catheter is advanced into the space. Solutions of a local anesthetic, opioids, or a combination of the 2 can now be administered through the catheter. For combined spinal-epidural analgesia (B), the lumbar epidural space is also identified with an epidural needle (1). Next, a very thin spinal needle is introduced through the epidural needle into the subarachnoid space (2). Correct placement can be confirmed by the free flow of cerebrospinal fluid. A single bolus of local anesthetic, opioid, or a combination of the 2 is injected through this needle into the subarachnoid space (3). Subsequently, the needle is removed and a catheter is advanced into the epidural space through the epidural needle (4). When the single-shot spinal analgesic wears off, the epidural catheter can be used for the continuation of pain relief. (*Reproduced from* Eltzschig HK, Lieberman ES, Camann WR. Regional anesthesia and analgesia for labor and delivery. N Engl J Med 2003;348(4):323; with permission.)

technique is often done. This technique is performed by first identifying the epidural space using a 17-gauge or an 18-gauge epidural needle. A longer spinal needle is then inserted in a needle-through-needle technique to reach the subarachnoid space and deposit the intrathecal dose of medication (see **Fig. 2**B). An epidural catheter is then placed into the epidural space, which allows for subsequent dosing with additional local anesthetic or opioid medication, if necessary. In women who have an epidural catheter in situ for labor analgesia and later require a cesarean delivery, the epidural can be extended to surgical anesthesia by using a higher potency local anesthetic such as 2% lidocaine. Additional advantages of using regional anesthesia for cesarean delivery include the ability of the mother to be awake and alert for the infant delivery, the presence of a partner in the operating room, and the ability to include a long-acting opioid such as morphine in the subarachnoid or epidural injection to provide up to 18 to 24 hours of postoperative pain relief.

Regional Anesthesia for Labor and Vaginal Delivery

Labor pain is caused by uterine contractions and cervical dilation. These pain impulses are transmitted through the lower thoracic, lumbar, and sacral nerve roots and are amenable to epidural blockade (**Fig. 3**).[20] In 2006, the American College of Obstetricians and Gynecologists (ACOG) and the ASA issued a joint statement indicating that maternal request is a sufficient medical indication for pain relief.[21] An increasing number of women are choosing lumbar epidural to alleviate labor pain, which allows for the continuous infusion of a dilute local anesthesia solution, opioid, or both into the lumbar epidural space.[15,19,20] The use of epidural analgesia during childbirth varies from region to region, but approximately 60% of women in the United States and the United Kingdom choose this form of pain relief.[1] Studies have confirmed the increased analgesic efficacy of epidurals compared with parenteral opioids.[22] Although the use of labor analgesia can prolong the duration of labor by approximately 1 hour, concerns about the use of epidurals during labor leading to increased incidence of cesarean delivery have not been substantiated.[20,23,24] The 2006 ACOG opinion statement reaffirms the notion that "the fear of unnecessary cesarean delivery should not influence the method of pain relief that women can choose during labor".[21] Contraindications to the use of regional anesthesia include patient refusal, increased intracranial pressure, some preexisting neurologic disorders, hemodynamic instability, local or systemic infection, frank coagulopathy, and the use of anticoagulant or antithrombotic medications. The latter two hematologic contraindications are the focus of this article.

Alternative Methods of Pain Control for Labor and Vaginal Delivery

Labor pains can lead to increased maternal blood pressure, increased catecholamine release, and hyperventilation. Although epidural analgesia has been shown to be the most effective form for pain relief in labor, some women may choose alternative forms of pain control. The other modalities of pain control include psychoprophylaxis (Lamaze method), transcutaneous electric nerve stimulation (TENS), inhalational analgesia using nitrous oxide (rarely used in the United States but popular in other countries), systemic opioids,[25] various hypnotic techniques, and immersion in water. The administration of intravenous opioid using a PCA system has been associated with higher patient satisfaction compared with intermittent opioid boluses given by the provider.[25] Parenteral opioids rapidly cross the placenta and appear in fetal circulation. The potential for neonatal respiratory depression must be considered if parenteral opioids have been administered.

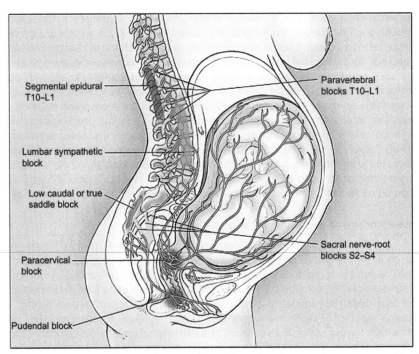

Fig. 3. Pathways of labor pain. Labor pain has a visceral and a somatic component. Uterine contractions may result in myometrial ischemia, causing the release of potassium, bradykinin, histamine, and serotonin. In addition, stretching and distention of the lower segments of the uterus and the cervix stimulate mechanoreceptors. These noxious impulses follow sensory nerve fibers that accompany sympathetic nerve endings, traveling through the paracervical region and the pelvic and hypogastric plexus to enter the lumbar sympathetic chain. Through the white rami communicantes of the T10, T11, T12, and L1 spinal nerves, these impulses enter the dorsal horn of the spinal cord. The pathways of the impulses could be mapped successfully by a demonstration that blockade at different levels along this path (sacral nerve root blocks S2 through S4, pudendal block, paracervical block, low caudal or true saddle block, lumbar sympathetic block, segmental epidural blocks T10 through L1, and paravertebral blocks T10 through L1) can alleviate the visceral component of labor pain. (*Reproduced from* Eltzschig HK, Lieberman ES, Camann WR. Regional anesthesia and analgesia for labor and delivery. N Engl J Med 2003;348(4):320; with permission.)

Complications of Neuraxial Analgesia and Anesthesia

Epidural analgesia and anesthesia are generally safe, but serious complications can occur. The complications of nerve injury, postdural puncture headache, epidural abscess, and meningitis are not reviewed in this article. Epidural hematoma is a rare complication, but patients with underlying hematologic disorders are at an increased risk and the sequelae are potentially catastrophic. Management of obstetric patients with impaired clotting function can therefore be challenging for the anesthesiologist and the hematologist.

Epidural hematoma

Symptoms of acute spinal hematoma include sharp radiating back pain with a radicular component and sensory and motor deficits that outlast the expected duration of spinal or epidural anesthesia.[26] Neuraxial hematologic complications in the obstetric population are rare. A retrospective study of severe neurologic complications after the use of central neuraxial anesthetic technique in Swedish obstetric patients between 1990 and 1999 estimated the risk of hematoma after obstetric epidural to be 1:200,000.[17] Ruppen and Derry[27] identified 27 studies including a total of 1.4 million obstetric patients and determined the rate of epidural hematoma to be 1 in 168,000 and the risk of persistent neurologic injury to be 1 in 237,000. None of the cases with persistent neurologic injury were clearly attributed to epidural hematoma.[27] A UK prospective study noted that the incidence of complications of epidural and CSE anesthesias were at least twice those of spinal and caudal anesthesias.[28] In another comprehensive literature review, Loo and Dahlgre[29] identified 7 cases of spinal hematoma after labor epidural (through 1998) and 3 patients with risk factors for bleeding, including 1 patient with abnormal activated prothrombin time (aPTT) and 1 with cholestasis of pregnancy and abnormal coagulation profile. Although anticoagulation therapy with low-molecular-weight-heparin (LMWH) is considered a risk for development of epidural hematoma, there are no case reports of epidural hematoma in an obstetric patient on enoxaparin or other anticoagulant medications.[29] However, spontaneous epidural hematoma has been described in the obstetric population, including 1 case in a patient being treated with enoxaparin, 60 mg subcutaneously twice daily, for antiphospholipid syndrome.[30]

Anesthesia for Patients with Hemoglobinopathies

Sickle cell disease and thalassemias are the 2 largest and most significant groups of hemoglobinopathies.[31] The perioperative management of patients with sickle cell disease includes confirmation of preoperative diagnosis, clinical assessment, prevention, and management of postoperative complications. Acute sickle cell crises have been reported to occur in 16.9% of patients after cesarean delivery and hysterectomy.[31] Principles of anesthetic management include maintaining oxygenation, hydration, thermoregulation, and acid-base regulation. The use of regional anesthesia may reduce pain-induced respiratory splinting and improve oxygenation in these patients.[32] Adequate lateral tilt positioning is critical in these patients because venous stasis owing to vena caval compression by the gravid uterus may contribute to a sickle cell crisis.[33]

Patients with thalassemia are classified by whether the α or β chain production is affected. Clinical severity varies with differing genotypes. For those with severe anemia and extramedullary hematopoiesis, bony abnormalities of maxillofacial area can complicate airway access.[31] Most patients with thalassemia carrier state present with mild microcytic anemia, and their anesthetic care is uneventful.

Anesthesia for Patients with Preexisting Coagulopathy

Thrombocytopenia

Following injury to blood vessels, platelets play an important role in establishing the initial hemostatic plug and subsequent activation of the coagulation cascade. A low platelet count may impair surgical hemostasis, leading to an increased risk of hemorrhage and anesthetic complications, such as epidural hematoma. The most common causes of thrombocytopenia in pregnancy include gestational thrombocytopenia, preeclampsia, disseminated intravascular coagulation (DIC), idiopathic thrombocytopenic purpura, and collagen vascular disorders. Other rare causes include May-Hegglin anomaly, Bernard-Soulier syndrome, and Glanzmann thrombasthenia.[34]

Anesthesia management of patients with thrombocytopenia The prevalence of mild thrombocytopenia (a platelet count $<150 \times 10^9$/L) was recorded in 6.6% of patients in a large obstetric center over a 7-year period.[35] The approach to a patient with thrombocytopenia begins with a thorough review of history that may reflect a bleeding disorder, such as symptoms of menorrhagia, epistaxis, prolonged bleeding following dental procedures, and previous history of unanticipated blood transfusion. It is also important to elicit medication use that may affect platelet function, including nonsteroidal antiinflammatory drugs, aspirin, and some herbal medications.[36] The physical examination may be significant for mucocutaneous bleeding, splenomegaly, petechiae, ecchymoses, or excessive bleeding around the peripheral intravenous sites. However, pregnancy may make the physical examination somewhat unreliable because some signs, such as epistaxis, bleeding gums, or easy bruising, may be associated with normal physiologic effects of pregnancy. A high index of suspicion for DIC should exist in obstetric situations including placental abruption, massive hemorrhage and transfusion, intrauterine fetal demise, and amniotic fluid embolism (AFE).[18]

There is a wide range of opinion, with little actual evidence, regarding the safe lower limit of platelet count for neuraxial anesthetic techniques. In a survey in 1996, all respondents stated that they would insert an epidural if the platelet count was greater than 100×10^9/L, only 16% of academic and 9% of private anesthesiologists would do so if the platelet count was 80 to 99×10^9/L, and only 2% and 0% would if the platelet count was 50 to 79×10^9/L.[37] The most recent (2007) ASA practice guidelines for obstetric anesthesia do not comment on a specific platelet count that is considered safe for neuraxial anesthesia.[15] There are insufficient data to assess whether a routine platelet count can predict anesthesia-related complications in uncomplicated parturients.[15] Platelet count is clinically useful for those with suspected pregnancy-related hypertensive disorders or other disorders associated with coagulopathy.[15]

In addition to the absolute platelet count, adequate platelet function should be considered in determining if neuraxial anesthesia can be delivered safely. In preeclampsia, platelet function has been shown to be abnormal despite a normal platelet count, the mechanism of which remains unclear.[38] Yuen and colleagues[38] reported on a case of epidural hematoma for a patient with severe preeclampsia after epidural placement for cesarean delivery. Her platelet count at the time of anesthetic intervention was 71×10^9/L, an increase from 49×10^9/L from the time of admission. One hour after cesarean delivery under epidural anesthesia, the patient developed hypertension and an unusual tonic-clonic seizure that was generalized but spared her lower limbs (which had a motor and sensory deficit from the L1 dermatome downward). A 4-mL clot extending from T12 to L2 level was discovered on computed tomographic scanning. When thrombocytopenia occurs in the context of preeclampsia, other coagulation parameters may also be abnormal.[39] Conversely, in a case series of 7 deliveries in 3 sisters with the May-Hegglin anomaly, no adverse neurologic sequelae were noted.[40] Neuraxial techniques (5 epidurals and 2 spinals) were used in deliveries in all 7 patients with platelet counts ranging from 14×10^9/L to 100×10^9/L. Several case series have documented the use of neuraxial techniques in patients who had thrombocytopenia (platelet count $<100 \times 10^9$/L) without any adverse neurologic effects.[41–43] However, these individual experiences cannot be extrapolated to all patients, and the overall clinical picture, rather than the absolute platelet count, is important in determining the risk of epidural hematoma in these patients.[44]

There is no single test of coagulation that can be used to predict the bleeding risk. As a bedside test of whole blood anticoagulation, thromboelastography (TEG) may become a useful tool in helping the anesthesiologist determine the coagulation and fibrinolysis function in certain obstetric situations (**Fig. 4**). TEG was first established

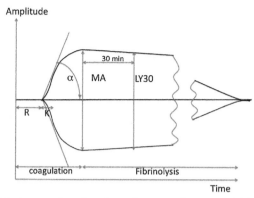

Amplitude

Fig. 4. TEG trace. R is the reaction time from the start of test to initial clot formation. The R time is prolonged with clotting factor deficiencies and heparin. K is the clot formation time, and α angle, the speed of clot onset. The α angle is decreased with clotting factor deficiencies, platelet dysfunction, thrombocytopenia, and hypofibrinogenemia. MA is the maximum clot amplitude. The widest point of the trace of MA represents clot strength and is reduced with platelet dysfunction. LY30 is the percentage of clot lysis at 30 minutes. It measures the rate of amplitude reduction 30 minutes after MA.

in 1941 and popularized for the use of coagulation monitoring during cardiac and liver transplant surgeries.[45] TEG has been used to demonstrate the hypercoagulable state of normal pregnancy as well as the impaired coagulation that develops in the setting of severe preeclampsia.[46,47] A significant correlation was found between the maximum amplitude (an indicator of clot strength) and platelet count in healthy term parturients.[48] Preliminary studies suggest that TEG may be a sensitive test to detect the decline of enoxaparin in patients after stopping therapy, with an in vitro correlation of increased TEG R-time (time to initial clot formation) and anti-Xa activity.[49] The platelet function analyzer (PFA-100, Dade Behring, Deerfield, IL, USA) is an alternative bedside assay of coagulation that specifically evaluates platelet function and may be a superior assay for the detection of abnormal platelet function in severe preeclamptic patients.[50] The information obtained from TEG or PFA-100 may be used in conjunction with usual coagulation tests to determine if adequate coagulation is present before any surgical or anesthetic intervention.

If a neuraxial technique is chosen for patients with thrombocytopenia, a single-shot spinal technique using a small-gauge needle is safer than a large epidural needle,[17,28] although labor analgesia generally requires the use of the epidural catheter. The use of a soft flex-tip epidural catheter compared with stiffer catheters is also associated with less venous cannulation and may be safer in these patients.[51]

The timing of epidural catheter removal is as important as the timing of placement because epidural hematoma can occur at either time. When thrombocytopenia is associated with hypertensive disorders of pregnancy, the nadir of platelet count can occur 24 to 48 hours after delivery and may be abnormal for several days. Therefore, in these patients, it is prudent to remove the epidural catheter as soon as it is no longer needed, provided there is no clinical evidence of coagulopathy.[18] Patients at a higher risk of epidural hematoma should be closely monitored for neurologic symptoms of spinal cord compression after any neuraxial technique.

Factor deficiencies

Hemophilia A and B are X-linked recessive bleeding disorders caused by mutations in the genes for factors VIII (FVIII) and IX (FIX). In most cases, the female carrier produces sufficient FVIII or FIX such that the overall factor levels exceed 50 IU/L (50%).[34] Epidural analgesia has been used in obstetric patients with hemophilia A and B without neurologic sequelae.[52] In this series, 5 of the 6 patients had factor levels greater than 50% and 1 patient was diagnosed postnatally.[52] Neuraxial anesthesia can usually be performed if factor levels are greater than 50 IU/L and the remaining coagulation profile is normal, and factor replacement should be considered if these levels are less than 50 IU/L before delivery or neuraxial anesthesia.

Factor XI (FXI) deficiency is a rare inherited bleeding disorder predominantly seen in the Ashkenazi Jewish population. The bleeding risk in these patients is unpredictable and does not correlate with low plasma FXI levels. Singh and colleagues[53] reported on a case series of obstetric patients with FXI deficiency in which 9 of 13 women were managed with neuraxial anesthesia without complications. Women with severe FXI deficiency and prolonged aPTT can be managed with fresh frozen plasma (FFP) transfusion (10–20 mL/kg) before neuraxial anesthesia.[53]

von Willebrand disease

von Willebrand disease (vWD) is a familial bleeding disorder associated with a deficiency of von Willebrand factor (vWF) and a comparable reduction of FVIII activity. Acquired vWD is associated with certain lymphoproliferative disorders, plasma cell dyscrasias, and autoimmune disorders such as systemic lupus erythematosus and can present similarly.[54] During pregnancy, most women with type 1 vWD show an improvement in their FVIII and vWF levels to normal and neuraxial anesthesia has been performed without requiring desmopressin (DDAVP).[55,56] Because the hypercoagulable state of pregnancy diminishes after delivery, any indwelling epidural catheter should be removed shortly after delivery. Activities of FVIII and FVIII ristocetin cofactor (RiCoF) and the vWF antigen (vWF:Ag) level should be within the normal range before spinal or epidural needle placement.[34] DDAVP is generally effective for the treatment of type 1 vWD and should be considered before neuraxial anesthesia. The goal is to maintain vWF:Ag and RiCoF assay levels greater than 50 IU/L. Patients with other vWD subtypes (types 2 and 3), or those not responsive to DDAVP, require antihemophilic factor (human) (Humate-P) to increase levels of FVIII. Administration of Humate-P before neuraxial anesthesia has been described in a patient with vWD.[57] If normalization of vWF:Ag and FVIII levels cannot be demonstrated, avoidance of regional anesthesia is generally recommended.

Anesthesia for Patients on Anticoagulant and Antithrombotic Medications

Indication for anticoagulant and antithrombotic medications

Venous thromboembolism is the leading cause of maternal morbidity and mortality in the developed world.[58] Pregnancy is a hypercoagulable state, which increases the risk of embolic complications. There are many situations that would necessitate the use of anticoagulant or antithrombotic medications in the parturient. Recent guidelines from the Pregnancy and Thrombosis Working Group and the American College of Chest Physicians have highlighted the importance of anticoagulant therapy in the prophylaxis and treatment of venous thromboembolism in pregnancy and in patients with mechanical heart valves.[59] Women who have an underlying thrombophilia or a previous history of thromboembolism are often treated with prophylactic doses of unfractionated heparin (UFH) or LMWH.[60] Common thrombophilias encountered in the parturient include Factor V Leiden mutation, activated protein C resistance, antiphospholipid syndrome, methylenetetrahydrofolate reductase mutation, and prothrombin mutation.[60] Recurrent first trimester pregnancy losses are sometimes associated with an underlying thrombophilia. These women may represent another group of patients who are treated with thromboprophylaxis during pregnancy to reduce the risk of spontaneous abortion. For the anesthesiologist, the indication for anticoagulation is extremely important because it directly affects whether or not the temporary cessation of anticoagulation during the peripartum period would be recommended for the safe initiation of regional anesthesia.

Regional technique in patients on anticoagulant and antithrombotic medications

For patients who have had a documented history of venous thromboembolism, the risk of stopping anticoagulation in order to safely initiate neuraxial anesthesia must be weighed against the risk of epidural hematoma as well as the requirement to use less-effective (ie, nonepidural) forms of pain relief in the event of abnormal coagulation at the time of labor. One case report describes a patient with antithrombin III deficiency and a history of deep vein thrombosis (DVT) and pulmonary embolism during her previous pregnancy who developed DVT during her subsequent pregnancy despite thromboprophylactic treatment with subcutaneous heparin.[61] Therapeutic dose subcutaneous LMWH was initiated and continued until the time of delivery. She received intravenous nalbuphine (an opioid agonist-antagonist), as well as nitrous oxide–oxygen mixture for labor analgesia.[61]

The presence of a thrombophilia and the use of thromboprophylaxis does not automatically negate the possibility of neuraxial anesthesia in these patients. If possible, these patients can be transitioned from LMWH to UFH at 38 weeks' gestation in anticipation of labor and delivery. UFH has a shorter half-life, and its action can be monitored by testing the aPTT before performing a neuraxial technique. This approach has been used successfully in the management of a series of patients with Factor V Leiden mutation in which 16 of 17 patients underwent epidural or spinal anesthesia without any neurologic sequelae.[58] Another series reviewed 20 patients with antiphospholipid syndrome of whom 3 received an epidural for cesarean delivery and 7 for labor analgesia. There were no neurologic deficits in any of these women. None of these patients received any form of heparinization for at least 24 hours before epidural placement.[62]

Guidelines from various national anesthesia societies are summarized in **Table 1**. Most recommendations reflect expert opinion based on case reports and pharmacokinetic and pharmacodynamic data. The incidence of spinal hematoma after neuraxial techniques in the obstetric population receiving anticoagulants is unknown but is thought to be extremely low.[59]

The American Society of Regional Anesthesia guidelines The American Society of Regional Anesthesia and Pain Medicine (ASRA) recently published the third edition of evidence-based guidelines regarding the use of regional anesthesia in patients receiving antithrombotic or thrombolytic therapy (see **Table 1**). For patients on a prophylactic dose of UFH, such as 5000 U administered subcutaneously twice daily, neuraxial techniques are not contraindicated.[63] The safety of neuraxial techniques in patients receiving doses greater than 10,000 U daily or more frequently than twice-daily dosing has not been established. Pharmacokinetic data have shown that obstetric patients may require thrice-daily dosing to achieve therapeutic drug levels because of increased volume of distribution as well as increased glomerular filtration rate.[59] Because of the variation in dose and frequency among obstetric patients, a normal aPTT level should be obtained before any neuraxial technique.

LMWH compared with UFH is the drug of choice for prophylaxis and treatment of thrombophilia because of a superior bioavailability, reduced dosing interval, more predictable pharmacology, and reduced incidence of side effects such as

Table 1
Guidelines from national anesthetic societies for the timing of neuraxial anesthesia in patients receiving anticoagulant and antithrombotic drugs

	Antiplatelet Medications		GPIIb/IIIa Inhibitors		UFH		LMWH	
	Aspirin/NSAIDs	Thienopyridines	Abciximab	Tirofiban or Eptifibatide	Subcutaneous	Intravenous	Prophylactic	Therapeutic
Austria								
Before[a]	2 d spinal	Clopidogrel 7 d	48 h	8 h	4 h	4 h	12 h	24 h
After[b]	3 d epidural	Ticlopidine 10 d	4 h	4 h	1 h	1 h	4 h	4 h
Belgium								
Before[a]	No CI	Clopidogrel 7 d	24–48 h	8–10 h	—	—	12 h	24 h
After[b]		Ticlopidine 10 d	2–4 h	2–4 h	1 h	1 h	4 h	4 h
France								
Before[a]	No CI	CI	24–48 h	8–10 h	12 h	4 h	10–12 h	24 h
After[b]			—	2–4 h	6–8 h	6–8 h	4–12 h	24 h
Germany								
Before[a]	No CI	Clopidogrel 7 d	—	24 h	4 h	4 h	12 h	24 h
After[b]		Ticlopidine 10 d	—	—	1 h	1 h	2–4 h	2–4 h
Netherlands								
Before[a]	—	—	—	—	No CI	4–6 h	10 h	24 h
After[b]		—	—	—	—	1 h	2 h	24 h
Spain								
Before[a]	No CI	NR	24 h	8 h	No CI	4 h	12 h	24 h
After[b]		—	—	—	—	1 h	6 h	6 h
United States								
Before[a]	No CI	Clopidogrel 7 d	48 h	8 h	No time interval	—(NB)/2–4h(CW)	10–12 h	24 h
After[b]		Ticlopidine 14 d	—	—	1 h	1 h	6–8 h	24 h (NB)/2 h (CW)

	Warfarin	Fondaparinux	Direct Thrombin Inhibitors			Fibrinolytics
			Hirudins	Melagatran	Argatroban	
Austria						
Before[a]	INR<1.4	36 h	10 h	8 h	—	Not indicated
After[b]	Restart after CW	4 h	4 h	4 h	—	
Belgium						
Before[a]	INR<1.4	36 h	8–10 h	8–10 h	—	CI
After[b]	Restart after CW	12 h	2–4 h	2–4 h	—	
France						
Before[a]	INR<1.5	Not recommended	CI	CI	CI	CI
After[b]	—					
Germany						
Before[a]	INR <1.4	36–42 h	8–10 h	8–10 h	4 h	CI
After[b]	Restart after CW	6–12 h	2–4 h	2–4 h	2 h	
Netherlands						
Before[a]	INR<1.8	—	—	—	—	CI
After[b]	Restart after CW	—	—	—	—	
Spain						
Before[a]	INR≤1.5	36 h	24 h	8–10 h	—	24–36 h (before NB/CW)
After[b]	Restart after CW	6–12 h (NB)/12 h (CW)	6 h	2–4 h	—	4 h (after NB/CW)
United States						
Before[a]	—(NB)/INR<1.5 (CW)	—	—	—	—	NR
After[b]	Restart after CW	—	—	—	—	

Abbreviations: CI, contraindication; CW, catheter withdrawal; GP, glycoprotein; INR, international normalized ratio; NB, neuraxial block; NR, not recommended; NSAIDs, nonsteroidal antiinflammatory drugs.

[a] Before refers to time interval before NB or CW.

[b] After refers to time interval after NB or CW before anticoagulation should be reinitiated.

Data from Butwick AJ, Carvalho B. Neuraxial anesthesia in obstetric patients receiving anticoagulant and antithrombotic drugs. Int J Obstet Anesth 2010;19:193–201.

osteoporosis and heparin-induced thrombocytopenia. At present, ASRA does not recommend using anti-Xa levels to predict the risk of bleeding because there are no studies to document its utility. In patients who are on prophylactic dose of LMWH, neuraxial techniques should be avoided for at least 10to 12 hours after the last dose of LMWH. At therapeutic doses of subcutaneous LMWH (eg, enoxaparin, 1 mg/kg every 12 hours or 1.5 mg/kg daily; dalteparin, 120 U/kg every 12 hours, or dalteparin, 200 U/kg day; or tinzaparin, 175 U/kg), needle insertion should be delayed for at least 24 hours.[63]

For patients on oral anticoagulants (eg, warfarin), the ASRA recommends stopping them before 4 to 5 days and ensuring a normal international normalized ratio (INR) before proceeding with neuraxial block. However, warfarin is not commonly used during pregnancy because of its fetal teratogenic effects.

The recommendations for patients on antiplatelet medication and thrombin inhibitors are summarized in **Table 1**. Low-dose aspirin alone is generally considered safe for neuraxial techniques.[64]

Obstetric Hemorrhage and Transfusion

Patients with hematologic disorders are at an increased risk of postpartum hemorrhage if they have any uncorrected coagulation abnormalities, although massive hemorrhage can occur in the obstetric patient even in the absence of a coagulation disorder. Anesthesia care involves acute resuscitation of these patients, which sometimes necessitates massive transfusion of blood products. The use of cell salvage in the obstetric population has been controversial because of the theoretical risk of administering blood that contains amniotic fluid components, which can lead to AFE.[65,66] Aside from AFE, cell salvage can also introduce other problems such as equipment malfunction, coagulopathy, and air embolism.[67] With the current techniques of cell salvage, red blood cells (RBCs) are washed and filtered through a leukocyte filter, which reduces the amniotic fluid contaminant level to that found in maternal blood after normal placental separation.[65] This technique should be considered in situations in which massive transfusion is required or anticipated or in Jehovah Witness patients who decline the use of autologous blood products, assuming they will accept cell salvage blood. However, more recent case reports regarding the use of cell salvage in obstetrics have suggested that the use of negatively charged, leukocyte reduction filters may lead to cytokine release (ie, bradykinin), causing significant hypotension.[68–70] Further studies are required to elucidate the true safety of cell salvage and the recommended use of leukocyte reduction filters in this population.[71]

The appropriate ratio of blood products to manage postpartum hemorrhage in obstetrics is unknown, but we can draw on massive transfusion experiences in trauma resuscitation. Data from trauma and combat-related literatures suggest that the use of RBCs, FFP, and platelets in a 1:1:1 ratio is associated with improved survival to hospital discharge and reduced death from hemorrhage.[72–74] This idea is increasingly being applied to massive transfusion scenarios in the obstetric population as well.[75] A preliminary in vitro model for dilutional coagulopathy during postpartum hemorrhage resuscitation suggests that a 1:1 RBC:FFP ratio is more efficacious than the traditional 3:1 RBC:FFP ratio.[76] Emerging strategies to manage postpartum hemorrhage include the use of activated recombinant factor VII (rFVII) in massive obstetric hemorrhage.[77,78] At present, the use of rFVII is limited because of the extremely high cost of this medication. Patients with abnormal placental implantation (placenta accreta, increta, percreta) or other risk factors for postpartum hemorrhage may benefit from preemptive uterine artery embolization or balloon placement by interventional radiologists to minimize blood loss and preserve fertility.[79,80] Prevention of maternal mortality from hemorrhage is improved with careful multidisciplinary care involving anesthesiologists, obstetricians, interventional radiologists, and hematologists. Hospitals should develop and incorporate into practice a massive transfusion protocol and provide multidisciplinary education for all obstetric care providers, including both physicians and nurses.[81] Examples of such protocols can be found at resources such as the California Maternal Quality Care Collaborative website www.cmqcc.org.

SUMMARY

The management of patients with hematologic disorders in pregnancy involves a multidisciplinary approach involving specialists from hematology, obstetrics, and anesthesiology. It is important to involve the anesthesiologist early in gestation so that a safe anesthetic plan can be devised. Endotracheal intubation of obstetric patients can be technically difficult, and every effort should be made to use a regional technique, if possible. Patients with underlying coagulopathy or on anticoagulant and antithrombotic medications pose a special risk for the rare complication of an epidural hematoma after neuraxial anesthesia. The timing of cessation of these medications before and during labor and the appropriate timing for anesthetic intervention need to balance the risk of thrombosis versus that of hemorrhage. Consensus statements from anesthesia societies may guide in the decision process, but the ultimate plan has to be made on an individual basis after discussion with the obstetric and hematology teams.

REFERENCES

1. Gatt S, Camann W. Principles of obstetric anesthesia. In: Powrie RO, Greene MF, Camann W, editors. De Swiet's medical disorders in obstetric practice. 5th edition. Chichester (West Sussex): Wiley-Blackwell; 2010. p. 625–32.
2. Tsen LC, Kodali BS. Can general anesthesia for cesarean delivery be completely avoided? An anesthetic perspective. Expert Rev Obstet Gynecol 2010;5(5): 517–24.
3. Ross BK. ASA closed claims in obstetrics: lessons learned. Anesthesiol Clin North America 2003;21(1):183–97.
4. Hawkins JL, Koonin LM, Palmer SK, et al. Anesthesia-related deaths during obstetric delivery in the United States, 1979–1990. Anesthesiology 1997;86: 277–84.
5. Davies JM, Posner KL, Lee LA, et al. Liability associated with obstetric anesthesia: a closed claims analysis. Anesthesiology 2009;110:131–9.
6. Cormack RS, Lehane J. Difficult tracheal intubation in obstetrics. Anaesthesia 1984;39(11):1105–11.
7. Davies JM, Weeks S, Crone LA, et al. Difficult intubation in the parturient. Can J Anaesth 1989;36(6):668–74.
8. Barnardo PD, Jenkins JG. Failed tracheal intubation in obstetrics: a 6 year review in a UK region. Anaesthesia 2000;55:685–94.
9. Saravanakumar K, Cooper GM. Failed intubation in obstetrics: has the incidence changed recently? Br J Anaesth 2005;94(5):690.
10. Pilkington S, Carli F, Dakin MJ, et al. Increase in Mallampati score during pregnancy. Br J Anaesth 1995;74(6):638–42.
11. Kodali BS, Chandrasekhar S, Bulich LN, et al. Airway changes during labor and delivery. Anesthesiology 2008;108:357–62.
12. Wong CA, McCarthy FJ. Gastric emptying of water in obese pregnant women at term. Anesth Analg 2007;105(3):751–5.

13. Wong CA, Loffredi M. Gastric emptying of water in term pregnancy. Anesthesiology 2002;96(6):1395–400.
14. Ali RA, Egan LJ. Gastroesophageal reflux disease in pregnancy. Best Pract Res Clin Gastroenterol 2007;21(5):793–806.
15. ASA. Practice guidelines for obstetric anesthesia: an updated report by the American Society of Anesthesiologists Task Force on Obstetric Anesthesia. Anesthesiology 2007;106(4):843–63.
16. Practice guidelines for preoperative fasting and the use of pharmacologic agents to reduce the risk of pulmonary aspiration: application to healthy patients undergoing elective procedures: a report by the ASA task force on pre-op fasting guidelines. Anesthesiology 1999;90(3):896–905.
17. Moen V, Dahlgren N. Severe neurological complications after central neuraxial blockades in Sweden 1990–1999. Anesthesiology 2004;101(4):950–9.
18. Douglas MJ. Platelets, the parturient and regional anesthesia. Int J Obstet Anesth 2001;10(2):113–20.
19. Bucklin BA, Hawkins JL, Anderson JR, et al. Obstetric anesthesia workforce survey: twenty-year update. Anesthesiology 2005;103:645–53.
20. Eltzschig HG, Lieberman ES, Camann WR. Regional anesthesia and analgesia for labor and delivery. N Engl J Med 2003;348(4):319–32.
21. Analgesia and Cesarean Delivery Rates. ACOG committee opinion No.339. Obstet Gynecol 2006;107:1487–8.
22. Hawkins JL, Gibbs CP, Orleans M, et al. Obstetric anesthesia work force survey. 1981 versus 1992. Anesthesiology 1997;87:135–43.
23. Wong CA, Scavone BM, Peaceman AM, et al. The risk for cesarean delivery with neuraxial analgesia given early versus late in labor. N Engl J Med 2005;352(7): 655–65.
24. Wang FZ, Shen XF, Guo XR, et al. Epidural analgesia in the latent phase of labor and the risk of cesarean delivery. Anesthesiology 2009;111:871–80.
25. Douglas MJ. Alternatives to epidural analgesia during labour. Can J Anaesth 1991;38:421–4.
26. Vandermuelen EP, van Aken H. Anticoagulants and spinal-epidural anesthesia. Anesth Analg 1994;79(6):1165–77.
27. Ruppen W, Derry S. Incidence of epidural hematoma, infection, and neurological injury in obstetric patients with epidural analgesia/anaesthesia. Anesthesiology 2006;105(2):394–9.
28. Cook TM, Counsell D. Major complications of central neuraxial block: report on the third national audit project of the Royal College of Anaesthetists. Br J Anaesth 2009;102(2):179–90.
29. Loo CC, Dahlgre G. Neurological complications in obstetric regional anesthesia. Int J Obstet Anesth 2000;9(2):99–124.
30. Forsnes E, Occhino A, Acosta R. Spontaneous spinal epidural hematoma in pregnancy associated with using low molecular weight heparin. Obstet Gynecol 2009; 113:532–3.
31. Firth PG. Anesthesia and hemoglobinopathies. Anesthsiol Clin 2009;27:321–36.
32. Firth PG, Head CA. Sickle cell disease and anesthesia. Anesthesiology 2004; 101(3):766–85.
33. Dunn A, Davies A, Eckert G, et al. Intraoperative death during Caesarian section in a patient with sickle-cell trait. Can J Anaesth 1987;34(1):67–70.
34. McLintock C, Repke JT, Bucklin B. Hematologic disease in pregnancy. In: Powrie RO, Greene MF, Camann W, editors. De Swiet's medical disorders in obstetric practice. 5th edition. Chichester (West Sussex): Wiley-Blackwell; 2010. p. 48–81.

35. Burrows RF, Kelton HK. Pregnancy in patients with idiopathic thrombocytopenic purpura: assessing the risks for the infant at delivery. Obstet Gynecol Surv 1993;48:781–8.

36. Hepner DH, Harnett M, Segal S, et al. Herbal medicine use in parturients. Anesth Analg 2002;94:690–3.

37. Beilin Y, Bodian CA, Haddad EM, et al. Practice patterns of anesthesiologists regarding situations in obstetric anesthesia where clinical management is controversial. Anesth Analg 1996;83:735–41.

38. Yuen TS, Kua JS, Tan IK. Spinal haematoma following epidural anaesthesia in a patient with eclampsia. Anaesthesia 1999;54:350–71.

39. Leduc L, Wheeler JM. Coagulation profile in severe preeclampsia. Obstet Gynecol 1992;79(1):14–8.

40. Fishman EB, Connors JM, Camann WR. Anesthetic management of seven deliveries in three sisters with the May-Hegglin Anomaly. Anesth Analg 2009;108(5):1603–5.

41. Rolbin SH, Abbott D. Epidural anesthesia in pregnant patients with low platelet counts. Obstet Gynecol 1988;71(6):918–20.

42. Rasmus KT, Rottman RL. Unrecognized thrombocytopenia and regional anesthesia in parturients: a retrospective review [abstract only]. Obstet Gynecol 1989;73(6):943–6.

43. Beilin Y, Zahn J. Safe epidural analgesia in thirty parturients with platelet counts between 69000 and 98000 mm(-3). Anesth Analg 1997;85(2):385–8.

44. Frenk V, Camann W, Kodali BS. Regional anesthesia in parturients with low platelet counts. Can J Anaesth 2005;52:114.

45. Luddington RJ. Thrombelastography/thromboelastometry. Clin Lab Haematol 2005;27(2):81–90.

46. Sharma SK, Philip K. Assessment of changes in coagulation in parturients with preeclampsia using thromboelastography. Anesthesiology 1999;90(2):385–90.

47. Sharma SK, Vera RL, Stegall WC, et al. Management of a postpartum coagulopathy using thromboelastography. J Clin Anesth 1997;9:243–7.

48. Beilin Y, Arnold I, Hossain S. Evaluation of the platelet function analyzer (PFA-100) vs. the thromboelastogram (TEG) in the parturient. Int J Obstet Anesth 2006; 15(1):7–12.

49. Farber MK, Segal S, Dorfman D, et al. Comparison of ACT, TEG, and anti-Xa in detecting decline of therapeutic enoxaparin concentration. Park Ridge (IL): American Society of Anesthesiologists; 2008 [abstract: A573].

50. Davies JR, Fernando R, Hallworth SP. Hemostatic function in healthy pregnant and preeclamptic women: an assessment using the platelet function analyzer (PFA-100) and thromboelastograph. Anesth Analg 2007;104(2):416–20.

51. Banwell BR, Morley-Forster P, Krause R. Decreased incidence of complications in parturients with the arrow (FlexTip Plus) epidural catheter. Can J Anaesth 1998; 45:370–2.

52. Kadir RA, Economides DL, Braithwaite J, et al. The obstetric experience of carriers of haemophilia. Br J Obstet Gynaecol 1997;104:803–10.

53. Singh AJ, Harnet MJ, Connors MJ, et al. Factor XI deficiency and obstetrical anesthesia. Anesth Analg 2009;108(6):1882–5.

54. Cuker A, Connors JM, Katz JT, et al. A bloody mystery. N Engl J Med 2009;361: 1887–94.

55. Milaskiewicz RM, Holdcroft A. Epidural anaesthesia and von Willebrand's disease. Anaesthesia 1990;45(6):462–4.

56. Stedeford JC, Pittman JA. Von Willebrand's disease and neuraxial anaesthesia. Anaesthesia 2000;55(12):1228–9.

57. Cohen S, Zada Y. Neuraxial block for von Willebrand's disease. Anaesthesia 2001;56(4):397.
58. Harnett MJ, Walsh ME, Tsen LC. The use of central neuraxial techniques in parturients with Factor V Leiden mutation. Anesth Analg 2005;101(6):1821–3.
59. Butwick AJ, Carvalho B. Neuraxial anesthesia in obstetric patients receiving anticoagulant and antithrombotic drugs. Int J Obstet Anesth 2010;19:193–201.
60. Kupferminc MJ. Thrombophilia and pregnancy. Reprod Biol Endocrinol 2003;1: 111–23.
61. Pattee CL, Penning DH. Obstetrical analgesia in a parturient with antithrombin III deficiency. Can J Anaesth 1993;40(6):507–10.
62. Ringrose DK. Anaesthesia and the antiphospholipid syndrome: a review of 20 obstetric patients. Int J Obstet Anesth 1997;6(2):107–11.
63. Horlocker TT, Wedel DK, Rowlingson JC, et al. Regional anesthesia in pt receiving antithrombotic or thrombolytic therapy. American Society of Regional Anesthesia and Pain Medicine Evidence-Based Guidelines (Third Edition). Reg Anesth Pain Med 2010;35(1):64–101.
64. Sibai BM, Caritis SM, Thom E, et al. Low-dose aspirin in nulliparous women: safety of continuous epidural blocks and correlation between bleeding time and maternal-neonatal bleeding complications. Am J Obstet Gynecol 1994;172:1553–7.
65. Waters JH, Biscotti C, Potter PS, et al. Amniotic fluid removal during cell salvage in the Cesarean section patient. Anesthesiology 2000;92:1531–6.
66. Catling SJ, Williams S, Fielding AM. Cell salvage in obstetrics: an evaluation of the ability of cell salvage combined with leucocyte depletion filtration to remove amniotic fluid from operative blood loss at caesarean section. Int J Obstet Anesth 1999;8(2):79–84.
67. Camann WA. Cell salvage during cesarean delivery: is it safe and valuable? Maybe, maybe not! Int J Obstet Anesth 1999;8(2):75–6.
68. Sreelakshmi TR, Eldridge J. Acute hypotension and leucocyte depletion filters. Anaesthesia 2010;65:742–4.
69. Kessack LK, Hawkins N. Severe hypotension related to cell salvaged blood transfusion in obstetrics. Anaesthesia 2010;65:745–8.
70. Hussain S, Clyburn P. Cell salvage-induced hypotension and London buses. Anaesthesia 2010;65:659–63.
71. Geoghegon J, Daniels JP, Mooer PA, et al. Cell salvage at caesarean section: the need for an evidence-based approach. BJOG 2009;116:743–7.
72. Borgman MA, Spinella PC, Perkins JG, et al. The ratio of blood products transfused affects mortality in patients receiving massive transfusions at a combat support hospital. J Trauma 2007;63:805–13.
73. Sperry JL, Ochoa JB, Gunn SR. An FFP: PRBC transfusion ratio ≥1:1.5 is associated with a lower risk of mortality after massive transfusion. J Trauma 2008;65: 986–93.
74. Maegele M, Lefering R, Paffrath T, et al. Red blood cell to plasma ratios transfused during massive transfusion are associated with mortality in severe multiply injury: a retrospective analysis from the Trauma Registry of the Deutsche Gesellschaft fur Unfallchirurgie. Vox Sang 2008;95:112–9.
75. Burtelow M, Riley E, Druzin M, et al. How we treat: management of life-threatening primary postpartum hemorrhage with a standardized massive transfusion protocol. Transfusion 2007;47:1564–72.
76. Sadana N, Farber MK, Kaufman R, et al. Traditional vs. new transfusion protocols for obstetric hemorrhage: which is better? San Antonio (TX): Society for Obstetric Anesthesia and Perinatology; 2010 [abstract: 6].

77. Welsh A, McClintock C. Guidelines for the use of recombinant activated factor VII in massive obstetric hemorrhage. Aust N Z J Obstet Gynaecol 2008;48(1):12–6.
78. Thorarinsdottir HR, Sigurbjournsson FT, Hreinsson K, et al. Effects of fibrinogen concentrate administration during severe hemorrhage. Acta Anaesthesiol Scand 2010;54:1077–82.
79. O'Rourke N, McElrath R, Baum R, et al. Cesarean delivery in the interventional radiology suite: approach to obstetric hemostasis. Anesth Analg 2007;104: 1193–4.
80. Kodali BS. Bloodless trilogy? Anesthesia, obstetrics and interventional radiology for cesarean delivery. Int J Obstet Anesth 2010;19:131–2.
81. Skupski DW, Lowenwirt IP, Weinbaum FI, et al. Improving hospital systems for the care of women with major obstetric hemorrhage. Obstet Gynecol 2006;107: 977–83.

Index

Note: Page numbers of article titles are in **boldface** type.

Hematol Oncol Clin N Am 25 (2011) 445–455
doi:10.1016/S0889-8588(11)00027-X
0889-8588/11/$ – see front matter © 2011 Elsevier Inc. All rights reserved.

hemonc.theclinics.com

Moving?

Make sure your subscription moves with you!

To notify us of your new address, find your **Clinics Account Number** (located on your mailing label above your name), and contact customer service at:

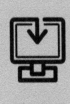

Email: **journalscustomerservice-usa@elsevier.com**

800-654-2452 (subscribers in the U.S. & Canada)
314-447-8871 (subscribers outside of the U.S. & Canada)

Fax number: **314-447-8029**

Elsevier Health Sciences Division
Subscription Customer Service
3251 Riverport Lane
Maryland Heights, MO 63043

*To ensure uninterrupted delivery of your subscription, please notify us at least 4 weeks in advance of move.